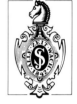

Bronchial Carcinoma

An Integrated Approach
to Diagnosis and Management

Edited by
Michael Bates

Foreword by Sir Thomas Holmes Sellors

With 104 Figures, including 8 in colour

Springer-Verlag
Berlin Heidelberg New York Tokyo
1984

Michael Bates, FRCS, FACS
Bays Hill House, Barnet Lane, Elstree, Hertfordshire, England

ISBN 3-540-13234-1 Springer-Verlag Berlin Heidelberg New York Tokyo
ISBN 0-387-13234-1 Springer-Verlag New York Heidelberg Berlin Tokyo

Library of Congress Cataloging in Publication Data
Main entry under title:
Bronchial carcinoma.
Includes bibliographies and index. 1. Bronchi – Cancer. 2. Lungs – Cancer. I. Bates,
Michael, 1917–   . [DNLM: 1. Carcinoma, Bronchogenic – diagnosis. 2. Carcinoma,
Bronchogenic – therapy. 3. Lung Neoplasms – diagnosis. 4. Lung Neoplasms –
therapy. WF 658 B869] RC280.B9B74 1984 616.99'423 84-5576
ISBN 0-387-13234-1 (U.S.)

Filmset by Herts Typesetting, 84 Fore Street, Hertford.
Printed by Page Bros. (Norwich) Limited, Mile Cross Lane, Norwich.

2128/3916-543210

Preface

In a condition of such complexity as bronchial carcinoma and at a time when the scientist's understanding of malignant disease is still incomplete, it is inevitable that views within the medical profession will proliferate. This book is an attempt to assemble these views in the light of 33 years of surgical experience and is intended for those specialists who will be concerned with the diagnosis and treatment of lung cancer in the foreseeable future.

The wide clinical experience of the contributing authors has enabled every aspect of this disease to be considered, with emphasis being placed on diagnostic techniques such as CT scanning and fine needle transpleural biopsy, as well as on the latest method of treatment by lasers.

Bronchial carcinoma remains the major cause of cancer death in the United Kingdom, accounting for 6% of all deaths. While the incidence has decreased slightly in the male population, there has been an equivalent increase in the female population.

For the last 40 years surgical removal has been advised as the treatment offering the best hope of a cure. During this time, excision by radical pneumonectomy has gradually given way to more conservative surgical procedures with improved long-term results. There has also been a growing realisation of the importance of the patient's own immunity to the disease. Artificial means of stimulating this immunity have been tried; however, recent studies using intrapleural injection of BCG both in America and in the United Kingdom have failed to confirm any improvement in the survival rate.

Since the introduction of the cobalt unit, and more recently of linear accelerators, many of the disadvantages and the morbidity previously associated with radiotherapy have been removed. The results of treatment with radiotherapy alone and in combination with surgery have been more encouraging. Oat or small cell carcinoma, in particular, has been resistant to successful treatment by surgery, radiotherapy or chemotherapy alone, but considerably improved results have been obtained by combining these methods of treatment. The success achieved with chemotherapy in the treatment of Hodgkin's disease and other lymphomas is being extended into the field of therapy for bronchial carcinoma.

Improved diagnostic techniques have greatly changed the management of this disease. The demonstration of subclinical metastases in the brain, liver or bones by isotope scanning has helped to avoid surgery when other treatment would be more appropriate. Computerised axial tomography can reveal mediastinal node involvement and small pulmonary or pleural tumours not detected on routine tomography.

In 1974 pre-operative TNM staging became a routine assessment of the size of the primary tumour and the presence of metastases in intrathoracic lymph nodes and in distant organs.

The introduction of the flexible endoscope extended the limits of the rigid bronchoscope. The rigid instrument remains essential for assessing the state of the carina and the mobility of the main bronchi, while the flexible instrument allows a histological diagnosis to be made from peripheral and subsegmental lesions. If not obtained at bronchoscopy, sufficient material to effect a diagnosis can often be provided by transpleural biopsy under radiographic control.

Techniques of cell identification are improving, and individual cell types can be isolated with increasing accuracy from the neoplastic cells found in sputum and pleural fluid. There is the added advantage that this investigation can be carried out in the out-patient department. The routine screening of middle-aged males who are also smokers can result in a management problem when neoplastic cells are found in the sputum and yet the chest radiograph remains clear.

All these methods of investigation have significantly increased our appreciation of the need for different treatments for tumours of different cell types.

Mediastinoscopy has been performed as a routine procedure concurrent with bronchoscopy in many units. However, non-invasive CT scanning now can provide much of the information previously obtained at mediastinoscopy.

There has been little or no change in the common thoracic mode of clinical presentation of bronchial carcinoma, but there is now a wider appreciation of the extrathoracic manifestations, particularly of hormone disturbances shown by patients suffering from small cell carcinoma.

During recent years laser beams have been directed along the biopsy channel of a flexible endoscope to burn a path through a malignant bronchial obstruction. Potentially exciting work is being done with two types of laser: the Nd-YAG laser, which kills tumour cells through heat; and the argon rhodamine dye laser, used to activate haematoporphyrin given intravenously to label tumour cells and increase their absorption of laser energy.

Probably 60% of all thoracotomies for pulmonary conditions are performed on patients suffering from bronchial carcinoma. Now that secretions and suppuration are no longer major problems, the anaesthetic management of thoracic resection is relatively straightforward. However, post-thoracotomy pain remains a source of distress in the recovery period. Considerable success in relieving this pain is reported to follow the epidural injection of methadone and the application of a cryoprobe to the intercostal nerves adjacent to the thoracotomy incision. Less dramatic but more generally applicable is the use of intercostal or paravertebral blocks, and continuous parenteral infusion of narcotic analgesics.

The chapters in this book deal with these subjects in detail, and because of the many disciplines represented it is hoped that they will provide a comprehensive study from which further progress against lung cancer can evolve.

Acknowledgements

I am particularly indebted to my wife, who enabled the publishers to continue with the production of this book by correcting the galley and page proofs during the prolonged period of my serious indisposition.

I am pleased to acknowledge the special help and advice given to me by Dr. Stewart Clarke.

I wish to thank Mr. Charles Drew for allowing me to reproduce his photographs of Mr Morriston Davies and Dr. Evarts Graham. Dr. Walford Harrison kindly provided the histological photomicrographs (Figs. 6 and 7) shown on pp. 169 and 170. Mr. C. J. Vardey of Glaxo Ltd. generously supplied financial help towards the cytology colour photographs. Dr. Georgina Bates provided the explanatory drawing of a specimen photograph (Fig. 9a) on p. 172.

I am grateful to the following physicians who not only have referred their patients for surgical treatment, but by continuing with the long-term assessments have produced invaluable clinical information: *North Middlesex Hospital and Edmonton Chest Clinic* — Dr. J. Vernon Davies, Dr. R. S. Francis, Dr. R. H. Elphinstone, Dr. E. N. O'Brien, Dr. Wendy Scott, Dr. S. E. Josse, Dr. T. M. Macken, Dr. A. Pringle, Dr. I. Ramsay and Dr. I. Woolf. *Tottenham Chest Clinic* — Dr. J. H. Pratt-Johnson, Dr. R. H. Hirst, Dr. R. A. Grande and the late Dr. T. A. McQuiston. *Broomfield Hospital, Chelmsford* — Dr. M. Duffy, Dr. J. Utting and Dr. G. Pyne. *Essex County Hospital, Colchester* — Dr. F. Kellerman, Dr. P. Kennedy and Dr. R. C. Hudson. *Ilford Chest Clinic* — Dr. D. Adler. *Thurrock Chest Clinic* — Dr. J. T. Brown. *Waltham Abbey Hospital* — Dr. E. Rhys Jones. *East Herts Hospital* — the late Dr. A. Pines. *Chase Farm Hospital* — Dr. J. D. Kinloch, Dr. S. Freedman and Dr. N. Peters. *Barking Chest Clinic* — Dr. R. A. Storring. *Chingford Hospital* — Dr. M. Morris. *St. Margarets Hospital, Epping* — Dr. J. P. Warren.

I am most grateful for invaluable secretarial help which was given over a long period of time by Mrs Daphne Brint of the North Middlesex Hospital, Mrs Daphne Ketley of Broomfield Hospital, Chelmsford, and Mrs Margaret Brett of Essex County Hospital, Colchester.

London, 1984   Michael Bates

Foreword

Bronchial carcinoma has, within the last few decades, been increasing with alarming frequency until it has gained the unenviable reputation of being the most common form of cancer in man. Of the many predisposing and possible factors, cigarette smoking stands out as a major cause, though hormonal and immunological influences are receiving consideration.

This present work brings together all facets of the disease with each section being contributed by an experienced and recognised expert in his or her field and has been edited by a distinguished and highly experienced thoracic surgeon in Mr. Michael Bates. In a multi-disciplinary field, the balance and authority that has been achieved will make this a 'classic' for all those interested in and practising in the subject.

Bronchial carcinoma is not a single cell disease; its behaviour varies with the predominant cell involved, and when it comes to treatment, the course of action varies. Some cell forms give rise to early invasion of regional glands while others remain localised; it is these latter cases which can respond to excisional surgery. In the past the standard and early treatment was pneumonectomy when an absence of distant metastases and only local invasion could be proved, but unhappily only a small proportion of the patients diagnosed as having the disease could meet these criteria. The trends in surgical practice and results are fully described with the Editor's wide experience and show a tendency towards a more conservative approach where possible – lobectomy rather than pneumonectomy. Radiotherapy, alone or in conjuction with surgery, has generally proved disappointing except in palliation, but recent experiences with radiation combined with chemotherapy are showing promise.

When one thinks of the accounts given in text books of not too many years ago – a few paragraphs expressing little hope – the present work is a credit to those authors who have contributed so successfully to the understanding of the many problems that face us in contending with this unhappy disease.

Aylesbury, Buckinghamshire   Sir Thomas Holmes Sellors
August, 1984

Contents

Contributors

Alan Bailey, MB, BS, MRCP
Director of BUPA Medical Research Centres, Bristol and
Birmingham

Michael Bates, FRCS, FACS
Thoracic Surgeon to the North Middlesex, Royal Northern and
Royal Free Hospitals

Gordon Canti, MB, BS, FRCP
Department of Cytology, St. Bartholomew's Hospital, London

Stewart Clarke, MD, FRCP
Physician to the Royal Free and Brompton Hospitals, London

Robert Dick, MB, BS (Sydney), MRACR, FRCR
Department of Diagnostic Radiology, Royal Free Hospital,
London

Professor Dr. Peter Drings
Innere Abteilung, Krankenhaus Rohrbach, Klinik für
Thoraxerkrankungen, 6900 Heidelberg 1, West Germany

Allen R. Gibbs, MRCPath
Senior Lecturer in Pathology, University Hospital of Wales, Cardiff

Stephen J. Golding, MB, BS, LRCP, DMRD, FRCR
Lecturer in Radiology, University of Oxford, and Consultant in
Administrative Charge, Oxford Regional CT Unit

Hilary Howells, FFARCS
Director, Department of Anaesthesia, The Royal Free Hospital,
London

Philip Hugh-Jones, MA, MD (Camb), FRCP
Physician in Charge of the Chest Unit in the Department of
Medicine, King's College Hospital, London

Edna Matthews, DMRT, FRCR
Consultant in Radiotherapy and Oncology, North Middlesex and
Bartholomew's Hospitals, London

Michael Meredith Brown, RD, MB, BChir, FRCS
Thoracic Surgeon to the Royal Surrey County Hospital, Guildford

John A. Meyer, MD, FACS
Associate Professor of Surgery, State University of New York,
Upstate Medical Center, Syracuse, U.S.A.

Nicholas Plowman, MD, MRCP, FRCR
Consultant Radiotherapist, St. Bartholomew's and Great Ormond
Street Hospitals, London

Brian Porter, FFARCS
Senior Registrar in the Department of Anaesthesia, The Royal Free
Hospital, London

Sally J. Ratter, PhD
Senior Biochemist in the Department of Endocrinology, St.
Batholomew's Hospital, London

Lesley H. Rees, MSc, MD, MB, BS (Hons), MRCPath, FRCP
Professor of Clinical Endocrinology, St. Bartholomew's Hospital,
London

Barry Ross, MB, BS, FRCS
Thoracic Surgeon, Norfolk and Norwich Hospital, Norwich

Roger M.E. Seal, FRCP, FRCPath
Consultant Pathologist, Llandough Hospital, Penarth

Bryan H.R. Stack, MB, ChB, FRCP
Consultant in Respiratory Medicine, Western Infirmary, Glasgow

Maurice Sutton, FRCS, FRCR
Director, Department of Radiotherapy and Oncology, North
Middlesex Hospital, London

Benjamin Timmis, MRCP, FRCR
Department of Diagnostic Radiology, Royal Free Hospital, London

Adrian Timothy, MB, BS, MRCP, FRCR
Consultant in Radiotherapy, St. Thomas Hospital, London

Professor Dr. Ingolf Vogt-Moykopf
Thoraxchir. Abteilung, Krankenhaus Rohrbach, Klinik für
Thoraxerkrankingen, 6900 Heidelberg 1, West Germany

Chapter 1

Historical Survey

Michael Bates

It is accepted universally that the first successful removal of a proven bronchial carcinoma was performed by Morriston Davies (Fig. 1) in 1912 and reported the following year. In the short intervening period of 70 years since the date of that operation, bronchial carcinoma has changed from a rare disease into one which has become the scourge of the modern world. Most of this increase has occurred during the last 50 years; thus in his book on *Surgery of the Thorax* written in 1933, Holmes Sellors was able to state that 'true pulmonary cancer is rare' and devoted only two pages to the pathology and X-ray appearances.

Morriston Davies' patient was a man aged 44 with a radiological shadow in his right lower lobe. He was coughing up prune-juice sputum in which malignant cells were identified. Right lower lobectomy was performed for a breaking-down squamous cell carcinoma, with individual ligation of the vessels at the hilum, and suturing of the bronchus. Unfortunately the patient died on the 8th post-operative day from an empyema. At autopsy the bronchus was found to be intact. The operation was

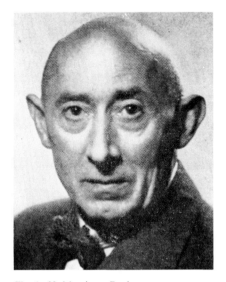

Fig. 1. H. Morriston Davies.

performed under ether anaesthesia and this was the first recorded occasion on which X-rays were used to identify the shadow in the lung.

During the previous 200 years there had been isolated reports of patients undergoing partial removal of cancerous growths from the lung. Many of these reports undoubtedly were of operations performed to deal with the consequences of chest injuries, tuberculosis, lung abscess or bronchiectasis. When fractured ribs allowed the lung to herniate, an intercostal incision was made, the edges of the pleura were sutured to the chest wall and the portion of herniated lung was removed by the cautery. Sloughs removed from lung abscess cavities also could have been misdiagnosed as 'growths'.

The rarity of this disease was emphasised in 1912 by Adler, who was able to collect only 374 cases reported before the year 1900. In 1930 Davidson wrote a book on cancer of the lung in which he gave some interesting statistical figures on the relative and absolute increases in this disease between the years 1900 and 1930. He quoted figures from hospitals in Germany and France and also from the Brompton and London Hospital in England.

In spite of Morriston Davies' successful lobectomy in 1912, further advances in chest surgery were delayed, partly by the advent of the First World War, but largely by the dangers of infection and fear of the open pneumothorax during surgery. Gask, in a Lettsomian Lecture in March 1921, drew attention to the lack of major thoracotomies on the operating lists of the London hospitals and commented on the pre-war methods of Sauerbruch of Munich and Meyer of New York who, in 1904 and 1909 respectively, had operated in negative pressure chambers large enough to contain both the patient and the surgical team (Gask 1950, pp. 167, 168). Apart from the very considerable expense of these chambers, they provided cramped operating conditions for the surgeon. Modern thoracic surgery was not possible until endotracheal anaesthesia with positive pressure ventilation was introduced by Meltzer and Auer in 1910. In an anaesthetic symposium held in New York in 1910 Meltzer paid tribute to Sauerbruch and reminded the audience of the importance of his original description of differential pressures and the development of his negative pressure chamber. However, the next important advance in thoracic anaesthesia did not occur until 1928, when Guedel and Waters first described the closed endotracheal technique with cuffed tubes. This method finally overcame many of the supposed dangers of operation with an open pneumothorax.

In his textbook on laryngeal surgery, published in 1914, Chevalier Jackson drew attention to the importance of bronchoscopy as an aid to the diagnosis of bronchial carcinoma, and in 1925, in conjunction with other authors, he pointed out that bronchoscopy gave one the opportunity not only to prove the diagnosis by biopsy but also to consider the possibility of limiting surgery to a lobectomy. The use of the bronchoscope for the diagnosis of lung cancer was infrequent before 1932, when Vinson reported his experience with 71 patients.

In 1928 the role of radiotherapy in the treatment of bronchial carcinoma was first considered by Paterson, and in an extensive review of the literature he was unable to find any evidence of a cure by irradiation. He reviewed 19 cases treated in the Mayo Clinic between 1921 and 1926 and all had died. He did find that the palliation obtained was worthwhile and resulted in a more merciful type of death; life, however, was not prolonged. In the following year, 1929, Stanford Cade confirmed this in his book on the *Radium Treatment of Cancer*. Prior to 1929 there had been very few reports of radium treatment for bronchial carcinoma, one exception being a short chapter in a book by de Nabias published in 1928. Cade considered surface or distance application to be the method most likely to succeed in the treatment of bronchial carcinoma as it would allow a larger quantity of radium to be used over a longer period of time.

Nineteen thirty-three was the most important year in the development of modern thoracic surgery, for it was then that Evarts Graham successfully removed the left lung in one stage from a physician, aged 48, who subsequently survived for many years — even longer than his surgeon, who died in 1957.

Evarts Graham (Fig. 2) dealt with the hilar vessels by mass ligation. The mucosa of the bronchial stump was cauterised and then transfixed with chromic catgut, before the insertion of seven radon seeds into various parts of the stump. In order to eliminate the large pleural space, the 3rd to 9th ribs inclusive were resected and the chest closed without drainage. Subsequently an empyema developed which required drainage on repeated occasions. The 1st and 2nd ribs were then also resected in order to reduce further the size of the empyema. Meade, who wrote a most comprehensive history of thoracic surgery in 1961, stated during a discussion on a clinical meeting reported by Burford in 1958, that he had had the good fortune to be present when Evarts Graham reported this case.

Following this successful operation many other surgeons reported series of successful resections during 1933. However, some were still afraid of the possible complications of an open pneumothorax during surgery. Both Churchill and Reinhoff reported in 1933 the use of a pre-operative pneumothorax to determine whether or not the patient could tolerate the loss of one lung, but this practice was short-lived.

In 1932 Shenstone and Janes of Toronto performed a series of lobectomies in which the hilar structures were divided between the thick cords of two tourniquets

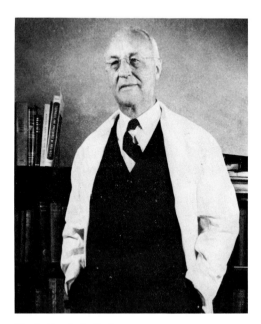

Fig. 2. Evarts A. Graham.

and the stump oversewn with thick continuous chromic catgut. In 1933 Roberts and Nelson reported ten lobectomies from St. Bartholomew's Hospital performed in a similar way, two of the lobectomies being for bronchial carcinoma. Unfortunately this method resulted in a high incidence of postoperative haemorrhage and bronchial fistulae, and it was not long before ligation of the individual hilar vessels and suture of the bronchus became a routine procedure. In the same year Churchill stressed the importance of using absorbable sutures for closing the bronchus, which should not be traumatised by crushing as this would invite infection in devitalised tissue. He also appreciated the ease with which growth could be spread through one or both lungs by bronchial embolism, and the possibility of malignant cells being disseminated into the general circulation by extension from the pulmonary veins.

In an article on the incidence of malignant disease of the lung at the Brompton Hospital, Tudor Edwards noted in 1934 that the disease was increasing both as a result of better methods of diagnosis, and by an absolute incidence. In cases which were inoperable at thoracotomy owing to main bronchial obstruction, he inserted radon seed introducers which were left in a main bronchus for up to 7 days, the growth receiving a gamma radiation equivalent to 1.795 mgh of radium. At the same thoracotomy he inserted radon seeds directly into the growth.

In 1935 Shield of Toronto reported the use of high spinal anaesthesia for patients undergoing thoracotomy. The main advantage was that the patient could expectorate sputum during the operation, but the disadvantages were lowered blood pressure, dyspnoea and cyanosis. Magill (1936) in London supported Shield's views and favoured this form of anaesthesia in reviewing 23 cases of lobectomy and pneumonectomy performed under high spinal anaesthesia.

In 1938 Crafoord in Stockholm published a monograph on the technique of pneumonectomy, and as well as stressing the importance of individual ligation of hilar vessels and suturing and burying the bronchial stump, he showed that anaesthesia by regular rhythmical inflation was far superior to Sauerbruch's negative pressure chamber.

In 1946 Charlotte Auerbach and Robson produced evidence that mustard gas could induce true mutations in animals. This followed research into nitrogen mustard as a chemical warfare agent and led to the development of drugs to treat cancer. Two years later Karnofsky et al. reported on the use of nitrogen mustard as a palliative treatment for carcinomas.

After the Second World War, blood transfusion services had improved and antibiotics were available. Patients undergoing thoracotomy could expect to benefit from a smoother and shorter postoperative course.

Allison (1946) introduced the term 'radical pneumonectomy' to describe the removal of the whole lung together with the mediastinal nodes and lymphatics, with intrapericardial ligation of the vessels. It was considered that partial removal of the lung for operable cases of lung cancer was inadequate and had little chance of success. In 1955 Brock and Whytehead supported radical pneumonectomy as the treatment of choice and quoted a lower operative mortality of 11% as against 18% for simple extrapericardial pneumonectomy. However, other surgeons found an increased operative morbidity of bronchial fistulae and cardiac arrhythmias with the intrapericardial procedure, and it was soon appreciated that lobectomy gave equally good results without the greater mortality of pneumonectomy.

In America Robinson et al. (1956) favoured a policy of lobectomy, and this view was confirmed by Belcher (1959) when quoting a 37% survival rate in a series of 264 lobectomies. In 1958 Churchill et al. reported a 5-year survival rate of 33% among

93 patients who had undergone lobectomy, and 24% among 127 patients treated by pneumonectomy. From Pennsylvania University, also in 1958, Johnson et al. reported 100% blood vessel invasion in cases of undifferentiated carcinoma and concluded that radical pneumonectomy did not improve the outcome. Therefore the policy of performing lobectomy whenever it is technically feasible has been continued since that time and is accepted universally as the treatment of choice.

In 1949 Daniels introduced the surgical investigation of scalene node biopsy performed at the same time as bronchoscopy. He and a minority of surgeons considered that the finding of malignant cells in non-palpable scalene nodes indicated inoperability.

The 1950s saw further advances in aetiology, diagnosis and treatment. In America Wynder and Evarts Graham suggested tobacco smoking as a possible aetiological factor in lung cancer, and Doll and Hill (1956) initiated an investigation into the smoking habits of British doctors. They reported in 1956 that the death rate for those who continued to smoke 25 or more cigarettes a day from 1951 onwards was 40 times higher than for the non-smokers.

In 1951 Brooks et al. reported on 306 patients treated with radiotherapy between 1944 and 1948 at the Joint Consultative Clinic of the Brompton and Royal Cancer Hospitals. They found that considerable palliation was achieved for troublesome haemoptysis, superior vena caval obstruction and bone metastases. They also noted some improvement in patients who had received pre- or post-pneumonectomy radiotherapy.

In 1956 Bignall compared the results in a series of 207 patients with lung cancer treated with varying doses of radiotherapy, with those in 215 patients who had no treatment and survived for 2 months. He decided that the results were the same with or without treatment, and that a larger dose of radiotherapy was no more effective than a smaller one.

In 1956 Smart and Hilton wrote an interesting and important paper from University College Hospital in which they confirmed that radiotherapy was of little value in inoperable cases, but that it could be of greater value in those patients in good general health and with operable lesions. Having had considerable success with three patients who survived between 5 and 13 years following treatment, they decided to treat a group of 33 patients, all of whom had proven carcinomas, with primary radiotherapy. Those patients with undifferentiated growths received 4000–4500 rads, and those with squamous cell growths, 5000–5500 rads. Twelve of these patients survived for 5 or more years, giving a 5-year survival rate of 33%. They pointed out that the poor results of radiotherapy were associated with poor clinical material, but where radiotherapy was given to fitter patients with operable growths the results were exactly comparable with surgery, but without the operative death rate. It seems strange that this policy was not pursued, and surgical treatment remained the treatment of choice.

The concept of combination therapy came into being, and in 1955 Bromley and Szur reported the results in 66 patients treated with pre-operative radiotherapy using the 250 kV machine followed by pneumonectomy. Sadly this resulted in a 27% incidence of postoperative empyema and bronchial fistula, and the treatment had to be abandoned.

In 1956 Price Thomas introduced a major surgical advance in an article on conservative resection of the bronchial tree. The operation of sleeve resection was designed for those patients with poor respiratory reserve who would not tolerate pneumonectomy. A growth situated at the origin of an upper lobar bronchus could be removed by lobectomy. This entails the removal of a cylinder of the main bronchus, the middle and lower lobes on the right side or the lower lobe on the left side then being anastomosed to the trachea at carinal level. This procedure could also be performed on the pulmonary artery. Price Thomas reported that this operation had been performed previously by Allison, but gave no date.

About this time it was realised that the prognosis following surgical treatment was related to the specific histological variety of tumour concerned, an observation made by Holmes Sellors in 1955 in a personal series of 689 thoracotomies in which he found the prognosis for adenocarcinoma to be as poor as for the oat cell tumour.

In 1957 Morrison and Deeley reported improved results with megavoltage X-ray therapy for inoperable cases. Unlike the 250 kV machine, megavoltage X-ray allows deeper penetration of malignant tissue without damage to the skin and surrounding structures, such as bones.

In 1959 Carlens introduced mediastinoscopy to inspect and obtain lymph node tissue for biopsy from the superior mediastinum. This method was given strong support in this country by Sarin and Nohl-Oser (1969), and in Canada by Pearson et al. (1972). The presence of a positive contralateral node certainly avoided unnecessary operatons. However, Sarin and Nohl-Oser advised radiotherapy when an involved ipsilateral node was found — a policy with which all did not agree. Pearson et al. felt that in certain selected cases of squamous cell growth, thoracotomy should be performed. In 1978 Abbey Smith analysed the incidence of mediastinal node involvement in 417 patients operated on between 1964 and 1969; he found node involvement in only 13.4% and a resectability rate of 97.4%. He therefore concluded that routine mediastinoscopy prior to surgery was not justified.

In 1962 Paulson et al. advised radiotherapy before embarking on surgical treatment for a Pancoast tumour. This tumour syndrome was first described in 1924 when Pancoast called it a superior sulcus tumour with a specific histological origin arising from an embryonal epithelial rest. The majority of tumours causing this syndrome are of the squamous cell variety, but adenocarcinomas may also be responsible. Surgical treatment on its own was not successful either in removing the whole tumour or in relieving pain. Paulson advised 3000 rads of ionising radiation to the lesion and surgical removal 3–6 weeks later. The involved ribs, chest wall muscles and intercostal nerves, the sympathetic chain and stellate ganglion, the lowest trunk of the brachial plexus and the upper lobe concerned would be removed 'en bloc'. In 1966 Paulson wrote a second paper in which 57 patients had received this treatment; 45 cases had been resected with only two postoperative deaths. Of 30 of these patients who had been operated upon 5 or more years before, 10 were alive and well.

In 1962 Watson and Berg were credited with one of the first descriptions of small cell carcinoma of the lung as a tumour type which differs from the other types of lung cancer. They also found a good response to nitrogen mustard, which was not so with other tumours. They suggested that these small cell carcinomas might be better treated with a combination of chemotherapy and supervoltage radiation. When Kern et al., in 1968, reported the histological varieties in 94 long-term survivors, there were no instances of small cell carcinoma.

In 1964 the Medical Research Council initiated a trial to investigate the possible advantage of giving either busulphan or cyclophosphamide in conjunction with surgical excision of carcinomas other than oat cell. The 5-year-old follow-up report by Miller in 1971 concluded that these drugs were of no benefit, and in fact busulphan was likely to cause severe thrombocytopenia.

In 1966 McNeill and Chamberlain introduced the further surgical investigation of mediastinotomy. The 2nd or 3rd costal cartilage was excised on either side, allowing a mediastinal node to be removed extrapleurally, or the pleura could be opened deliberately and a limited intrapleural exploration carried out.

The introduction of the flexible bronchoscope in 1968 by Ikeda of Japan has added greatly to the information previously supplied by the rigid bronchoscope. While the latter instrument is essential in assessing the operability of tumours in a main bronchus, the flexible instrument allows biopsy specimens to be obtained from small peripheral and segmental lesions, particularly when they lie in the apical segments of the upper lobes. This is of value in the so-called occult carcinoma, where the chest X-ray remains clear even though neoplastic cells have been found in the sputum. Bronchial brushings can be taken from subsegmental carinae until the source of the positive brush is identified.

In 1969 the Medical Research Council reported on a comparative trial of surgery and radiotherapy for the primary treatment of oat cell carcinoma. The results published by Miller et al. for both forms of treatment were disheartening: a 3% survival rate for surgery at 4 years and 7% for radiotherapy. This report had a very damaging effect on the development of surgical treatment for this particular growth over the next 10 years. In 1974 Bates et al., in a small series, reported improved results of 24% survival at 4 years by treating oat cell carcinoma with pre-operative radiotherapy — 1750 rads given by the Cobalt machine — immediately followed by pneumonectomy. The complications of bronchopleural fistula and empyema previously experienced by Bromley and Szur were not a problem.

In 1969 Green el al. reviewed the results of a randomised trial in which 946 patients from the Veterans' Administration Lung Cancer Study Group were treated with either nitrogen mustard or oral and intravenous cyclophosphamide. They found a better response with squamous cell to nitrogen mustard, and with small cell to cyclophosphamide. However, the overall influence on survival time was not remarkable.

In 1970 Dart et al. reported on 6 years' experience of using stapling machines for bronchial closure. This method greatly reduced the incidence of bronchopleural fistula.

Le Roux (1972) reported the first use of segmental resection for bronchial carcinoma and found the results to be no worse than after more extensive resections for small peripheral tumours. Such a limited resection is of particular benefit to those patients who develop a new primary growth. Abbey Smith et al. (1976) found this situation arising between 8 and 12 years after the first resection and only in patients who continued to smoke.

In 1973 computerised axial tomography was developed and Kreel commented in 1976 on its ability to reveal mediastinal lymph node involvement not seen on routine tomography. A further important development in 1973 was the endorsement of the TNM system of staging by the American Joint Committee for Cancer Staging, reporting through its Task Force on Carcinoma of the Lung; as a result this system is accepted universally.

In 1974 Earle Wilkins gave a masterly account of the extrathoracic manifestations of bronchial carcinoma, and subsequent workers have been able to show that the ectopic hormones responsible for these symptoms are produced by the oat cell carcinoma in 90% of instances.

Also in 1974 Selawry reviewed the response of the various histological types of lung cancer to different chemotherapeutic agents. In 1977 Cohen cited a prolonged remission in a patient with inoperable small cell carcinoma who had been treated with cyclophosphamide and methotrexate, the patient being alive and well 2 years after cessation of treatment.

In 1976 Price Evans focussed attention on the immunological aspects of the disease and showed that non-specific active immunisation can improve the survival rate. In the same year McKneally et al. reported on 60 patients injected with BCG intrapleurally following resection and found that some patients with limited disease had gained benefit. However, when Lowe et al. (1980) reviewed this claim, they were unable to support it.

In 1978 Toty et al. described the use of a laser beam directed along the flexible endoscope to relieve malignant bronchial obstruction. Since then there have been further exciting developments regarding the potential therapeutic value of lasers.

In his 1981 Honoured Guest's Address to the American Association for Thoracic Surgery, Abbey Smith speculated that any immunotherapy or chemotherapy found to be effective might have to be continued indefinitely after successful resection to overcome the problem of long-term recurrence.

The Mayo Lung Project has been the largest analysis of the value of close-surveillance screening to detect early lung cancer. The interim report (Woolner et al. 1981) suggested that the results may not justify the cost.

A realistic appraisal of this historical survey cannot avoid the conclusion that 50 years of dedicated effort has yet to be rewarded with the success which in 1933 Evarts Graham justifiably could have expected.

References

Abbey Smith R (1978) The importance of mediastinal lymph node invasion by pulmonary carcinoma in selection of patients for resection. Ann Thorax Surg 25:5–11

Abbey Smith R (1981) Examination of the long term results of surgery for bronchial carcinoma. J Thorac Cardiovasc Surg 82:325–333

Abbey Smith R, Nigam BK, Thompson JM (1976) Second primary lung carcinoma. Thorax 31:507–517

Adler I (1912) Primary malignant growths of the lungs and bronchi. Longmans Green, New York

Allison PR (1946) Intrapericardial approach to the lung root in the treatment of bronchial carcinoma by dissection pneumonectomy. J Thorac Surg 15:99–117

Auerbach C, Robson JM (1946) Chemical production of mutations. Nature 157:302

Bates M, Hurt RL, Levison V, Sutton M (1974) Treatment of oat cell carcinoma of the bronchus by pre-operative radiotherapy and surgery. Lancet I:1134–1135

Belcher JR (1959) Lobectomy for bronchial carcinoma. Lancet II:639–642

Bignall JR (1956) Bronchial carcinoma. Effect of radiotherapy on survival. Lancet I:876–879

Brock RC, Whytehead LL (1955) Radical pneumonectomy for bronchial carcinoma. Br J Surg 43:8–24

Bromley LL, Szur L (1955) Combined radiotherapy and resection for carcinoma of the bronchus with experiences with 66 patients. Lancet II:937–941

Brooks WDW, Davidson M, Price Thomas C, Robson K, Smithers DW (1951) Carcinoma of the bronchus. Thorax 6:1

Burford TH, Ferguson TB, Spjut HJ (1958) Results in the treatment of bronchogenic carcinoma. An analysis of 1008 cases. J Thorac Surg 36:316–328

Cade S (1929) Radium treatment of cancer. J & A Churchill, London

Carlens E (1959) Mediastinoscopy: a method for inspection and tissue biopsy in the superior mediastinum. Dis Chest 36:343–352

Churchill ED (1933) The surgical treatment of carcinoma of the lung. J Thorac Surg 2:254–266

Churchill ED, Sweet RH, Scannell JG, Wilkins EW Jr (1958) Further studies in the surgical management of carcinoma of the lung. J Thorac Surg 36:301–308

Cohen MD (1977) Small cell bronchogenic carcinoma. A prolonged remission following chemotherapy. JAMA 237:2528

Crafoord C (1938) On the technique of pneumonectomy in man. Tryckeri Aktiebolaget Thule, Stockholm

Daniels AC (1949) Method of biopsy useful in diagnosing certain intrathoracic diseases. Dis Chest 16:360–366

Dart CH Jr, Scott SM, Takaro T (1970) Six-year clinical experience using automatic stapling devices for lung resections. Ann Thorac Surg 9:535–550

Davidson M (1930) Cancer of the lung and other intrathoracic tumours. Wm Wood, New York

de Nabias S (1928) Le traitement par le radium de quelques neoplasms. Chahine, Paris

Doll R, Hill AB (1956) Lung cancer and other causes of death in relation to smoking. Br Med J II:1071–1082

Edwards AT (1934) Malignant disease of the lung. J Thorac Surg 4:107–134

Gask G (1950) Essays in the history of medicine. Butterworths, London

Graham EA, Singer JJ (1933) Successful removal of the entire lung for carcinoma of the bronchus JAMA 101:1371–1374

Green RA, Humphrey E, Close H, Patno ME (1969) Alkalating agents in carcinoma of bronchus. Am J Med 46:516–529

Guedel AE, Waters RM (1928) A new intratracheal catheter. Anaesth Analg 7:238–239

Holmes Sellors T (1933) Surgery of the thorax. Constable, London

Holmes Sellors T (1955) Results of surgical treatment of carcinoma of the lung. Br Med J I:445–448

Ikeda S, Yanai N, Ishikawa S (1968) Flexible fibrescope. Keio J Med 17:1

Jackson C (1914) Peroral endoscopy and laryngeal surgery textbook. Laryngoscope Publishing Co., St. Louis, Mo.

Jackson C. Tucker G, Lukens RM, Moore WF (1925) Bronchoscopy as an aid to the thoracic surgeon. JAMA 84:97–102

Johnson J, Kirby CK, Blakemore WS (1958) Should we insist on radical pneumonectomy as a routine procedure in the treatment of carcinoma of the lung? J Thorac Surg 36:309–315

Karnofsky DA, Abelmann WH, Craver LF et al. (1948) The use of nitrogen mustards in the palliative treatment of carcinomas. Cancer 1:634–656

Kern WH, Jones JC, Wiles DC (1968) Pathology of bronchogenic carcinomas in long term survivors. Cancer 21:772–780

Kreel L (1976) The EMI whole body scanner in the demonstration of lymph node enlargement. Clin Radiol 27:421–429

Le Roux BT (1972) Management of bronchial carcinoma by segmental resection. Thorax 27:70–74

Lowe J, Iles PB, Shore DF, Langman MJS, Baldwin RW (1980) Intrapleural BCG in operable lung cancer. Lancet I:11–13

Magill IW (1936) Anaesthesia in thoracic surgery with special reference to lobectomy. Proc R Soc Med 29:643–653

McKneally MF, Mauer C, Kausel HW (1976) Regional immunotherapy of lung cancer with intrapleural BCG. Lancet I:377–379

McNeill TM, Chamberlain JM (1966) Diagnostic anterior mediastinotomy. Ann Thorac Surg 2:532–539

Meade RH (1961) A history of thoracic surgery. Charles C Thomas,Springfield, Ill.

Meltzer SJ (1910) The method of respiration by intratracheal insufflation, the scientific principle and the practical availability in medicine and surgery. Med Record New York 77:477–483

Meyer W (1909) Pneumonectomy with the aid of differential pressure: an experimental study. JAMA 53:1978–1987

Miller AB, Fox W, Tall R (1969) Five year follow-up of the Medical Research Council comparative trial of surgery and radiotherapy, for the primary treatment of small or oat celled carcinoma of the bronchus. Lancet II:501–505

Miller AB (1971) A Medical Research Council working party study of cytotoxic chemotherapy as an adjuvant to surgery. Br Med J II:421–428

Morrison R, Deeley TJ (1957) Treatment of inoperable carcinoma of the bronchus by megavolt X-ray therapy. Lancet II:907–909

Morriston Davies H (1913) Recent advances in the surgery of the lung and pleura. Br J Surg 1:228–258

Pancoast HK (1924) The importance of careful Roentgen-ray investigations of apical chest tumours. JAMA 83:1407

Paterson R (1928) Roentgen-ray treatment of primary carcinoma of the lung. Br J Radiol i.NS:90–96

Paulson DL (1966) The survival rate in superior sulcus tumours by presurgical irradiation. JAMA 196:342

Paulson DL, Shaw RR, Kee JL, Mallams JT, Collier RE (1962) Combined preoperative irradiation and resection for bronchogenic carcinoma. J Thorac Cardiovasc Surg 44:281–294

Pearson FG, Nellems JM, Henderson RD, Delarve NC (1972) The role of mediastinoscopy in the selection of treatments for bronchial carcinoma with involvement of superior mediastinal nodes. J Thorac Surg 64:382–390

Price Evans DA (1976) Immunology of bronchial carcinoma. Thorax 31:493–506

Price Thomas C (1956) Conservative resection of the bronchial tree. J R Coll Surg Edin 1:169–186

Reinhoff WF Jr (1933) Pneumonectomy. A preliminary report of two successful cases. Bull Johns Hopkins Hosp 53:390

Roberts JEH, Nelson HP (1933) Pulmonary lobectomy. Technique and report of ten cases. Br J Surg 21:227–301

Robinson JL, Jones JC, Meyer BW (1956) Indications for lobectomy in the treatment of carcinoma of the lung. J Thorac Surg 32: 500–507

Sarin CL, Nohl-Oser HC (1969) Mediastinoscopy: a clinical evaluation of 400 consecutive cases. Thorax 24:585–588

Sauerbruch F (1904) Über die Ausschaltung der schädlichen Wirkung der Pneumothorax bei intra-thorakalen Operationen. Zentralbl Chir 31

Selawry OS (1974) The role of chemotherapy in the treatment of lung cancer. Semin Oncol 1:259

Shenstone NS, Janes RM (1932) Experiences in pulmonary lobectomy. Can Med Assoc J xxvii:138

Shield HJ (1935) Spinal anaesthesia in thoracic surgery. Anaesth Analg 14:193–198

Smart J. Hilton G (1956) Radiotherapy of cancer of the lung. Results in a selected group of cases. Lancet 1:880–881

Task Force on Carcinoma of the Lung (1973) Clinical staging system for carcinoma of the lung. American Joint Committee for Cancer Staging and End Results Reporting, Chicago

Toty L, Personne C, Hertzog P et al. (1978) Utilisation d'un Faiscean Laser (YAG) a conducteur souple, pour le traitements endoscopique de certains lesions tracheobronchique. Rev Fr Mal Respir 7:57–60

Vinson PP (1932) Primary carcinoma of the bronchi: report of 71 cases in which the diagnosis was made by bronchoscopy. Minn Med 15:15–17

Watson W, Berg J (1962) Oat cell lung cancer. Cancer 15:759–768

Wilkins EW Jr (1974) Extrathoracic manifestations of thoracic neoplasms. In: Smith RE, Williams WG (eds) Surgery of the lung — the Coventry Conference. Butterworth, London pp 69–85

Woolner LB, Fontana RS, Sanderson DR, et al. (1981) Mayo lung project evaluation of lung cancer screening through December 1979. Mayo Clin Proc 56:544–555

Wynder EL, Graham EA (1950) Tobacco smoking as a possible etiologic factor in bronchogenic carcinoma. JAMA 143:229–336

Chapter 2

The Epidemiology of Bronchial Carcinoma

Alan Bailey

Introduction

Lung cancer is now the commonest malignant disease affecting civilised man and is competing with breast cancer to become the commonest in women. If it is not yet a common problem in the developing world, it soon will be. At the beginning of this century it was rare. By the 1930s it accounted for 0.5% of the certified causes of death in men and 0.2% in women, and by the beginning of the 1980s these proportions had increased to over 6% for men and approaching 2% for women. Undoubtedly some of this increase can be ascribed to the better diagnostic facilities made available to an ageing population. But that a true increase in the incidence is still occurring can be seen from the annual registration rates in Table 1. In men this continuing increase is in the 65 and over age group; the rates are beginning to fall in other age groups. In women the rates are still increasing in most age groups over 45. Lung cancer now accounts for nearly one-third of all male cancer registrations (28%) and just under one-tenth of female registrations (9%). The comparable figures (standardised mortality ratios: SMR) for certified causes of death (as a proportion of all malignant disease) are 37% for men and 14% for women.

Further refining of the crude figures given above leads to three epidemiological conclusions. First, there has been an increase in incidence — some of it representing a true increase in this disease. Secondly, the disease is far commoner in men, but the incidence in women is rising faster. Thirdly, it carries a poor prognosis. These points are further elaborated below.

Table 1. Registrations for lung cancer by sex and specific age groups (England and Wales)

	Rates per 100 000 population										
	1970	1971	1972	1973	1974	1975	1976	1977	1978	1979[a]	1980[a]
Males											
All ages	101	109	108	111	114	113	116	118	114	115	113
45—50	62	61	58	54	58	57	53	51	45		
80—85	367	484	502	538	614	597	625	697	745		
Females											
All ages	21	23	24	25	27	28	29	30	32	33	35
65—70	68	75	80	81	88	92	95	104	108		
70—75	70	82	79	90	90	94	102	104	118		

[a] Provisional figures (age breakdown not available)
Source: OPCS Medical Statistics: Cancer surveillance — trachea, bronchus and lung (various years)

Incidence

The proportion of increased incidence that can be attributed to improved diagnosis will largely have occurred between the wars, when chest X-rays and bronchoscopy became common diagnostic tools. Even so, many cases of lung cancer would be obscured by the pneumonia that they would present with and which would often kill the patient, so it was not until the antibiotic era that the true incidence of lung cancer could be determined. Although there has been some improvement in diagnostic technique since 1945, there is general agreement that the post-war rise in the disease is real. The rise in incidence is mainly related to squamous and oat cell varieties of carcinoma of the bronchus. This is discussed further later.

Sex and Age Differences

Sex and age differences in lung cancer are considered in greater detail later on, in relation to smoking habits. In England and Wales there are three times as many deaths from lung cancer in men as women. In men, although the overall registration rate seems to be declining, the death rate is still increasing in the elderly population, but in women the increase is most noticeable under the age of 65.

Prognosis

The survival rate for all forms of lung cancer is poor and there is no appreciable difference between the sexes. The crude and relative survival rate (that is the survival rates after correcting for the patient's probability of dying from a cause other than lung cancer) are given in Table 2. There is a slight suggestion that patients under 55 have higher survival than others — but this is the only area for optimism.

Table 2. Crude and relative survival rates: Cancer of bronchus and lung (England and Wales)

Sex	Registration years	Number of cases	Crude % survival		Relative % survival	
			1 yr	5 yrs	1 yr	5 yrs
Males	1971–73	71 525	19	6	20	8
Females	1971–73	16 340	17	6	18	7

Source: Trends in Cancer Survival in Great Britain (1982)
          Cancer Research Campaign, London

Geographical Distribution

We have so far considered statistics for England and Wales. International comparisons must be treated with caution because of differences in death certification and diagnostic criteria. However, the United Kingdom heads the league table of SMR for lung cancer, with a rate almost double that of white Americans and about five times that of the Japanese.

Social Class Differences

In men, the change in SMR by social class (I–V as defined by the Registrar General) has become more marked over the years. In 1931 no gradient was present but the latest figures show a marked gradient (Fig. 1). Thus if lung cancer is caused by some environmental agent, as seems likely because of its changing incidence, then this agent affected all classes equally in the 1930s but more selectively now. In fact, the agent is tobacco smoke. and the evidence linking smoking and lung cancer in man is reviewed below.

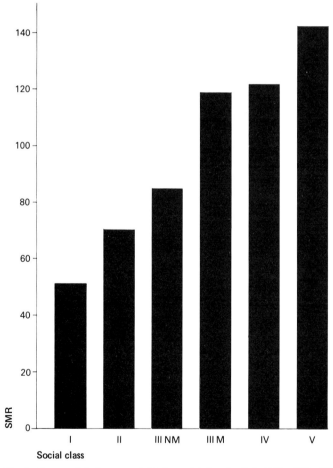

Fig. 1. Cancer of the lung: mortality by social class (males), 1970—1971. (Office of Population Censuses and Surveys/Cancer Research Campaign Cancer Registration Statistics. No. 43. Studies on Medical and Population Subjects. ICD 162. H.M.S.O., p 49)

The Smoking Habit

Tobacco was imported into Europe during the sixteenth century for medicinal purposes, doctors regarding it as a cure-all. Sir Walter Raleigh made it fashionable, so that by the first half of the seventeenth century there was a booming tobacco trade in London. However, the King, James I, was firmly against the habit. He recognised its mood altering qualities and its addictive nature, calling it "a stinking, loathsome thing, and so is hell"! He imposed a special tobacco tax, on the grounds that it was impairing the workers' health, of six shillings and tenpence per pound (the importation duty was originally twopence a pound). Soon the sale of tobacco became a royal monopoly and the King grew rich on its tax. Despite the expense, smoking became more popular during the seventeenth century and was generally recommended as an antiseptic at the time of the plague; physicians attending the sick smoked freely. For a time in France tobacco could only be obtained on prescription.

For the next 200 years the habit grew of smoking tobacco in clay pipes. As it was an expensive habit, the bowls of the pipes were small. It was not until the Crimean war (1854–1856) that the cigarette was introduced. About this time a movement grew up in England wanting to banish smoking completely, and special smoking compartments were introduced on trains in 1868. During the early part of this century smoking in public was generally frowned upon. Cigarettes overtook pipes as the commonest way of consuming tobacco, but after the First World War fashion changed again. Smoking became respectable and women smoked in public.

The 1950s marked a new era in the smoking story. By then four-fifths of all tobacco consumed was in the form of cigarettes. The filter-tipped, lower tar producing cigarette was introduced (Fig. 2). Doll and Bradford Hill in Britain and Wynder in America produced, independently, retrospective evidence that linked smoking (mainly cigarette smoking) with death from lung cancer. This has since been confirmed by a number of prospective studies. Although the risk of lung cancer is slightly increased in pipe and cigar smokers, this risk is substantially less than it is for cigarette smokers.

Important Factors in the Relationship Between Smoking and Lung Cancer

Tumour-Producing Contents of Cigarette Smoke

At least 500 different chemicals have been isolated from cigarette smoke. Table 3 lists a number of compounds known to initiate or cause cancer in animals. The concentration of these compounds in cigarette smoke is such that if cigarettes had been invented today they would be regarded as potentially too 'toxic' for sale to the public! The chemicals responsible for human cancer are most likely to be carried in the 'tar', the portion of smoke which is trapped on a glass fibre filter. If tar containing the polynuclear aromatic hydrocarbons is removed, tumourgenic activity is reduced by up to 50%. Despite the presence of animal cancer initiators in smoke, most of the evidence that smoking produces lung cancer in man is still epidemiological.

Table 3. Potential cigarette poisons

Tar	Tumour initiator
Nicotine	General toxin
Carbon monoxide (CO)	Toxin (? atherogenesis)
Hydrogen cyanide	Cilia and general toxin
Benzo(a)pyrene	Tumor initiator
Nitrosamines	Carcinogens
Phenol	Co-carcinogen
Acrolein	Cilia toxicity
Polonium–210	Carcinogen
Nickel compounds	Carcinogens
Cadmium compounds	Carcinogens

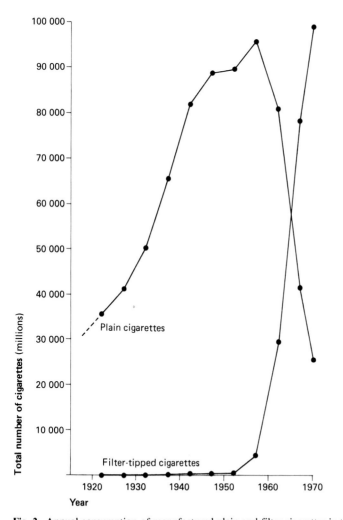

Fig. 2. Annual consumption of manufactured plain and filter cigarettes in the United Kingdom. [Wald NJ (1976) Mortality from lung cancer and coronary heart disease in relation to changes in smoking habits. Lancet I:136—138]

Quantity Smoked

The risk of developing lung cancer is directly proportional to the amount smoked. In men, smoking up to 10 cigarettes per day increases the risk of lung cancer about fivefold over the non-smoker. At 20 per day it is more than a tenfold increase. More details are given in Fig. 3 from Doll's study on British doctors and in Table 4.

At present the mortality ratios for women are less than for men (Table 5). This reflects differences in smoking habits between the sexes, the fact that women have mostly smoked filter-tipped cigarettes and the length of exposure mentioned above.

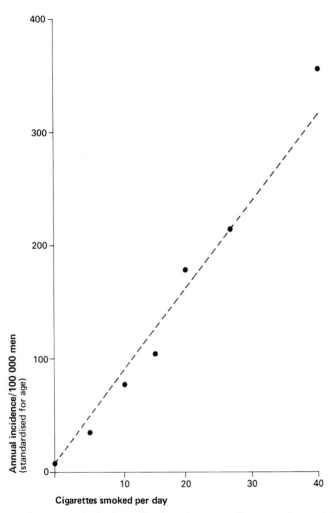

Fig. 3. Age-standardised mortality from lung cancer in non-smokers and cigarette smokers (U.K. male doctors) by amount smoked. [Doll R (1970) Practical steps towards the prevention of bronchial carcinoma. Scott Med J 15:433–447]

Table 4. Male lung cancer mortality by age and cigarette consumption

| Smoking category | Age (years). | | | | | | | | | | | |
| | 35–54 | | | 55–69 | | | 70+ | | | All ages | | |
	Death rate[a]	No. of deaths	Mortality ratio	Death rate[a]	No. of deaths	Mortality ratio	Death rate[a]	No. of deaths	Mortality ratio	Death rate[a]	No. of deaths	Mortality ratio
Never	6	11	1.00	19	27	1.00	25	11	1.00	12	49	1.00
Current smokers												
1–9/day	38	9	6.33	68	12	3.58	134	5	5.36	56	26	4.67
10–19/day	24	15	4.00	168	57	6.84	234	10	9.72	90	82	7.50
20–39/day	58	138	9.67	264	218	13.89	446	27	17.84	159	381	13.25
40+/day	47	26	7.83	334	50	17.58	754	6	29.84	201	82	16.75

[a]Annual death rate per 100 000
Source: Hammond EC (1966) Smoking in relation to the death rates of one million men and women. Natl Cancer Inst Mongr 19:127–204

Table 5. Male and female lung cancer mortality ratios by cigarette consumption

| | Number of cigarettes smoked daily | | | |
	1–9	10–19	20–30	40+
Men	4.7	10.0	16.7	21.0
Women	1.1	2.4	4.9	5.3

Source: Hammond EC (1972) Smoking habits and air pollution in relation to lung cancer. In: Lee HK (ed) Environmental factors in respiratory disease. Academic Press, London New York, pp 172–198

Cigarette Smoking vs Other Types of Tobacco Product

Lung cancer mortality ratios for pipe and cigar smokers are a fraction of that for cigarette smokers: in the US studies about one-eighth, and in the UK studies about one-quarter. Cigar and pipe tobacco is alkaline and more irritating to the respiratory mucosa. Nicotine is absorbed rapidly through the mouth and the necessity to inhale deeply is reduced. Using carboxyhaemoglobin (COHb) as a marker of inhalation depths, it is found that cigar and pipe smokers generally have lower COHb levels than cigarette smokers for the same amount of tobacco smoked. This may not apply to secondary cigar and pipe smokers, i.e. those who have changed from cigarette smoking to pipe or cigar smoking and who may inhale deeply. In this case the nature of the inhaled cigar or pipe smoke may be more dangerous than cigarette smoke.

Studies based on self-reported inhaling habits have produced conflicting results. Again, using COHb as a marker for inhalation habit is unreliable. Most early surveys of inhaling habit are based on the type of question "Do you inhale?" with answers classified into 'No' or 'Yes — slight', 'Yes — moderate' etc.

Depth of inhalation is very much part of the whole smoking habit and will vary from individual to individual according to his or her physical and psychological needs and the type of material smoked. Most studies on inhaling have been too superficial for firm conclusions to be drawn.

Ex-smokers

The early work on British doctors showed that the relative risk of lung cancer fell soon after giving up the smoking habit. Prospective studies all show a reduction in risk proportionate to the length of time since quitting. After 10 years of abstinence the risk of lung cancer approximates to that in non-smokers of the same age.

Filter-Tipped Cigarettes

Filter-tipped cigarettes have been available for most of this century, but only became popular in the late 1950s and early 1960s. By 1970 four out of five cigarettes smoked in the United Kingdom were filter-tipped. They are designed to produce less tar, and people who smoke filter cigarettes have lower rates of lung cancer than those who continue to smoke plain cigarettes. There have been many attempts at producing a 'safe' cigarette but without success. The latest venture using NSM (non-smoking materials) failed to attract smokers — and it is doubtful whether its health risks would have been substantially lower anyway.

International Epidemiology

The United Kingdom has a higher death rate from lung cancer than any other country. For most other countries where statistics are available, the lung cancer death rate correlates with the mean number of cigarettes smoked per adult per year 30 years before the study year. Three countries, the United States, Japan and Ireland, have a lower rate than would be expected.

International comparisons must be regarded with caution because of differences in death certification, smoking habits (including the type of tobacco smoked) and the pattern of disease generally. For instance, in the United States the death rate from ischaemic heart disease in the middle-aged group was almost 50% higher than in the United Kingdom in the 1960s. This meant that fewer susceptible men in the United States were at risk from lung cancer than in the United Kingdom (the majority of premature deaths from ischaemic heart disease occur in smokers).

The lower rate of lung cancer in Japanese men is thought to be due to different inhaling habits and the fact that smoking consumption fell in Japan during World War II, whereas it rose in the United Kingdom; the level in Japan did not rise again until the 1950s.

Occupational Factors

A number of substances used in industry have been shown to be carcinogenic for man. As far as lung cancer is concerned, the number of occupationally induced tumours is a small proportion of the whole. Some agents are probably synergistic with tobacco smoke.

Coal Dust. Percival Pott first described cancer of the scrotum in chimney sweeps — implicating coal dust as the carcinogen — in 1775 (Pott 1775). An increased mortality from lung cancer has been shown in gas retort workers and coke oven workers. The carcinogen is benzopyrene, present in coal tar.

Asbestos. It has been known since the 1930s that lung cancer occurs with pulmonary asbestos. Some controls on types of asbestos used in industry were introduced then but these have been shown to be far from adequate. It is now thought that even light exposure to asbestos dust is dangerous and new regulations were drawn up in the 1970s. There is also an increasing recognition of an association between blue asbestos (crocidolite) and pleural mesothelioma. Cigarette smokers seem to be more at risk to asbestos-related disease than non-smokers.

Ionising Radiation. Increases in lung cancer have been seen in Japan following the atomic bomb explosions and in patients irradiated for ankylosing spondylitis. There is a suggestion that miners of uranium and other radioactive materials have an increased risk for lung cancer. More recently, work from the United States has suggested an increased incidence in nuclear power workers (Bross and Driscoll 1981). In uranium workers there again appears to be synergy with cigarette smoking.

Other Agents. A number of agents have been implicated and are being studied. These include arsenic, used in various industrial processes and the manufacture of pesticides (Ott et al. 1974), chrome and nickle ore (Machle and Gregorious 1948; Bidstrup and Case 1956; Doll et al. 1970), mustard gas (Wada et al. 1968) and possibly vinyl chloride (Monson et al. 1974).

Air Pollution and Other People's Smoke

Urban air contains more coal tar and other pollutants that might be carcinogenic — but studies of lung cancer in urban and rural areas are not easy to interpret. On balance there seems to be an 'urban factor' associated with lung cancer. A study from Liverpool showed the age-standardised lung cancer mortality in the town to be double the rate in the North Wales rural areas, but this has not been confirmed elsewhere in the British Isles. Factors such as migration, better diagnosis in the towns and retirement to the country confuse the issue.

One question raised recently by several studies is how does other people's smoke affect the non-smoker. It has been shown that bronchitis and pneumonia are more common (as measured by the prevalence of cough) in children with smoking parents than in those with non-smoking parents. A Japanese study (Hirayama 1981) showed that the wives of heavy smokers had double the risk of lung cancer compared with the wives of non-smokers. Most of the cancers were adenocarcinoma, rather than the cigarette-related squamous cell carcinoma. This and other factors have led experts to question whether, despite highly significant statistics, this is a causal relationship. However, a Greek study (Trichopolous et al. 1981) much smaller than the Japanese one supported the latter's results. In a smaller number of cases the relative risk of lung cancer was more than three times that expected in wives of heavy smokers. Adenocarcinoma was specifically excluded from this study, although about one-third of cases did not have cytological examination. Further studies from North America have confirmed the relationship (Garfinkel 1981; Correa et al. 1983), and the balance of evidence suggests that other people's smoke may harm the non-smoker.

Vitamin A

Vitamin A deficiency enhances susceptibility of animals to cancer. In vitro vitamin A analogues are effective anti-cancer agents. In a study from Norway (Bjelke 1975) the incidence of histologically proven lung cancer was nearly five times higher in men classified as having a low vitamin A intake. Other retrospective studies have shown low vitamin A levels, measured as serum retinol, in patients with cancer compared with controls without cancer. A prospective study based on BUPA's health screening operation in England showed that serum retinol levels had a predictive value for subsequent cancer, low levels being most clearly associated with an increased risk of lung cancer (Wald et al. 1980). So far vitamin A is the only nutritional element to be epidemiologically related to lung cancer. It is possible that cigarette smokers might be able to protect themselves from lung cancer by ensuring an adequate vitamin A intake (but not excessive, as vitamin A is toxic in large doses), but this is by no means proven. Dietary differences where they affect vitamin A intake may contribute to the social class and urban/rural difference in lung cancer rates.

Susceptibility

Despite the constant relationship between smoking and lung cancer, it must be remembered that only a minority of smokers die of lung cancer. More will die of other smoking-related disease such as ischaemic heart disease or chronic bronchitis. Nevertheless, there is reason to believe that some people are more susceptible to developing tobacco-related lung cancer than others. This could be genetically determined but to date there is no convincing evidence. In twin studies not enough cases have been reported for conclusions to be drawn. Enzyme chemistry may throw light on the question of susceptibility, but more research is needed.

The Decline in Lung Cancer

Doll and Bradford Hill's original study on doctors provided good evidence that giving up smoking reduced the risk of lung cancer. On average an ex-smoker reduces his chance of developing lung cancer to that of a non-smoker in about 10 years. A 10-year randomised study of antismoking advice (Rose et al. 1982) showed a 23% reduction in lung cancer deaths in the intervention group. On a national scale there has been a decline in the death rate from lung cancer during the 1970s in the middle age groups of men (35–60 years). This decline is more marked in the higher social classes and can be accounted for by their reduced consumption since World War II, by the reduction of tar yield of cigarettes (starting in 1950) and by the change to filter-tipped cigarettes. The tar yield is thought to be a particularly important factor. In the United States, where tar yields remained high through the 1960s and 1970s, there has been no fall in lung cancer rates.

Prevention of Lung Cancer

More is known about the cause of lung cancer than about almost any other major malignant disease. World-wide there are probably some 400 000 preventible deaths a year from lung cancer, and the figure is rising.

In Britain the number of cigarette smokers is gradually falling, particularly among professional and managerial males. At present the strategy for prevention consists of health education and government warnings on the cigarette packets. This is unlikely to have a major effect on the disease since promotion, particularly to the Third World, is at a high level.

The government in Britain could act by increasing the tax on tobacco, just as did James I! The percentage drop in smoking is about half the percentage increase in price when small increments in tax are made. Governments are subject to various lobbies against punitive taxation from groups with a commercial interest in the multi-million pound tobacco industry, and others who feel that swingeing increases might affect the poorer sections of the community adversely. In addition, it looks as if the Treasury has decided that it is 'cost effective' to allow people to smoke themselves to death, rather than to look after them in their old age.

The role of prevention is therefore left to the medical and allied professions. In Britain the Health Education Council has a minute budget compared with the amount spent on promoting smoking. In a busy general practice, helping smokers to give up and organising health education for school children generally gets low priority. However, it has been shown that people need the general practitioner's advice on smoking more than anyone else's. We also find in the BUPA Medical Centre's health screening operation that doctors who do not smoke have a greater success rate in getting patients to quit smoking than doctors who smoke themselves.

In the community, some local authorities have set up anti-smoking clinics and a variety of private agencies and paramedical practitioners claim reasonable success rates for helping people to give up smoking. In hospital practice there has been some success in making wards into smoke-free areas — particularly medical wards with their high proportion of patients suffering from smoking-related diseases. Unfortunately, smoking is still very prevalent among hospital nurses.

Action on Smoking and Health (ASH), a College of Physicians' pressure group and information agency, has helped in the preventive field by summarising scientific work, by disseminating newsletters highlighting the dangers of smoking and by commenting on the politics involved. Meanwhile, as the rest of this book demonstrates, health services will continue to use scarce resources attempting to cure and palliate a largely preventible disease.

References

Bidstrup PL, Case RAM (1956) Carcinoma of the lung in workmen in the bichromates-producing industry in Great Britain. Br J Ind Med 13:260–264

Bjelke E (1975) Dietary vitamin A and human lung cancer. Int J Cancer 15:561–565

Bross IDJ, Driscoll DL (1981) Direct estimates of low-level radiation risks of lung cancer at two NRC-compliant nuclear installations: Why are the new risk estimates 20 to 200 times the old official estimates. Yale J Biol Med 54:317–328

Correa P, Williams Pickle L, Fontham E, Lin Y, Haenszel W (1983) Passive smoking and lung cancer. Lancet II: 595–597

Doll R, Morgan LG, Speizer FE (1970) Cancers of the lung and nasal sinuses in nickel workers. Br J Cancer 24: 623–632

Garfinkel L (1981) Time trends in lung cancer mortality among non-smokers and a note on passive smoking. J Natl Cancer Inst 66:1061–1066

Hirayama T (1981) Non-smoking wives of heavy smokers have a higher risk of lung cancer: a study in Japan. Br Med J 282: 183–185, and 283:1466

Machle W, Gregorius F (1948) Cancer of respiratory system in United States chromate-producing industry. Public Health Rep 63:1114–1127

Monson RR, Peters JM, Johnson MN (1974) Proportional mortality among vinyl-chloride workers. Lancet II:397–398

Ott MG, Holder BB, Gordon HL (1974) Respiratory cancer and occupational exposure to arsenicals. Arch Environ Health 29:250–255

Pott P (1775) Chirurgical observations relative to the cataract, polypus of the nose, the cancer of the scrotum, the different kinds of ruptures and the mortification of the toes and feet. London.

Rose G, Hamilton PJS, Colwell L, Shipley MJ (1982) A randomised controlled trial of anti-smoking advice: 10-year results. J Epidemiol Community Health 36:102–108

Trichopoulos D, Kalandidi A, Sparros L, MacMahon B (1981) Lung cancer and passive smoking. Int J Cancer 27:1–4

Wada S, Miyanishi M, Nishimoto Y, Kambe S, Miller RW (1968) Mustard gas as a cause of respiratory neoplasia in man. Lancet I:1161–1163

Wald N, Idle M, Boreham J, Bailey A (1980) Low serum vitamin A and subsequent risk of cancer. Lancet II:813–815

Chapter 3

Hormone Production by Bronchial Tumours

Sally J. Ratter and Lesley H. Rees

Introduction

The production of polypeptide hormones and various 'tumour-associated' proteins by neoplasia occurring in non-endocrine tissues such as the lung is classically referred to as 'inappropriate' or 'ectopic' hormone production. The detection of ectopic hormone synthesis and release and the appreciation of the role this may play in associated endocrine syndromes has led to their extensive study, which has had particular relevance for clinical diagnosis, treatment of the endocrine syndromes, monitoring tumour therapy and the search for tumour markers. More recently they have been used as an important aid to the understanding of the biosynthetic pathways of peptide hormones and their precursors.

One of the earliest reports of a non-endocrine tumour causing an endocrine syndrome occurred in 1928 when Brown published the case history of a patient with adrenocortical hyperactivity, diabetes, raised blood pressure, hirsutism and a bronchial carcinoma. At the time no correlation was made between the tumour and the endocrine syndrome, though we can now realise that the clinical features were those of Cushing's syndrome due to inappropriate ACTH secretion from a bronchial carcinoma. Subsequently there were various reports of endocrine syndromes in patients with tumours of the lung and other non-endocrine tissues which could be relieved by removal of the tumour, when that was possible. However, confirmation that these tumours were actually synthesising and secreting hormones awaited the development of methodologies sufficiently sensitive to permit the detection of these peptides in plasma and tumour tissues.

The advent of the new techniques of radioimmunoassay (RIA) in the 1960s (Berson and Yalow 1964) introduced the sensitivity and specificity required to detect these hormones at their relatively low levels in the circulation. Thus, Liddle et al. (1969) were able to publish their important study on inappropriate ACTH release from non-endocrine tumours causing Cushing's syndrome, where they coined the term 'ectopic humoral syndrome'.

The development of these sensitive assays has since enabled detection of hormone release by some tumours at levels which do not cause an overt syndrome or obvious clinical symptoms, a feature which introduced the exciting possibility of peptides as tumour markers. It was hoped that specific tumour markers might aid early diagnosis, provide a means of monitoring the activity of such tumours during treatment and supply early indication of recurrence. However, the search for specific tumour markers has not yet been so fruitful as was originally hoped. It is now also becoming apparent that some of these peptide hormones may be present in small amounts in normal tissues traditionally regarded as 'non-endocrine', including the lung, where peptides such as ACTH, bombesin and somatostatin have all been detected (Holdaway et al. 1977; Wood et al. 1981). The function of these peptides — if any — in such small quantities in this tissue remains unknown and it has not been established that their presence is due to de novo synthesis rather than uptake from the circulation. However, if these peptides are found to be present in normal tissues, the use of the term 'ectopic' will become redundant.

Criteria for Ectopic Hormone Production

The diagnosis of an ectopic humoral syndrome can be complex since the clinical symptoms and biochemical features do not always fit the classically described pattern and frequently the very small amounts of hormone released cause no apparent physiological change. Unfortunately this has resulted in a number of rather inconclusive and badly authenticated case reports and thus a critical appraisal of the literature is mandatory. In order to try and overcome this problem a number of validation criteria have been proposed, one or more of which must be substantiated to confirm a tumour as the source of inappropriate hormone production. These include:

1. Association of a tumour with an endocrine syndrome and/or inappropriately raised levels of circulating hormone(s).
2. Regression of an endocrine syndrome and/or a fall in hormone levels after removal of the tumour.
3. Persistent endocrine abnormality after the removal of the gland normally associated with synthesis and release of the hormone.
4. Presence of an arteriovenous gradient across the vascular bed of the tumour.
5. Demonstration of hormone in tumour tissue in amounts greater than in adjacent non-involved tissue.
6. Demonstration of hormone synthesis in vitro and/or extraction of appropriate mRNA from the tumours.

These criteria, however, are not all sufficient on their own to prove ectopic hormone production. The first is the weakest since the simultaneous presence of a tumour with elevated circulating hormone levels does not identify that tumour as the source of the hormone. It is possible that a patient could have two separate pathologies or that the tumour might actually be producing a substance which is stimulating the release of that hormone from its normal gland. In this regard, the well known, although rare, association of bronchial carcinoids with acromegaly, caused by the elaboration of a growth hormone releasing factor(s) by the tumour, is of interest (see below). Furthermore, the secretion of some hormones, such as ACTH and GH, is very labile in normal subjects, and elevated levels can occur in the presence of anxiety and pain, both of which may be associated with advanced malignancy. Removal of the tumour as required by criterion 2 is often either impossible or not indicated clinically, and for obvious reasons criterion 3 is rarely met. The taking of arteriovenous samples across a tumour is often difficult and again usually not clinically relevant, and furthermore the possibility of the well described episodic hormone secretion makes interpretation of any data obtained difficult. However, there have been some well documented reports of successful demonstrations of hormone gradients across tumours (Ratcliffe et al. 1972; Rees et al. 1974), and these demonstrations have proved of diagnostic value in the localisation of some occult ectopic hormone secreting neoplasia (Rees et al. 1977; Drury et al. 1982). When considering the tumour content of a hormone (the fifth criterion) one must consider the possibility of hormone uptake from the circulation; furthermore, hormone levels are often very low and may not differ greatly from apparently normal tissue (Holdaway et al. 1974). However, despite all these reservations, at least the demonstration of de novo synthesis of the hormone by tumour cells in vitro provides definite proof of ectopic hormone production. Unfortunately, the specialised techniques involved and the lack of availability of suitable fresh tissue have restricted opportunities for such full documentation. Thus, evidence of ectopic hormone production is frequently based on limited data — usually the clinical symptoms and plasma hormone levels; caution should therefore be exercised in accepting this as conclusive proof.

Mechanisms of Ectopic Hormone Production

The concepts which have been developed to explain the mechanism(s) of ectopic hormone production have been reviewed at length by Baylin and Mendelsohn (1980).

1. *The Sponge Theory.* This suggests that there is a selective tumour uptake of the hormone(s) from the circulation to be later released on necrosis of the cells (Unger et al. 1964). Although there is good evidence that some tumour cells can bind specific peptides (Schorr et al. 1972), this theory does not hold for most instances of ectopic hormone production, where good evidence exists for in vivo and in vitro peptide synthesis.

2. *Mutation and Abnormal Genes.* It has been proposed that mutant genes are responsible for ectopic hormones. However, if this were so it would be expected that there would be a random association of any hormone with tumour types or tissue sites and also that there would be differences in primary peptide structure. This is not the case since there certainly is specificity. Thus specific hormones are associated only with certain tumour types, e.g. ACTH and ADH with small cell tumours of the lung and humoral hypercalcaemia with squamous cell lung tumours. Also there is considerable evidence to show that the ectopic hormones are structurally very similar or even identical to normal hormones (Coombes et al. 1974; Morton et al. 1978), although larger molecular precursor forms may predominate, some of which may appear in the plasma (Ratter et al. 1980). This is probably due to altered post-translational processing rather than to altered DNA sequence.

3. *Derepression of Genes.* This theory proposes that a portion of DNA not normally available for transcription becomes derepressed in the tumour cell.

Although this would explain the similarity of structure between the ectopic and the eutopic hormones, it does not explain tumour specificity and there has, as yet, been no direct evidence for such a process. However, the presence of the very small amounts of hormones in normal cells suggests that these gene transcriptions are never completely repressed (Odel et al. 1977) whilst in the tumour cells they are amplified.

4. *Dedifferentiation*. Finally, it has been suggested that there is a return of the gene expression of the tumour cell to that of its parent embryological tissue and thus this also includes possible gene derepression. This proposal is supported by the frequency of secretion, by these tumours, of those peptides and proteins normally associated with the fetus or placenta, such as human chorionic gonadotrophin (HCG), human placental lactogen (HPL), A-fetoprotein (AFP) and carcinoembryonic antigen (CEA). However, both the normal and the neoplastic pathways of cellular differentiation remain to be described.

Incidence of Ectopic Hormone Production

The introduction of RIA, with its capacity to measure peptides in much smaller concentrations than had been possible previously, demonstrated that the incidence of peptide hormone synthesis by bronchial tumours was far more frequent than had been thought. It became apparent that many tumours released hormones in small amounts or in a form possessing reduced bioactivity. In the latter case the very low circulating levels could not be detected by the insensitive bioassays used for hormone assay prior to the introduction of RIA. Furthermore, release of biologically inactive hormones would obviously not result in any clinical syndrome. It has been suggested that almost all lung cancer patients exhibit the secretion of at least one ectopic hormone (Krauss et al. 1981) whereas other studies propose that the incidence is nearer to 60% (Gropp et al. 1980). Cushing's syndrome, inappropriate antidiuresis and humoral hypercalcaemia are the commonest clinical syndromes, with calcitonin being the commonest 'silent' peptide released by bronchial tumours. Although other hormones, e.g. growth hormone and insulin, have been reported to be produced ectopically by lung tumours, these claims have not been fully validated. The incidence of an actual overt endocrine syndrome is much lower, with figures of some 10% for all types of lung tumour (Azzopardi et al. 1970). This discrepancy between the incidence of ectopic hormone release, when actively sought, and the observed overt incidence of clinical syndromes may be due to several factors, including release of biologically inactive hormones, episodic hormone secretion and multiple ectopic hormone secretion with the typical manifestations of one hormone excess being masked by another.

The specificity of occurrence of ectopic hormones with the particular histological types of lung tumour is of considerable interest. Thus, in his 1981 review of the literature of tumours of the bronchus, Bondy quoted an incidence of 36% for elevated circulating ACTH levels in patients with small cell tumours, 25% in patients with adenocarcinomas and none in patients with squamous cell tumours, although an association with squamous cell tumours has been reported by others (Yesner 1978). Clinical evidence of Cushing's syndrome was found in only 5% of patients with small cell tumours and was not associated with the other tumour types. Secretion of calcitonin, however, is observed in 20% with squamous cell tumours, 51% with small cell tumours, 33% with adenocarcinoma and 33% with large cell tumours, whilst humoral hypercalcaemia is almost exclusively associated with the squamous cell tumours. It is possible that more than one hormone may be released by a tumour (Rees et al. 1974). The most commonly associated hormones are ACTH and antidiuretic hormone (ADH), some 20% of patients with the ectopic ACTH syndrome also having ectopic ADH secretion (Merrill and Bondy 1982). Yesner (1978) suggested that the range of ectopic hormones secreted superimposed on the spectrum of lung histopathology suggests that the degree rather than the kind of hormone secretion may be associated with the level of maturation of the tumour, from small cell to squamous cell to adenocarcinoma.

Adrenocorticotropic Hormone (ACTH)

Since the first published case report of adrenocortical hyperactivity in association with a non-endocrine tumour (Brown 1928), the ectopic ACTH syndrome has become the best documented of all the ectopic endocrine syndromes. Small cell tumours of the lung are the most frequent cause of ectopic Cushing's syndrome, and together with endocrine tumours of the foregut they account for more than 90% of all cases of the ectopic ACTH syndrome (Azzopardi and Williams 1968). ACTH is detectably released from some 30%–40% of small cell lung tumours, although only 2%–5% are associated with the clinical syndrome. Ectopic ACTH has also been found in adenocarcinomas, some large cell and a very few squamous cell tumours (Krauss et al. 1981), although it is generally accepted that these tumours are not associated with overt Cushing's syndrome.

The metabolic effects seen with ectopic production of ACTH are mainly due to the very high glucocorticoid output by the adrenals under the continual stimulus of the relatively high levels of ACTH. They are encountered, most typically, in middle-aged men and include severe hypercortisolaemia and hypokalaemic alkalosis with muscle weakness and wasting, carbohydrate intolerance with glycosuria, hypertension and oedema. The characteristic facies of the pituitary disease are not usually seen, although this may be due to the short history of the disease, the mean survival time without treatment being approximately 3 months.

There is a range of diagnostic tests to aid the differential diagnosis of ectopic ACTH syndrome from pituitary-dependent Cushing's disease, as illustrated in Table 1. It is very important to stress that all the criteria are not necessarily fulfilled in every case and often the clinical symptoms and biochemical results are confusing and contradictory, making diagnosis difficult without any overt evidence of a tumour. The association of hypokalaemic alkalosis with ACTH levels in excess of 200 ng/litre is strongly suggestive of the ectopic syndrome, although the previously accepted level of 200 ng/litre as being the dividing line between pituitary-dependent Cushing's disease and the ectopic syndrome should be treated with great caution (personal observation). In most cases ACTH secretion by these tumours does not respond to any sort of dynamic stimulation or suppression test, such as the administration of a large dose of dexamethasone or metyrapone, although again

Table 1. Differential diagnosis of Cushing's syndrome

	Normal	Ectopic ACTH syndrome	Pituitary-dependent Cushing's disease
Plasma cortisol	Normal	Elevated	Elevated
Plasma ACTH			
9.00 h	Normal (< 10–80 ng/l)	Elevated — may be highly elevated	Normal or elevated
24.00 h	< 10 ng/l	Elevated	Elevated
Dexamethasone			
2 mg/24 h	Suppression	No suppression	No suppression
8 mg/24 h	Suppression	No suppression	Suppression
Insulin tolerance test	Stimulation	No stimulation	No stimulation
Metyrapone	Stimulation	No stimulation	Stimulation
K^+	Normal (3.3–5.0 mmol/l)	< 3.0 mmol/l	Normal
HCO_3	Normal (20–28 mmol/l)	> 30 mmol/l	Normal

paradoxical results have been obtained (personal observation). Such results are most often observed when ectopic ACTH production is due to a bronchial carcinoid tumour. This group of patients often present with Cushing's syndrome long before there is any radiological evidence of a tumour and are more likely to be diagnosed as having pituitary-dependent Cushing's disease. There is no sex bias and the age of presentation is lower than the age of presentation of the ectopic ACTH syndrome associated with bronchial carcinoma. Furthermore the body habitus and facies may resemble those of pituitary-dependent Cushing's disease. Frequently ACTH levels are only mildly elevated and hormone release may by cyclical in nature, such that the plasma ACTH may be within the normal range for long periods, ranging from hours to weeks (Bailey 1971; LH Rees, personal observation). Frequently ACTH secretion from bronchial carcinoids can be suppressed by high doses of dexamethasone (8 mg daily for 2 days) and some may respond by releasing ACTH after stimulation with metyrapone (Mason et al. 1972), thus presenting a picture more akin to pituitary-dependent Cushing's disease. However, the presence of hypokalaemia and peripheral oedema as well as the more rapid onset may help distinguish the ACTH-secreting lung carcinoid from a pituitary source of ACTH.

There is another group of patients who present with no clinical evidence of abnormal adrenal function, but who show an absent circadian rhythm of cortisol levels not suppressed by dexamethasone, although the plasma ACTH levels are apparently normal. Thus, Bondy and Gilby (1982) found that 77% of the patients in their study of small cell tumours had one abnormal test of adrenal function and that 37% had two or more abnormal results. They suggested that this could be due to the release of very small amounts of ectopic ACTH from the lung tumours which then suppress normal pituitary secretion. As this ACTH is not under feedback control or subject to diurnal variation, the normal diurnal rhythm and response to the circulating adrenal steroid levels is blunted, though without causing sufficient steroid secretion to produce the clinical features of Cushing's syndrome.

The discrepancy between the number of lung tumour patients who have elevated plasma levels of ACTH and the comparatively low incidence of overt Cushing's syndrome led to speculation that the ectopic ACTH was biologically inactive compared with pituitary ACTH. Thus Gewirtz et al. (1974) described a 'big ACTH' which had only 4% of the bioactivity of pituitary ACTH (1–39 ACTH) and which on trypsinisation released 1–39 ACTH. However, the chromatography techniques used in these studies were later shown to be inappropriate for plasma ACTH (Mains and Eipper 1976; Ratter et al. 1980) and subject to artefacts of plasma protein binding of the ACTH giving apparently large molecular weight material — the 'big ACTH'. It has since been shown that large molecular weight ACTH does appear in the plasma in the ectopic ACTH syndrome, having a molecular weight of some 22 000 daltons (22 K) (Ratter et al. 1980).

ACTH is normally synthesised in the corticotrophs of the anterior pituitary as a large common precursor for ACTH, β-LPH and pro-γ-MSH known as pro-opiomelanocortin (Nakanishi et al. 1979; Seidah et al. 1980). This precursor has also been shown to be present in cell cultures of ectopic ACTH-secreting lung tumours (Bertagna et al. 1978) and to be cleaved to release ACTH, β-LPH, β-endorphin and γ-MSH (Ratter et al. 1983). It was suggested that the 22-K form of ACTH, found in the plasma of patients with the ectopic syndrome, represents the N-terminal portion of the precursor, which for some reason has not been fully cleaved to release 1–39 ACTH (Ratter et al. 1980). The bioactivity of this 22-K ACTH is some 10% of 1–39 ACTH (SJ Ratter, PhD thesis). It was hoped that this 22-K ACTH could be a marker for lung tumours. However, it is also released by ectopic ACTH-secreting tumours in sites other than the lungs and recently has been shown to be released from a large and aggressive atypical pituitary tumour (Ratter et al. 1983).

Since the ACTH is concomitantly synthesised with β-LPH and γ-MSH as pro-opiomelanocortin, it is not surprising to find that the levels of these other peptides are elevated, similarly to that of ACTH, in ectopic Cushing's syndrome (Jeffcoate et al. 1978; Hope et al. 1981; Hale et al. 1983). Differences in the relative degree of elevation of these peptides as detected in the plasma are probably introduced through differences in half-life and clearance rates. The hyperpigmentation frequently associated with Cushing's syndrome is probably due to the MSH activity found in these peptides. Any effects of β-LPH, β-endorphin or γ-MSH released from ectopic tumours must await the elucidation of their bioactive functions in the normal state. However, it has been shown that γ-MSH can have a potentiating effect on ACTH-induced steroidogenesis (Pedersen and Brownie 1980; Al Dujaili et al. 1981), and this may be one of the reasons for the profound metabolic disorders associated with the ectopic syndrome.

There has been some evidence for the ectopic secretion of a CRF-like substance from lung tumours causing inappropriate ACTH release from the pituitary (Amatruda and Upon 1974; Suda et al. 1977). The recent isolation and synthesis of a synthetic CRF (CRF-41) (Vale et al. 1981) has made it available for the development of an RIA which hopefully will be able to confirm or refute the presence and release of CRF from any similar tumours found in the future. The prognosis of ectopic ACTH syndrome associated with bronchial small cell tumours is poor and often the patient suffers more from the effects of the severe hypercortisolaemia than from those of the tumour itself. Bondy and Gilby (1982) found that in patients undergoing chemotherapy for small cell lung tumours, those who had evidence of abnormal adrenal function — though not necessarily overt Cushing's syndrome — had a shorter median survival (267 days) than those with normal adrenal control (362 days). Drugs such as metyrapone, aminoglutethimide and op'DDD which block adrenal corticosteroid synthesis will alleviate the clinical symptoms in the short-term, if radiotherapy or chemotherapy is not indicated, and should be used concomitantly when appropriate. These drugs alone do not significantly improve the long-term prognosis. However, patients who have bronchial carcinoids as the source of ectopic ACTH apparently can be cured by removal of these much lower grade malignancies. Drug treatment to relieve or control the symptoms of Cushing's syndrome (Jeffcoate et al. 1977) is usually used to prepare these patients for surgery and thus reduce operative risk.

Since ACTH levels can be elevated for many reasons, including in normal individuals subjected to stress, plasma ACTH measurement has no function as a tumour marker. However, the disappearance and reappearance of inappropriate levels can be used to monitor a tumour undergoing treatment.

Antidiuretic Hormone

Ectopic ADH, like ACTH, is most commonly associated with bronchial small cell tumours where the incidence is of about 30% (Bondy and Gilby 1982). The release of inappropriate ACTH and ADH seems to be related in these tumours since they are reported to be present together in 84% of small cell tumours secreting these hormones (Bondy and Gilby 1982). There have also been some reports of ADH release by adenocarcinomas (Vorherr et al. 1974), but it is not thought to be associated with squamous cell tumours (Bondy 1981).

The secretion of ADH by these tumours often produces a clinical syndrome of mild hyponatraemia which is asymptomatic and only detected when routine plasma electrolytes are determined, showing a plasma sodium level of less than 130 mmol/litre. However, in more severe cases the sodium level may fall below 120 mmol/litre and is then associated with water intoxication, lethargy, weakness, hyperirritability, confusion, depression, fits and coma, with a risk of cardiac arrhythmias and death when sodium levels fall below 110 mmol/litre. Diagnosis of the syndrome of inappropriate ADH is made on finding a hypotonic plasma associated with hypertonic urine and with the inability to excrete a water load in the presence of overhydration. The serum osmolality is usually less than 270 mOsm/kg whilst the urine osmolality is above 300 mOsm/kg and the plasma vasopressin (ADH; AVP) is above 2 μU/ml whereas it would normally be expected to be undetectable in relation to the low plasma osmolality. Urinary excretion of AVP is very high. It has also been found that the urinary excretion of AVP is increased in all patients with bronchial small cell tumours but not in those with adenocarcinomas or squamous cell tumours (Haefliger et al. 1977).

Normally, AVP is synthesised in the cells of the supra-optic and paraventricular nuclei and is associated with neurophysin, which acts as a carrier protein as AVP moves to the posterior pituitary. Neurophysin has also been detected in small cell lung tumours secreting AVP (Hamilton et al. 1972). The Herring bodies in which the neurophysin–AVP complex is normally stored in the posterior pituitary are not found in the tumours (Vorherr 1974), suggesting that the neurophysin and AVP are released as they are synthesised, and the tumour neurophysin seems to be less efficient in its binding of AVP. However, neurophysin is not always detectable in those tumours which are producing vasopressin. In a study of a group of patients with small cell lung tumours, North et al. (1980) reported finding elevated neurophysin levels in 62%. They suggested that this could be used as a marker to monitor response to therapy and possibly predict a relapse, as they had observed a fall in circulating neurophysin during therapy which was reversed several weeks before clinical evidence of recurrence of the tumours. The neurophysin acting as a carrier for oxytocin was also measured in this study, and a few cases of oxytocin production by small cell tumours have been described (Pettengill et al. 1977), although not in association with any clinical symptoms.

The incidence of AVP in tumours without neurophysin and the difference in the binding relationship of the AVP to neurophysin as compared with pituitary forms suggest that there may be different mechanisms in the synthesis of these tumour peptides. George and colleagues (1972) demonstrated incorporation of ^{3}H-phenyla-lanine into AVP-like peptides by undifferentiated lung tumour cells, whilst the chromatography of lung tumour AVP (Morton et al. 1970) showed 65% of the activity eluting in the same position of the synthetic pituitary AVP, with two peaks of larger molecular weight AVP-like material. This larger AVP showed reduced bioactivity. As yet there has been no further characterisation of these peptides to clarify the possibility that they may be large molecular weight precursors for AVP.

The mild form of the clinical syndrome can be successfully treated by water restriction alone, although if the patient is receiving cyclophosphamide this may cause drug-induced cystitis and is therefore contra-indicated. Intravenous hypertonic saline may be used acutely to treat convulsions but it can cause congestive heart failure. Administration of drugs which induce mild reversible nephrogenic diabetes insipidus can be used to dehydrate the overhydrated patient. However, the prognosis is related to the tumour itself and as this is so frequently a small cell tumour the prognosis is poor.

Having said that ectopic AVP secretion can occur, in many instances the water retention in patients with lung tumours may be due to other mechanisms. In a detailed study using hypertonic saline infusions, Robertson (1978) looked at osmoreceptor responsiveness in these patients and defined several different response patterns. He concluded that about half of the patients with lung cancer and inappropriate antidiuresis had excess vasopressin secretion resulting from posterior pituitary stimulation due to abnormal signals received from an altered or defective osmoreceptor, and suggested different mechanisms to explain this defect. Thus carcinomatous involvement of the vagus nerve could interfere with baroregulatory input, which was one of the hypotheses postulated by Schwartz et al. (1957) in the original publication on this subject. Furthermore, neoplastic disease resulting in inferior vena cava obstruction may cause hypovolaemia and/or hypotension, which can lower the threshold set point of the osmoregulatory system and stimulate vasopressin secretion. Finally, metastatic destruction of the hypothalamus could disturb posterior pituitary activity and, on a more speculative note, tumour production of substances capable of stimulating the posterior pituitary to secrete vasopressin remains a theoretical possibility.

Calcitonin

Inappropriately raised levels of calcitonin associated with lung tumours were first described by Coombes et al. (1974) in a study of 46 patients with non-thyroid cancer, 8 of whom had small cell bronchial tumours. Bondy, in his 1981 review of the literature, reported the incidence of calcitonin in lung tumours as 57% in small cell tumours, 20% in squamous cell tumours, 33% in adenocarcinoma and 33% in large cell tumours. These data were based on several studies using routine calcitonin RIA. However, Roos et al. (1980) demonstrated that the calcitonin immunoreactivity in the squamous and large cell tumours was artefactual and they quoted a figure of 27% for the incidence of calcitonin in small cell tumours and adenocarcinomas. This is a good example of the care required when interpreting results in attempts to identify sources of ectopic hormones.

The molecular size of calcitonin associated with lung tumours, as with ACTH and ADH, appears to be heterogeneous and generally of a larger size (40–100 K) than that associated with medullary carcinoma of the thyroid (Becker et al. 1978; Roos et al. 1980), which has a molecular weight of some 3.5 K. It has been suggested that these larger molecular weight forms could represent calcitonin precursors though this has not, as yet, been confirmed (Bertagna et al. 1978; Roos et al. 1980).

The levels of circulating calcitonin do not appear to relate to the tumour mass (Hansen et al. 1980), and although they are reported to fall during treatment they do not necessarily rise again as the tumour recurs and thus cannot be used satisfactorily to monitor treatment or as a tumour marker. There are no known clinical symptoms associated with the ectopic secretion of calcitonin from lung tumours and thus no specific treatment is necessary.

Finally, in some patients with lung cancer and elevated circulating calcitonin levels, the calcitonin is not ectopic but originates from the thyroid gland. Thus, in 75% of patients the elevated calcitonin levels decreased when therapy was directed at the primary tumour, and the actual level correlated with clinical status in 67% of patients. Interestingly, the incidence of hypercalcaemia was identical in two groups, and therefore did not correlate with raised calcitonin levels. Furthermore, hypercalcitoninaemia does not correlate with the presence of osseous metastases, which might be expected if thyroid calcitonin secretion was stimulated as a physiological response to their development (Silva et al. 1979).

Humoral Hypercalcaemia

Hypercalcaemia is a not uncommon accompaniment of cancer and is always associated with high morbidity and mortality. Cancer is the commonest cause of hypercalcaemia; the latter occurs in approximately 10%–20% of all patients suffering from cancer and in particular in those with tumours of the lung, breast or kidney, or with multiple myeloma. The accelerated bone resorption, which is usually the cause of the hypercalcaemia, is believed to be mediated by hormonal and/or metabolic mechanisms.

The symptoms of hypercalcaemia will not be elaborated, but their severity is usually related to the level of serum calcium. In most patients, regardless of the underlying pathology, the calcium is usually > 3.0 mmol/litre and the serum phosphate low or normal. When secondary renal damage ensues, hypokalaemic alkalosis may occur. The clinical features which help to distinguish this disorder from primary hyperparathyroidism include the rapidity of onset of symptoms and the absence of either periosteal bone resorption or nephrocalcinosis. Thus, it is usually easy to diagnose malignant hypercalcaemia, and from most series of patients studied it is generally agreed that malignancy only rarely presents as a problem of hypercalcaemia of unknown origin. Indeed, most surveys show that at least 75% of patients with hypercalcaemia of malignancy have overt metastatic disease and probably another 15% will have metastases if a careful search is instituted. This leaves a residue of about 10% of patients who have hypercalcaemia in association with localised neoplastic disease. Furthermore, these figures, which are generally accepted, are compatible with the poor prognosis of malignant hypercalcaemia since most patients will have advanced disease, with 50% dying within 3 months and 80% within 1 year of the onset of hypercalcaemia.

Cancer and primary hyperparathyroidism are common in the general population (cancer 1.4%; hyperparathyroidism approximately 0.7%), and in a review in 1976, Heath noted 118 cases of the coexistence of these two diseases and Dresner and Lebovitz (1978) proved primary hyperparathyroidism in 6 of 11 patients referred with hypercalcaemia and cancer. However, in practice differentiation between the diagnoses of primary hyperparathyroidism and malignant hypercalcaemia is rarely a problem. If doubt does exist, the hydrocortisone suppression test may be of value. If the test is performed as originally described (120 mg hydrocortisone per day for 10 days, correcting the serum calcium for haemodilution), it provides excellent discrimination, since significant suppression of serum calcium does not occur in primary hyperparathyroidism, whereas malignant hypercalcaemia is usually completely alleviated.

In patients with metastatic involvement of bone (usually from primary tumours of breast, bronchus or kidney), factors such as prostaglandin release by the tumour tissue may cause local bone resorption, resulting in liberation of calcium. However, most interest has been shown not in the mechanisms by which bony metastases cause hypercalcaemia (approximately 90% of patients), but in the mechanism by which hypercalcaemia occurs in the other 10% with localised tumours.

Hypercalcaemia in lung cancer without the presence of bone metastases was described initially by Connor et al. (1956), who observed that the calcium level returned to normal after resection of the tumour. Parathyroid hormone-like material was later extracted from a squamous cell lung tumour. Humoral hypercalcaemia is almost exclusively associated with squamous cell tumours. Thus, Bondy in his review (1981) quoted an incidence of 25% for squamous cell tumours, 0% for small cell tumours and adenocarcinomas and 6% for large cell tumours.

Although it was initially thought that this hypercalcaemia was due to ectopic parathyroid hormone (PTH) production, this has now been questioned and the actual mechanism of non-metastatic hypercalcaemia of lung cancer remains to be clarified. Closer examination of the PTH-like substance showed it to be immunologically different from that found in primary hyperparathyroidism (Benson et al. 1974). Two different biochemical pictures can be associated with cancer hypercalcaemia and tumours. One form resembles primary hyperparathyroidism and includes hypophosphataemia with increased excretion of nephrogenous cyclic AMP and tubular resorption of phosphate, whereas in the alternate form serum phosphate levels are normal and there is a lowered excretion of cyclic AMP and normal tubular resorption of phosphate (Stewart et al. 1980). Serum vitamin D levels are normal in both groups whilst they are elevated in primary hyperparathyroidism. Furthermore, plasma PTH levels may be undetectable or low whereas they are usually higher than normal in primary hyperparathyroidism. Extracts of tumour tissue have been shown to possess bone-resorbing activity which does not cross-react with any PTH antiserum (Powell et al. 1973). This evidence suggests that this non-metastatic hypercalcaemia is due to elaboration of some humoral substance(s) distinct from PTH itself (Skrabaneck et al. 1980). Thus, the nature of this possible humoral substance(s) remains to be elucidated.

The clinical features of humoral hypercalcaemia are the same as those associated with the hypercalcaemia of other aetiologies. Polyuria, thirst, dehydration and possible renal failure are the results of the effects on the kidney whilst anorexia, nausea, vomiting, constipation, abdominal pain, headaches, psychosis, drowsiness leading to fits and coma may also occur. Serum calcium is usually elevated above 4.0 mmol/litre and the disorder is distinguished from primary hyperparathyroidism by the more rapid onset, by the absence of radiological features of hyperparathyroidism such as periosteal erosions and nephrocalcinosis as well as by its responsiveness to high doses of glucocorticosteroids.

Apart from possible resection of the tumour or chemotherapy, treatment is the same as for other causes of raised calcium, including correction of the dehydration and increased oral intake of phosphate. Subcutaneous or intramuscular calcitonin or mithramycin can reduce the serum calcium but this effect tends to be short lasting.

Growth Hormone (GH) and Growth Hormone Releasing Factor(s) (GRF)

There have been a number of reports of growth hormone present in lung tumours and Beck and Burger (1972) found it in half of the lung tumours in their study. Elevated plasma growth hormone levels have also been found and these are associated with all the different histological types of tumour. Frequently the plasma GH shows a paradoxical rise, rather than the expected fall, during a glucose tolerance test (Sparagna et al. 1971). Growth hormone synthesis and release by large cell undifferentiated bronchial tumour cells in vitro was demonstrated by Greenberg et al. (1972), but other tumours apparently do not release their growth hormone into the circulation (Dabek 1974).

The secretion of ectopic growth hormone was thought to be the cause of hypertrophic pulmonary osteoarthropathy, which, with its clinical features of gross finger clubbing, painful symmetrical arthropathy and deep bone pain, was said to bear a resemblance to some features of acromegaly (although in the author's view no such similarity exists). However, there was no correlation between the occurrence or degree of hypertrophic pulmonary osteoarthropathy and the tumour and plasma growth hormone levels (Ennis et al. 1973). Evidence has also been presented for the release of a GRF by bronchial and other carcinoids which results in acromegaly by stimulating pituitary GH release (Beck et al. 1973; Dabek 1974; Sonksen et al. 1976). These tumour cell extracts were shown to stimulate the release of growth hormone from the pituitary (Beck et al. 1973), and removal of a bronchial carcinoid which was not itself secreting growth hormone resulted in cure of acromegaly.

More recently Frohman et al. (1980) have described three tumours with apparent GRF activity, one being a bronchial carcinoid. They were able to characterise the GRF activity partially, confirming that it was a peptide and that it could produce dose response curves for GH release from rat anterior pituitary cells in vitro. Since then Thorner et al. (1982) have isolated a 40 amino acid residue GH-releasing peptide from a pancreatic ectopic tumour causing acromegaly. This group have been able to sequence this peptide and characterise its GH-releasing properties, comparing it with the proposed hypothalamic GRF peptide (Rivier et al. 1982). Similar results have been reported with a 44 amino acid GRF active peptide isolated and sequenced from another pancreatic tumour by Guillemin et al. (1982). Full characterisation of a possible ectopic GRF from a bronchial neoplasm must await the availability of sufficient material.

Gonadotrophins

Ectopic gonadotrophin production is reported to occur in all the different histological types of lung tumour. Thus, Bondy in his review quotes 19% for small cell, 13% for squamous cell, 24% for adenocarcinoma and 9% for large cell bronchial tumours. The gonadotrophins, LH, FSH and HCG all consist of tetramers made up of two common α-subunits and two specific β-subunits. The development of RIA specific to the β-subunit of these hormones demonstrated that β-HCG is the gonadotrophin which is produced by the lung tumours (Hansen et al. 1980). In vitro β-HCG synthesis and release has been demonstrated from undifferentiated lung tumour cells which also released free α and β-HCG subunits, suggesting an altered synthesis by these cells (Rabson et al. 1973).

Clinically, gynaecomastia in males without galactorrhoea is the syndrome associated with ectopic HCG release, although it must be remembered that various types of benign thoracic disease may also cause this syndrome, including lung abscess or tuberculosis as well as starvation. The gynaecomastia may precede any radiological evidence of a tumour. It is usually bilateral and may or may not be associated with hypertrophic pulmonary osteoarthropathy, increased oestrogen production and testicular interstitial cell hyperplasia.

Human placental lactogen has also been detected in the plasma and tumour tissue of patients with gynaecomastia and increased oestrogen secretion but it is not thought to be responsible for the clinical symptoms (Weintraub and Rosen 1971). The highly sensitive HPL assay detected an incidence of approximately 50% in patients with lung cancer.

Other Hormones

There have been individual reports of possible ectopic production of other hormones by bronchial tumours, but the evidence does not, as yet, fulfil the criteria for true ectopic production.

More recently, interest has been focused on the family of neuropeptides localised in the gastrointestinal tract and nervous system — known as 'gut-hormones' — and their possible production by bronchial tumours. The physiological role of these peptides remains to be elucidated but it has been suggested that they could be responsible for such symptoms as anorexia, cachexia, hyperglycaemia and hypo-thermia in association with some lung tumours. Somatostatin has been measured in small cell and adenocarcinoma lung tumours (Penman et al. 1980; Wood et al. 1981), and neurotensin and bombesin in small cell, adenocarcinoma and squamous cell tumours (Wood et al. 1981).

Immunocytochemical and radioimmunological studies have demonstrated bombesin-like immunoreactivity (BLI) to be distributed in the mammalian central nervous system, with highest levels in the hypothalamus, and throughout the mammalian gut, where it is associated with nerve fibres. Although circulating levels of BLI have been reported in the rat, to date the evidence would indicate that if BLI is present in normal human circulation, levels are too low for detection by conventional RIA.

High levels of BLI have been found in human fetal and neonatal lung, where it is localised in the pulmonary neuro-endocrine cells of the bronchial and bronchiolar epithelium (Wharton et al. 1978; Track and Cutz 1982). BLI content of lung tissue appears to be highest at and immediately following birth, with low or undetectable levels reported in normal adult lung. This pattern is compatible with the age-dependent changes known to occur in the endocrine cells of the lung. The role of BLI in the human lung is unclear; however, it has been suggested that it may be involved in the control of pulmonary vessel and airway tone in response to airway gas composition. BLI has, however, been reported in extracts of small cell carcinoma of the lung and adenocarcinoma of the lung (Wood et al. 1981), as well as in a small cell line maintained in vitro (Moody et al. 1983; Sorenson et al. 1982).

Tumour cell lines in culture have been shown to secrete BLI continuously. However, it is still unclear whether BLI is exclusively related to small cell tumours and to what extent BLI is secreted into the peripheral circulation of patients suffering from such tumours. Pert and Schumacher (1982) could find no difference between circulating levels of BLI in patients with small cell tumours with limited stage disease and those with a variety of other neoplasia. Three patients with small cell tumours and extensive metastatic disease had very high levels. The authors state that BLI could be a likely tumour marker for small cell tumours. However, other workers have shown that only 7% of patients with small cell tumours had detectable levels of circulating BLI (Sorenson et al. 1982).

Conclusion

Modern methodological techniques, both clinical and biochemical, have introduced a more critical view of the incidence of ectopic hormones, with more stringent criteria to be fulfilled before there can be confirmation of tumour synthesis and release. The measurement of inappropriate circulating levels of a hormone or its presence in the tumour tissue cannot now be regarded as sufficient evidence and this should be remembered when reviewing the literature. This realisation has introduced some doubt as to the relationship of some hormones such as growth hormone or insulin with bronchial tumours, and to their clinical significance. However, there is no doubt of the association of ACTH, ADH and humoral hypercalcaemia with bronchial tumours or of the resulting clinical syndromes which can so profoundly affect the prognosis in a patient with lung cancer.

Much interest is now being focused on the presence of some of the neuropeptides, such as somatostatin and bombesin, in bronchial tumours, with particular reference to their possible clinical manifestations. However, the elucidation of the significance of these peptides in such tumours must parallel the elucidation of the biological actions of these peptides in the normal state.

The hope that some of these ectopic hormones could act as markers for lung tumours, introducing a possibility of 'at risk' screening, has yet to be realised. So far, none of the hormones have been found to be specific for any particular tumour type or site. However, they have been of some help in the monitoring of treatment of a tumour when elevated levels have fallen with successful reduction of tumour mass and when they have started to rise prior to recurrence of the tumour as detected by other means. The search for a specific tumour marker must continue.

References

Al Dujaili EAS, Hope J, Estivariz FE, Lowry PJ, Edwards CRW (1981) Circulating human pituitary pro-γ-melanotropin enhances the adrenal response to ACTH. Nature 291:156–159

Amatruda TT, Upton GV (1974) Hyperadrenocorticism and ACTH-releasing factor. Ann NY Acad Sci 230:168–180

Azzopardi JG, Williams ED (1968) Pathology of 'non-endocrine' tumours associated with Cushing's syndrome. Cancer 22:274–286

Azzopardi JG, Freeman D, Poole G (1970) Endocrine and metabolic disorders in bronchial carcinoma. Br Med J 4:528–530

Bailey RE (1971) Periodic hormogenesis. A new phenomenon. J Clin Endocrinol Metab 32:317–327

Baylin SB, Mendelsohn G (1980) Ectopic (inappropriate) hormone production by tumours: Mechanisms involved and the biological and clinical implications. Endocr Rev 1: 45–77

Beck C, Burger HG (1972) Evidence for the presence of immunoreactive growth hormone in cancers of the lung and stomach. Cancer 30:75–79

Beck C, Larkins RG, Martin TJ (1973) Stimulation of growth hormone release from superfused rat pituitary by extracts of hypothalamus and of human lung tumours. J Endocrinol 59:325–333

Becker KL, Snider RH, Silver OL (1978) Calcitonin heterogeneity in lung cancer and medullary thyroid cancer. Acta Endocrinol 89:89–99

Benson RC, Riggs RL, Richard BM, Arnaud CD (1974) Immunoreactive forms of circulating PTH in primary and ectopic hyperparathyroidism. J Clin Invest 54:175–181

Berson SA, Yalow RS (1964) Immunoassay of protein hormones. In: Pincus G, Thompson KV, Astwood EB (eds). The hormones, vol iv. Academic Press, New York, London, pp 557–630

Bertagna XY, Nicholson WE, Pettengill OS (1978) Ectopic production of high molecular weight calcitonin and corticotropin by human small cell carcinoma cells in tissue culture. Evidence for separate precursors. J Clin Endocrinol Metab 47:1390–1393

Bondy PK (1981) The pattern of ectopic hormone production in lung cancer. Yale J Biol Med 54:181–185

Bondy PK, Gilby ED (1982) Endocrine function in small cell undifferentiated carcinoma of the lung. Cancer 50:2147–2153

Brown WH (1928) A case of pluriglandular syndrome, 'diabetes of bearded women'. Lancet II:1022

Connor TB, Thomas WC Jr, Howards JE (1956) Etiology of hypercalcaemia associated with lung carcinoma. J Clin Invest 35:697 (Abstr)

Coombes RCC, Hillyard C, Greenberg PB, MacIntyre I (1974) Plasmaimmunoreactive calcitonin in patients with non-thyroid tumours. Lancet I:1080

Dabek JT (1974) Bronchial carcinoid tumour with acromegaly in two patients. J Clin Endocrinol Metab 38: 329–333

Dresner MK, Lebovitz HE (1978) Primary hyperparathyroidism in paraneoplastic hypercalcaemia. Lancet I:1004–1006

Drury PL, Ratter SJ, Tomlin S, Williams J, Dacie JE, Rees LH, Besser GM (1982) Experience with selective venous sampling in diagnosis of ACTH-dependent Cushing's syndrome. Br Med J (Clin Res) 284:9–12

Ennis GC, Cameron DP, Burger HG (1973) On the aetiology of hypertrophic pulmonary osteoarthropathy in bronchogenic carcinoma: Lack of relationship to elevated growth hormone levels. Aust NZ J Med 3:157–161

Frohman LA, Szabo M, Stachura ME, Berelowitz M (1980) Growth hormone-releasing activity from extrapituitary tumours in patients with acromegaly. J Clin Invest 65:43–54

George JM, Capen CC, Phillips AS (1972) Biosynthesis of vasopressin in vitro and ultrastructure of a bronchogenic carcinoma. J Clin Invest 51:151–158

Gewirtz G, Schneider B, Krieger DT, Yalow RS (1974) 'Big ACTH' conversion to biologically active ACTH by trypsin. J Clin Endocrinol Metab 38:227–230

Greenberg PB, Beck C, Martin TJ (1972) Synthesis and release of human growth hormone from lung carcinoma in cell culture. Lancet I:350–352

Gropp C, Haverman K, Scheuer A (1980) Ectopic hormones in lung cancer patients at diagnosis and during therapy. Cancer 46:347–354

Guillemin R, Brazeau P, Bohlen P, Esch F, Ling N, Wehrenberg WB (1982) Growth hormone-releasing factor from a human pancreatic tumour that caused acromegaly. Science 218:585–587

Haefliger JM, Dubied MC, Vallotton MB (1977) Excretion journaliere de l'hormone antidiuretiques lors de carcinome bronchique. Schweiz Med Wochensch 107:728–732

Hale AC, Lytras N, Ratter SJ, Tomlin S, Besser GM, Rees LH (1984) Immunoreactive γ-MSH in human plasma. Clin Endocrinol

Hamilton BPM, Upton GV Amatruda TT (1972) Evidence for the presence of neurophysin in tumours producing the syndrome of inappropriate antidiuresis. J Clin Endocrinol Metab 35:764–767

Hansen M, Hansen HH, Hirsch FR (1980) Hormonal polypeptides and amine metabolites in small cell carcinoma of the lung, with special reference to stage and subtypes. Cancer 45:1432–1437

Heath DA (1976) Hypercalcaemia and malignancy. Ann Clin Biochem 13:555–560

Holdaway IM, Bloomfield GA, Ratcliffe JG, Hinson KWF, Rees GM, Rees LH (1974) Adrenocorticotrophin levels in normal and neoplastic lung tissue. Taylor S (ed) Endocrinology 1973. Heinemann, London

Hope J, Ratter SJ, Estivariz FE, McLoughlin L, Lowry PJ (1981) Development of a radioimmunoassay for an amino-terminal peptide of pro-opiocortin containing the γ-MSH region. Measurement and characterisation in human plasma. Clin Endocrinol 15:221–227

Jeffcoate WJ, Rees LH, Tomlin S, Jones AE, Edwards CRW, Besser GM (1977) Metyrapone in the long-term management of Cushing's disease. Br Med J 2:215–217

Jeffcoate WJ, Tomlin S, McLoughlin L, Rees LH, Besser GM (1978) Plasma β-endorphin and adrenocorticotrophin in disease of the pituitary adrenal axis. J Enocrinol 80:6

Krauss S, Macy S, Ichiki AT (1981) A study of immunoreactive calcitonin (CT). Adrenocorticotrophic hormone (ACTH) and carcinoembryonic antigen (CEA) in lung cancer and other malignancies. Cancer 47:2485–2492

Liddle GW, Nicholson WE, Island DP, Orth DN, Abe K, Lowder SC (1969) Clinical and laboratory studies of ectopic humoral syndromes. Recent Prog Horm Res 25:283–314

Mains RW, Eipper B (1976) Biosynthesis of adrenocorticotropic hormone in mouse pituitary tumour cells. J Biol Chem 251:4115–4120

Mason AMS, Ratcliffe JG, Buckle RM, Stuart Mason A (1972) ACTH secretion by bronchial carcinoid tumours. Clin Endocrinal 1:3–25

Merrill WW, Bondy PK (1982) Production of biochemical marker substances by bronchogenic carcinomas. Clin Chest Med 3:307–320

Moody TW, Russell EK, O'Donohue TL, Lindon CD, Gazdar AF (1983) Bombesin-like peptides in small cell lung cancer: biochemical characterisation and secretion from a cell line. Life Sci 32:487–493

Morton JJ, Kelly P, Padfield PL (1978) Antidiuretic hormone in bronchogenic carcinoma. Clin Endocrinol 9:357–370

Nakanishi S, Akira A, Kita T, Nakamura M, Chang ACY, Cohen SN, Noma S (1979) Nucleotide sequence of a cloned cDNA for bovine corticotrophin-β-lipotropin precursor. Nature 278:423–427

North WG, Maurer LH, Valhn H, O'Donnell JF (1980) Human neurophysin as potential tumour markers for small cell carcinoma of the lung. Application of specific radioimmunoassays. J Clin Endocrinol Metab 51:892–896

Odell WD, Wolfsen A, Yoshimoto Y, Weitzman R, Fisher D, Hirose F (1977) Ectopic peptide synthesis: A universal concomitant of neoplasia. Trans Assoc Am Physicians 90:204

Pedersen RC, Brownie AC (1980) Adrenocortical response to corticotrophin is potentiated by part of the amino-terminal region of pro-corticotrophin/endorphin. Proc Natl Acad Sci USA 77:2239–2243

Penman E, Wass JAH, Besser GM, Rees LH (1980) Somatostatin secretion by lung and thymic tumours. Clin Endocrinol 13:613–620

Pert CB, Schumacher UK (1982) Plasma bombesin concentrations in patients with extensive small cell carcinoma of the lung. Lancet I:509

Pettengill OS, Faulkner CS, Wurster-Hill DH (1977) Isolation and characterisation of a hormone producing cell line from human small cell anaplastic carcinoma of the lung. J Natl Cancer Inst 58:511–518

Powell D, Singer FR, Murray TM, Mirkin C, Potts JT Jr (1973) Non-parathyroid humoral hypercalcaemia in patients with neoplastic disease. N Engl J Med 289:176–181

Rabson AS, Rosen SW, Tasjran AH (1973) Production of human chorionic gonadotrophin in vitro by a cell line derived from a carcinoma of the lung. J Natl Cancer Inst 50:669–674

Ratcliffe JG, Knight RA, Besser GM, Landon J, Stansfield AG (1972) Tumour and plasma ACTH concentrations in patients with and without the ectopic ACTH syndrome. Clin Endocrinal 1:27–44

Ratter SJ, Lowry PJ, Besser GM, Rees LH (1980) Chromatographic characterisation of adrenocorticotrophin in human plasma. J Endocrinol 85:359–369

Ratter SJ, Gillies G, hope J, Hale AC, Grossman A, Gaillard R, Cook D, Edwards CRW, Rees LH (1983) Pro-opiocortin related peptides in human pituitary and ectopic ACTH secreting tumours. Clin Endocrinol 18:211–218

Rees LH, Bloomfield GA, Rees GM (1974) Multiple hormones in a bronchial tumour. J Clin Endocrinol Metab 38:1090–1097

Rees LH, Bloomfield GA, Gilkes JJH, Besser GM (1977) ACTH as a tumour marker. Ann NY Acad Sci 297:603–620

Rivier J. Spiess J, Thorner MO, Vale W (1982) Characterisation of a growth hormone-releasing factor from a human pancreatic islet tumour. Nature 300:276–278

Robertson GL (1978) Cancer and inappropriate antidiuresis. In: Ruddon RW (ed) Biological markers of neoplasia: basic and applied aspects. Elsevier, New York

Roos BA, Lindall AW, Baylin SB, O'Neil JA, Frelinger JI, Birnbaum RS, Lambert PW (1980) Plasma immunoreactive calcitonin in lung cancer. J Clin Endocrinol Metab 50:659–666

Schorr I, Hinshaw HT, Cooper MA, Mahafee D, Ney RL (1972) Adenyl cyclase hormone responses of certain human endocrine tumour. J Clin Endocrinol Metab 34:447–451

Schwartz WB, Bennett W, Curelop S, Bartter FC (1957) A syndrome of renal sodium loss and hyponatraemia probably resulting from inappropriate secretion of antidiuretic hormone. Am J Med 23:529–542

Seidah NG, Benjannet S, Routhier R, DeSerres G, Rochemont J, Lis M, Chretien M (1980) Purification and characterisation of the N-terminal fragment of pro-opiocomelanocortin from human pituitaries: homology to the bovine sequence. Biochem Biophys Res Commun 95:1417–1424

Silva OL, Broder LE, Doppman JL, Snider RH, Moore CF, Cohen MH, Becker KL (1979) Calcitonin as a marker for bronchogenic cancer. Cancer 44:680–684

Skrabaneck P, McPartlin J, Powell D (1980) Tumour associated hypercalcaemia and 'ectopic hyperparathyroidism'. Medicine 59:262–282

Sonksen PH, Ayres AB, Braimbridge M, Corrin DR, Davies GM, Jeremiah SW, Oaten C, Lowy TET, West T (1976) Acromegaly caused by pulmonary carcinoid tumours. Clin Endocrinol 5:503–513

Sorensen GD, Bloom SR, Ghatei MA, Del Prete SA, Cate CC, Pettengill OS (1982) Bombesin production by human small cell carcinoma of the lung. Regul Pept 4:59–66

Sparagna M, Philips G, Hoffman C, Kucera L (1971) Ectopic growth hormone syndrome with lung cancer. Metabolism 20:730–736

Stewart AF, Horst R, Deftos LJ (1980) Biochemical evaluation of patients with cancer associated hypercalcaemia. Evidence for humoral and non-humoral groups. N Engl J Med 303:1377–1383

Suda T, Demura H, Demura R (1977) Corticotrophin-releasing factor-like activity in ACTH producing tumour. J Clin Endocrinol Metab 44:440–446

Thorner MO, Perryman RL, Cronin MJ, Rogol AD, Draynin M, Johanson A, Vale W, Horvath E, Kovacs K (1982) Somatotroph hyperplasia. Successful treatment of acromegaly by removal of a pancreatic islet tumour secreting a growth hormone-releasing factor. J Clin Invest 70:965–977

Track NS, Cutz E (1982) Bombesin-like immunoreactivity in developing human lung. Life Sci 30:1553–1556

Unger RH, Lochner JD, Eisentraut AM (1964) Identification of insulin and glucagon in a bronchogenic metastasis. J Clin Endocrinol Metab 34:823–831

Vale W, Spiess J, Rivier C, Rivier J (1981) Characterisation of a 41-residue ovine hypothalamic peptide that stimulates secretion of corticotrophin and beta-endorphin. Science 213:1394–1397

Vorherr H (1974) Para-endocrine tumour activity with emphasis on ectopic ADH secretion: Genetic, diagnostic, prognostic and therapeutic aspects. Oncology 29:382–416

Weintraub BD, Rosen SW (1971) Ectopic production of chorionic somatomammotrophin by non-trophoblastic cancers. J Clin Endocrinol Metab 32:94–101

Wharton J, Polak JM, Bloom SR, Ghatei MA, Solcia E, Brown M, Pearse AGE (1978) Bombesin-like immunoreactivity in the lung. Nature 273:769–770

Wood SM, Wood JR, Ghatei MA, Lee YC, O'Shaughnessy D, Bloom SR (1981) Bombesin, somatostatin and neurotensin-like immunoreactivity in bronchial carcinoma. J Clin Endocrinol Metab 53:1310–1312

Yesner R (1978) Spectrum of lung cancer and ectopic hormones. In: Sommers S, Rosen PP (eds) Pathology annual part 1. Appleton-Century-Crofts, New York, pp 217–240

Chapter 4

Bronchoscopy with Rigid and Flexible Instruments

Michael Meredith Brown

Indications

Bronchoscopy is indicated whenever symptoms, signs or findings arouse suspicion of a possible bronchial neoplasm. The appearances seen offer valuable diagnostic evidence to an experienced eye, and specimens for the laboratory can be obtained. On planning treatment, knowledge of the position and extent of the disease is valuable, and bronchoscopy is often aimed at determining both of these factors at one examination.

If surgical treatment is proposed, bronchoscopy is mandatory, and the surgeon will be wise to carry out the examination himself. If a previous bronchoscopy has been performed by a reliable colleague and the findings leave the possibility of resection scarcely in doubt, then the examination can be performed as the first stage of the definitive operation with a view to proceeding to thoracotomy, which will be abandoned if unexpected contra-indications are found. If radiotherapy is planned, particularly if radical treatment is proposed, bronchoscopy will give valuable information as to the site and proximal extent of the tumour. It may be wise to repeat bronchoscopy after a course of radiotherapy, particularly in those few patients with squamous cell carcinoma in whom a sequential operation is planned if the therapy has failed to obliterate the tumour.

The findings at bronchoscopy when the lesion is a small, truly peripheral tumour will usually be negative, and for such a lesion the procedure may not be indicated. However, useful information may be obtained. Brush cytology, especially under radioscopic guidance, may be positive; if thoracotomy is proposed, normal proximal bronchi will encourage a limited resection, and evidence of bronchitis will demand a careful consideration of respiratory function and preliminary treatment.

Rigid or Flexible?

Two complementary techniques are available for bronchoscopy. Many years' experience with rigid instruments established irrefutably that bronchoscopy is an essential aid to the management of bronchial carcinoma. The use of the flexible instrument during the last decade has reinforced its importance and has allowed many respiratory physicians to resume the practise of bronchoscopy, which had largely become a surgical prerogative.

Whoever performs a bronchoscopy must acquire and practise two skills: firstly that of manipulation, and secondly that of interpretation. He must know how to introduce the instrument in all types of patient of any age and of any build; he must be able to manoeuvre it to visualise all accessible bronchi to the full range that the instrument offers; he must know how to take biopsies and other specimens and how to take full advantage of the accessory equipment; and he must be aware at all times of the ways to ensure that the examination is conducted with the least possible hazard to the patient and with the minimum discomfort. Then he must know the meaning of what he sees so that he can interpret his findings; he must be aware of the normal anatomy and its variations so that he can appreciate structural changes associated with neoplasms; he must know the range of normal appearances of the mucosa and recognise the hypertrophic changes associated with carcinoma; and he must know of the many other alterations associated with disease. Both these skills, i.e. manipulation and interpretation, must be learnt, and both are equally important for either technique of bronchoscopy. Although clearly comparable, the needs for the two techniques are different. Written descriptions, diagrams and models are helpful but the skills are best acquired by observing and practising the procedures.

Many respiratory physicians perform bronchoscopy, usually using the flexible instruments, while most thoracic surgeons use the rigid instrument. Which method should be chosen? The decision will often depend on the convenience and availability of the necessary facilities and skilled personnel but other considerations are relevant:

The *flexible technique* offers an examination that can be performed almost anywhere with easily portable equipment. It can usually be performed without general anaesthesia and seldom causes the patient serious distress. The beautiful optics of the fibrescope provide a detailed view and the flexible tip a greater range than the rigid instrument with its telescopes can offer. The orifices of all the segmental bronchi and their subdivisions can nearly always be seen. The flexible instrument allows the collection of material for histological or cytological examination with great accuracy and from most parts of the lung, both central and peripheral. Bronchoscopy with the flexible instrument in selected patients and properly performed carries very little risk and complications are few. The flexible nature of the instrument allows its passage even in patients with a rigid deformity of the spine or an ankylosis of the jaw almost totally preventing opening of the mouth.

The *rigid technique* offers the operator a direct naked eye view, without the distortion that any optical device inevitably produces. Structural deformities and abnormal rigidity may be more easily appreciated. Aspiration of secretions or blood can readily be performed if necessary, using a large-bore sucker. With rigid telescopes, both direct and angled, the range of vision can be increased so that all segmental orifices are usually visible, but the range does not extend beyond this and so is significantly less than that of the flexible instrument. The excellent optics of rigid telescopes also present a beautiful enlarged image. The rigid bronchoscope gives an opportunity to take a relatively large biopsy, in practice only from areas accessible to the straight shafted biopsy forceps available. Bronchial carcinomas are often pleomorphic: the larger the biopsy specimen, the more likely it is to be representative, and the less likely the patient to be refused appropriate surgical treatment on a false suspicion of unsuitable histology. Carried out under general anaesthesia, rigid bronchoscopy allows the maintenance of full oxygenation throughout the procedure. The hazards for rigid bronchoscopy are also minimal, but there is perhaps a slightly greater danger of significant bleeding than with the flexible technique. The discomforts of the procedure, although perhaps a little different, are scarcely greater. The operator carrying out a rigid bronchoscopy can, if the equipment is available and he is familiar with its use and interpretation, pass the flexible bronchoscope through the rigid instrument and use it as a telescope to increase his range of vision and as a means of collecting pathological specimens beyond the range of the rigid instrument.

Most bronchoscopies performed by respiratory physicians will be with the flexible instrument using local anaesthesia; however, there are certain circumstances when the rigid instrument has advantages. Its better suction facilities make it preferred when there is copious secretion, when significant bleeding has occurred or is threatened, and when a large biopsy is demanded. Many surgeons when planning operative treatment prefer to use the rigid technique with the advantage of direct inspection. The state of the carina, its mobility and sharpness, and the rigidity of the main bronchi from infiltration can often be easily appreciated: these important indications of inoperability may be missed at a fibrescopic examination.

The Preparation

An up-to-date assessment that the patient is fit to undergo the procedure should be made. This should include at least a general examination with an examination of the lungs and the cardiovascular system. A superimposed infection or a cardiac arrhythmia may develop rapidly subsequent to the consultation at which the bronchoscopy was recommended, and may demand antibiotic cover or appropriate drugs. For similar reasons, an up-to-date chest X-ray is always desirable. In any case a recent film should always be to hand, and a lateral view should be available to localise the lesion. The patient's neck and jaw should be examined, particularly if rigid bronchoscopy is proposed, as deformity or ankylosis will be relevant. The teeth should be inspected and any loose ones noted. Severe caries or significant infection may demand preliminary dental treatment. Ideally, a recent blood count will be available; anaemia adds a hazard to the procedure both because the oxygen-carrying capacity of the blood is reduced and cyanosis may not become apparent, and because the procedure may cause blood loss, especially if a biopsy is taken, perhaps unsupportable. Severe anaemia consequently contra-indicates bronchoscopy until corrected.

There will always be reluctance to postpone a necessary investigation in a patient with malignant disease, and each case must be carefully considered, but sometimes the patient's safety will demand it.

The preparation usual before any anaesthetic should be carried out, whether a general or a local anaesthetic is proposed. Patients should starve for 4 hours before the examination but there is no virtue in a longer period, and excessive abstinence from all fluids may lead to undesirable dehydration. Appropriate premedication should be arranged and the proper consent form signed after the procedure has been explained to the patient. A careful explanation and reassurance are always valuable, and are essential to secure the patient's co-operation when local anaesthesia is used. If general anaesthesia is to be used, it may be wise to explain that the anaesthetic will be short; the advantages of early recovery sometimes make judgement of the exact dose of the barbiturate difficult, and the patient may be aware of the latter part of the proceedings although his muscles are still relaxed. No harm will come if he is aware of this possibility. He should also be warned that he may cough after the procedure, and perhaps bring up blood.

The Instruments and Venue

Instruments for Rigid Bronchoscopy

As the larynx, trachea and major bronchi lie in the same inclined frontal plane, which can be extended to the opened mouth, all that is required to examine the bronchi is a simple open-ended tube of the right dimensions and appropriately illuminated. A variety of instruments are available; those designed by Negus are highly recommended (Fig. 1). Various sizes of the same pattern, appropriate to patients of different ages and build, have dimensions based on cadaver measurements. The distal part of the straight tube is cylindrical and the proximal part conical or slightly flared. This ingenious variant gives the operator the impression of a larger image at the distal end. There are slots in the distal part to allow ventilation of the contralateral lung when the bronchoscope tip lies in a bronchus. Illumination is provided at the distal end by a small low-voltage bulb from a battery or by a fibre-light stem with a light source connected by a flexible cable.

Good suction equipment is essential for a satisfactory examination. It is necessary for removing secretions to obtain an adequate view and for laboratory examination, and for removing blood. Good suction may be life saving if fresh bleeding occurs. The source of suction must be of adequate power and the connecting tubing and connections of sufficient bore and rigidity. A variety of suction tubes to pass down the bronchoscope is available. For general use a slender tube is convenient (as it does not obstruct the view), with a slightly curved gum elastic tip that can be directed into the segments. This must be securely attached. Spares should be to hand, as should larger bore tubes or bronchial catheters. Care must be taken with metal tubes with

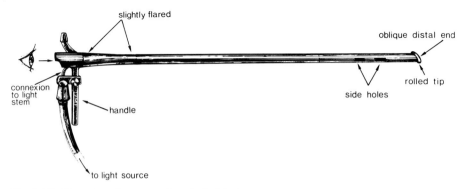

Fig. 1. The Negus bronchoscope — its principal features.

an unprotected distal end as this may easily cause bleeding. It is wise to have the whole suction system duplicated, in case of blockage or failure.

Rigid telescopes are available, some with illumination, allowing a magnified direct or angulated view. The fibrescope may also be used as a flexible telescope.

Swab carriers and a supply of swabs small enough to pass easily through the bronchoscope are useful for mopping secretions. It is essential that the little swabs are firmly secured in the carrier. If one becomes detached, it may be surprisingly difficult to find, especially if bleeding has occurred.

Equipment for collecting laboratory specimens include Luken's tubes or secretion collectors, a syringe to inject normal saline for bronchial washings, and biopsy forceps (Brock's angled forceps are the most useful).

Instruments for Flexible Bronchoscopy

The flexible bronchoscope, or bronchofibrescope, takes advantage of the optical properties of a flexible bundle of fine glass fibres to transmit light, both to provide illumination and to afford an image to view. Each glass fibre is coated with a layer of a second glass of a different refractive index. Light entering one end of the fibre is largely internally reflected and so emerges at the far end of the fibre with a large proportion of its original intensity. A bundle of many hundreds of fibres no more than a few millimetres in diameter will transmit the light from an intense source such as a projector bulb and provide at the far end of the instrument more than adequate illumination. With distal and proximal lenses, an image is returned to the operator's eye along another glass fibre bundle. The image received is naturally different from that observed by direct vision down an open rigid bronchoscope, but with experience the operator learns interpretation, and the magnification provided offers the opportunity of observing rather greater detail. The flexibility of the glass fibres allows an instrument whose distal end can be turned to enter lobar and segmental bronchi.

The fibrescope for bronchoscopy has a flexible shaft with distal objective lens and proximal eyepiece and controls. A range of instruments from several manufacturers is available; although they have different dimensions, there are only minor variations between them. The shaft is sufficiently long to reach the distal bronchi while the eyepiece remains conveniently outside the patient and is of small diameter, 7 mm or less. The shaft contains fibre bundles for illumination and viewing, and usually in addition a suction channel which can also be used for the passage of biopsy forceps or cytology brushes. The distal end is especially flexible and can be elevated or depressed in a single plane by fine wires attached to a control lever near the eyepiece; the angle can be fixed. This angulation, and the possibility of rotation of the whole instrument, allows a view in any direction. At the proximal end the eyepiece can be focused. In some instruments a convenient two-way channel allows control of suction while a biopsy forceps is passed. The instrument is usually equipped with its own light cable and connector. A compatible light source must be available, together with a suction apparatus.

Venue

Ideally, bronchoscopy by either method will be carried out in a properly designed endoscopy room or in an operating theatre. However, the examination can be conducted with satisfaction almost anywhere, provided electricity, suction and sufficient space are available. The room lighting is best equipped with arrangements for dimming. A bright light ahead of the operator must be avoided, but sufficient background illumination to observe the patient is essential.

The patient will usually lie on a firm surface. An operating table is ideal with a movable head flap preferably with a worm gear, but any firm surface will do, such as a patient trolley, with pillows to adjust the position of the head. Bronchoscopy can be performed with the patient in his bed, in which case, especially if local anaesthesia is used, a bedrest may be used to hold him in a sitting position, the operator looking over his shoulder; as a further alternative a dental chair may be used.

As well as the operator and anaesthetist, it is desirable to have at least two persons to assist at a bronchoscopy, one to present the instruments in an orderly fashion, the other to assist with this task and in the care of the patient.

If transbronchial biopsy is anticipated, facilities for radioscopy are desirable, preferably bi-plane: it may be best to conduct the examination in an X-ray department.

Technique

Rigid Bronchoscopy

Rigid bronchoscopy is usually performed with a general anaesthetic (see p.149).

The bronchoscope chosen should be of the largest size appropriate to the patient in question. This will usually be a standard adult bronchoscope for a man and a small adult bronchoscope for a woman. In a young patient with complete and prominent upper teeth an adolescent bronchoscope may be suitable.

The patient will usually be supine on a firm surface but he may lie in bed, with his shoulders held elevated. The rigid bronchoscope, being a straight tube, must be passed through the opened mouth aligned with the glottis and trachea (Fig. 2). Bearing in mind the inclined frontal plane in which the trachea normally lies, the operator must secure this alignment by adjusting the position of the patient's head relative to his trunk, keeping it in the midline without rotation, with the neck extended and the jaw raised. This can conveniently be done by using a single pillow of the right consistency, or by adjusting the movable head flap of an operating table; sometimes an assistant should hold the head. It is sometimes helpful to lift the tongue forwards and upwards so as to present the glottis. Taking the instrument by the handle and looking down the lumen, the operator places the instrument in the patient's mouth behind the tongue, with its beak forward. The patient's eyes should be protected, which may conveniently be achieved by a surgical towel folded round the head. The operator must be careful not to damage the patient's teeth, lips or gums; it is easy to injure the lower lip by catching it between the instrument and the

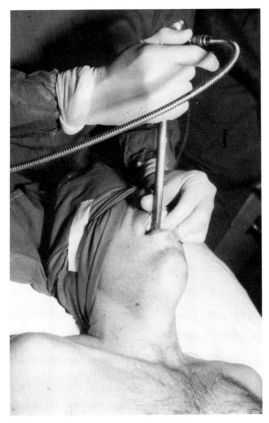

Fig. 2. Position of the patient's head in rigid bronchoscopy. The operator is using his thumb as a fulcrum and has protected the patient's teeth and lips with a swab, and his eyes with a folded towel.

teeth. The patient's upper jaw and gums may be protected by a swab, the retrieval of which must be checked at the end of the examination. The operator's thumb or forefinger laid along the upper jaw provides a fulcrum for the bronchoscope — the patient's teeth or gums should not be used for this purpose.

With the instrument in the mouth, the operator must find the glottis. The clue is the epiglottis, which is usually readily seen and must be raised forward with the beak of the instrument, if necessary using the digital fulcrum. He must then find the vocal cords that guard the glottis. Sometimes recognition of an arytenoid cartilage gives a lead to the glottis, which lies anterior and medial to it. The glottis is usually best found by keeping the head quite straight and the instrument strictly in the mid-line. When the glottis has been found and the vocal cords observed, the instrument should be rotated through 90° so that the beak will easily slip between them. Passing the instrument in this way is often a simple manoeuvre, especially in a patient with no upper teeth and with flexible cervical and mandibular joints. It can be difficult if there is a cervical deformity, an ankylosed jaw or prominent upper teeth, or copious secretions. Sometimes a gap in the teeth affords a convenient channel. During the introduction of the instrument, the relaxed patient is not receiving oxygen so if the operator does not quickly pass the glottis his efforts to find it must be interrrupted while the anaesthetist inflates the patient's lungs with oxygen using a mask. Once the bronchoscope tip lies in the trachea an excellent airway is established and further manoeuvres need not be hurried. The time available to the operator for his search reflects the patients's respiratory function.

The operator should examine the trachea, carina and bronchi, looking for the abnormalities described later in this chapter. He should examine all accessible parts of the bronchi of both sides. It may be wise to examine the side expected to be normal first so that it is not forgotten. Although unusual, simultaneous bilateral carcinoma and carcinoma without recognisable changes on a plain X-ray are sufficiently common to warrant a full examination at every bronchoscopy. If secretion is present it should be carefully aspirated with a sucker, avoiding damage to the mucosa, normal or abnormal, which might cause bleeding — always undesirable both for its hazard and because blood obscures the view. Direct vision should be supplemented by using telescopes.

Flexible Bronchoscopy

Bronchoscopy with the fibrescope can conveniently be performed under local anaesthesia on a day patient basis.

The preparation described above should be carried out. The patient may lie on a table, couch or bed, supine with pillows or with his back supported. The local anaesthetic can be given as for rigid bronchoscopy or more conveniently as outlined below. Supplementary intravenous sedation may be desirable.

The patient first sucks an anaesthetic lozenge or gargles with a solution. The operator may spray the pharynx, and apply surface anaesthetic to the chosen nostril.

The operator passes the tip of the fibrescope through the nostril or the mouth and will observe the posterior pharynx with the epiglottis, behind which he will see the vocal cords. Before advancing the instrument further he will inject through the suction channel more of the solution, e.g. 2 ml from a small syringe. This will spray the epiglottis and glottis. The patient is conscious and should be warned that he will cough. Coughing helps distribute the local anaesthetic. The vocal cords should be inspected and their movements on phonation observed. After a brief pause the tip of the fibrescope is steered between the vocal cords to enter the trachea. The manoeuvre is effected like other manipulations of the instrument, the operator slowly advancing the instrument held in one hand while the other hand controls the angulation of the tip by moving the lever near the eyepiece. The exact position of the tip with the objective lens is also established by rotation of the whole instrrument. More local anaesthetic should be injected into the trachea to anaesthetise its mucosa and that of the carina and main bronchi. The more peripheral bronchi are seldom sensitive. The examination can now proceed. It is sensible to examine all the bronchi in a systematic fashion. Secretion should be aspirated through the suction channel by placing a finger over the proximal control orifice. If the objective lens becomes obscured by secretion it can often be removed by suction or by wiping on the wall of a normal bronchus. A silicone anti-mist preparation reduces condensation on the distal lens. Pathological specimens should be collected as described below and the instrument removed gently when the examination is complete, maintaining observation during withdrawal.

Anaesthesia

General Anaesthesia for Rigid or Flexible Fibre-optic Bronchoscopy

The majority of bronchoscopies with the rigid instrument are performed under general anaesthesia, since the introduction of the Venturi jet has made this method so safe. Bronchoscopy with the use of the flexible instrument is generally carried out under sedation and local analgesia, but there may be indications for general anaesthesia (see p. 149).

Local Anaesthesia for Rigid or Flexible Bronchoscopy

Bronchoscopy with the rigid or flexible instrument can be performed under local anaesthetic with satisfaction, but great care must be taken in its administration and sufficient time allowed. Patient co-operation is essential and a full explanation of the procedure must be given.

Premedication similar to that for general anaesthesia is invaluable. It should alleviate anxiety and reduce secretion so that the surface anaesthetic is effective, and must not cause undue respiratory depression.

The patient may be seated, perhaps best in a dental chair, or lie supine on a couch, trolley or operation table with pillows available so that he can comfortably assume the necessary position.

A variety of agents for surface anaesthesia are available; lignocaine is widely used. A 4% solution is often recommended but a 2% solution is equally effective if time is allowed for it to act, and carries a lesser risk of toxic reaction. Such reactions, with loss of consciousness, fall of blood pressure and often convulsions are very rare, but can occur with alarming rapidity as the drug is quickly absorbed. Equipment for resuscitation and an intravenous barbiturate should always be to hand.

A local anaesthetic may be applied in various ways. It is wise to measure out the total dose proposed, perhaps in a minim glass. Time must be allowed for the premedication to take effect. The patient may suck an anaesthetic lozenge or gargle with a small quantity of the local anaesthetic. A swab soaked in the solution may be applied to the lip and the tongue and the pharynx sprayed. Great care should be taken to anaesthetise the larynx. This cannot be hurried. A laryngeal spray may be used, but perhaps the most effective method is surface application. Small swabs soaked in the anaesthetic solution and held in Krause's forceps are applied in turn to each pyriform fossa and then to the vocal cords, while the patient holds his tongue forward with the aid of a small cloth. Finally the lower trachea, carina and main bronchi can be anaesthetised after inserting the bronchoscope by injecting through a Clerf's spray.

Following local anaesthesia, the patient should not eat or drink until mucosal sensation has completely recovered.

Bronchial Anatomy

The bronchoscopist must clearly have a good knowledge of the anatomy of the normal bronchi (Brock 1946; Fig. 3) so that he can recognise the structural deformities and mucosal changes caused by carcinomata. He should be able to name the segmental branches (Thoracic Society 1950; Fig. 4) so that he can describe accurately the position of lesions observed. The study of diagrams and drawings, casts and models gives a good foundation to this knowledge which can only be secured by observing the bronchi of many patients.

The pattern (a) of the bifurcation of the trachea into main bronchi and (b) of the lobar bronchi seldom varies, but there are individual differences in the exact branching of the segmental bronchi. The structural appearances depend on the build and size of the patient and may be significantly modified by unrelated or previous disease such as scoliosis, goitres and fibrosis following pulmonary tuberculosis or a previous pulmonary resection. With advancing age the bronchial cartilages may become more prominent or calcified and the submucosal tissues atrophied so that the mucosa appears thinned.

Anatomy Seen with the Rigid Bronchoscope

The trachea is normally straight, inclining backwards in the mid-line, with a slight indentation on the left side where pulsation of the aortic arch can be observed. The cartilage rings are easily appreciated and their firm rigidity contrasts with the mobile soft posterior wall. The carina presents as a vertical keel between the two main

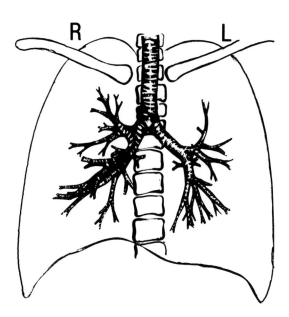

Fig. 3. The trachea and bronchi in relation to some of the structures seen in a chest X-ray.

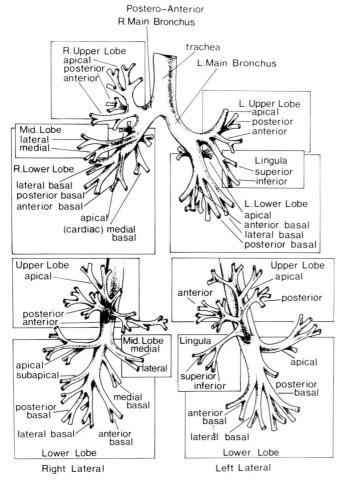

Postero–Anterior
R.Main Bronchus

trachea
L.Main Bronchus

R.Upper Lobe
apical
posterior
anterior

L.Upper Lobe
apical
posterior
anterior

Mid.Lobe
lateral
medial

Lingula
superior
inferior

R.Lower Lobe
lateral basal
posterior basal
anterior basal
apical
(cardiac) medial
basal

L.Lower Lobe
apical
anterior basal
lateral basal
posterior basal

Upper Lobe
apical
posterior
anterior

anterior

Upper Lobe
apical
posterior

apical
subapical

Mid.Lobe
medial
lateral

Lingula
superior
inferior

apical

posterior
basal

posterior
basal
lateral basal

medial
basal
anterior
basal

anterior
basal
lateral basal

Lower Lobe

Lower Lobe

Right Lateral

Left Lateral

Fig. 4 The bronchial tree, with the names of the segmental branches.

bronchi; the right bronchus continues the line of the trachea with only slight deviation so that the rigid bronchoscope looks directly into it, whereas the angulation of the left main bronchus means the operator must usually deviate the proximal end of his instrument to the right to obtain a direct view. These differences are reflected in a slight asymmetry of the normal carina, so that the keel may appear to lie a little to the left of the mid-line, but it is nearly always vertical and not distorted or irregular. Its sharpness varies considerably, reflecting the build and age of the patient.

The appearances of the main bronchi are similar to those of the trachea but on a smaller scale. This is well seen on the right, which is slightly larger than the left. The branching on the two sides is notably different. On the right, the upper lobe bronchus extends at right angles to the main bronchus with its orifice on the lateral wall, the upper lip lying a few millimetres below the carina or sometimes almost level with it. Within a short distance the upper lobe bronchus normally divides into three segmental bronchi, the orifices of which lie in the positions that their names indicate, i.e. apical, posterior and anterior. In about one-fifth of patients the upper lobe divides into four branches, all much the same size, or perhaps into two which each branch again; the fourth branch supplies the lateral segment. Occasionally two branches originate separately from the main bronchus, one closely above the other. A more interesting anomaly is found in less than 1% of patients, in whom part of the apical segment is supplied by a small accessory bronchus arising from the right lateral wall of the lower trachea, usually about 1 cm above the upper lobe bronchus proper. Beyond the upper lobe orifice the right main bronchus tapers to divide about 2 cm below into middle and lower lobe branches, with a more or less horizontal keel between them. The middle lobe bronchus, which varies a good deal in size, often looks like another segmental orifice, especially as it lies opposite to the opening of the apical branch of the lower lobe bronchus. It usually lies truly anterior at 12 o'clock but sometimes a little to the right, and can often be seen to divide into its two segmental branches, described as medial and lateral but not always truly in these positions. The lower lobe bronchus continues distally beyond its large apical branch, which may lie at 5 o'clock rather than the more usual fully posterior position. There is sometimes a subapical branch passing posteriorly and nearly always a medial basal branch from the left side. The remaining basal branches are variable in size and position, not always exactly corresponding with the standard anatomical description of posterior, anterior and lateral segmental branches.

On the left side, the main bronchus is unbranched for about 4 or 5 cm until it divides into upper and lower lobe bronchi. These are usually of more or less equal diameter, although the upper lobe may be larger. The left upper lobe bronchus proceeds at a more oblique angle than the right upper lobe bronchus and can often be seen into directly, as can its first branch to the lingula from its inferior wall. This again branches usually into two equal divisions described as superior and inferior. Beyond the lingula the upper lobe bronchus may curve upwards before dividing again into anterior and apico-posterior branches. The bifurcation of the latter is not always visible. The left lower lobe bronchus continues the line of the main bronchus or a little more medial. Its first branch, to the apical segment, lies posteriorly or slightly medially; there is no bronchial orifice opposite as the bronchus to the lingula, the analogue of the middle lobe, branches from the upper lobe bronchus. Nor is there a medial basal bronchus whereas the heart lies medially. Distally the left lobe bronchus divides into basal segmental branches; as on the right, the pattern is variable and nomenclature unimportant.

Respiratory movements can be observed in the bronchi, most readily when local anaesthetic is used and the patient is breathing naturally. Slight dilatation occurs on inspiration but the changes on expiration are more easily seen as the soft posterior wall bulges forward. These changes are marked if the patient coughs.

Pulsation is also seen in the normal bronchial tree, which is in close relationship with the heart and with large vessels. Aortic pulsation is best seen to the left of the trachea. The left ventricle is close to the left lower lobe bronchus. The left atrium lies beneath the carina and close to the right main bronchus, but its pulsation is seldom conspicuous. The right pulmonary artery is close to the upper lobe bronchus and basal branches on both sides are near the basal segmental bronchi. If the heart is hyperactive, marked pulsation can be seen in many parts.

The bronchial mucosa is of a uniform appearance and a pale pinkish colour which becomes still paler in old age. The mucosa is moist but the are no droplets or pools of mucus.

Anatomy Seen with the Flexible Bronchoscope

The bronchoscopist using the flexible bronchoscope, or fibrescope, sees the same anatomy as the bronchoscopist using the rigid bronchoscope, but from a different viewpoint, namely the objective lens of the fibrescope. This moves into the bronchi and so the observer is very close to the structures he is examining; thus he appreciates the angles at which the branches leave the main bronchus in a different way and is able to look directly into them, so the upper lobe bronchi may be seen directly ahead. The division of the segmental bronchi which bifurcate and divide again can be observed, often to the fourth division.

The Findings in Bronchial Carcinoma

A carcinoma may manifest itself in various ways: by mucosal changes or by structural alterations. Evidence of spread of the tumour may be found. In peripheral tumours there is often no abnormality. Signs of chronic bronchitis or of previous pulmonary disease assist in the assessment of the patient.

Inflammatory changes, namely oedema, hyperaemia and excess secretion, are often found adjacent to a carcinoma. If widespread, they may be due to an associated infection. This suspicion should be confirmed by bacteriology although culture is often negative.

Mucosal Changes

A great variety of changes may be seen. It is wise to compare a doubtfully abnormal area with another part, such as the corresponding contralateral bronchus, hopefully normal. A finely irregular proliferation of the mucosa is almost pathognomonic of squamous cell carcinoma. The mucosa is usually reddened but not often intensely so, and there may be associated ulceration. Haemoptysis may have occurred but even without this history blood clot or fresh bleeding are significant and should be noted. It is easy to cause bleeding from such a tumour, and care must be taken with the instrument and the sucker to avoid this as it is sometimes dangerous and can obscure the view. Proliferation is seldom seen in a small cell carcinoma, where the mucosa is oedematous and glistening, sometimes having a purplish colour and again being ulcerated. An appearance like the surface of a raspberry or mulberry may represent a carcinoid tumour, especially if the adjacent mucosa is perfectly normal. Mucosal proliferation can cause bronchial obstruction.

Bronchial Secretions

Most carcinomas do not secrete, although some adenocarcinomas may produce mucus. Normally produced mucus from the lung distal to a carcinoma may accumulate or be retained by the obstruction, and this can sometimes be observed.

Larger tumours become necrotic in the centre owing to their poor blood supply and may liquefy to form pus. Purulent secretion may also be evidence of an associated infection. Blood clot can liquefy to a brownish fluid.

Structural Changes

A carcinoma can cause alterations to the structure of the bronchial tree, distorting the normal anatomy. These changes may or may not be accompanied by mucosal abnormalities. A tumour can cause compression or distortion with displacement. The larger the tumour, the more marked the changes. Such changes are not specific to carcinoma, and may be seen with any bulky tumour or even with a large pleural effusion of any nature; but, particularly if accompanied by oedema, they must add to the suspicion of a carcinoma. A carcinoma can also cause significant deformity and distortion by infiltration of the bronchial wall. This change is accompanied by rigidity and by the loss of the normal minor changes in the bronchial calibre with respiration. This can most easily be appreciated in the larger bronchi, where the mobility of the soft membranous posterior wall can easily be seen in the normal patient to open up on inspiration, or, during general anaesthetic, on positive pressure ventilation. This sign of mucosal rigidity is valuable evidence of a bronchial carcinoma and a useful indicator of its proximal extent.

Direct Extension

There may be visible evidence of submucous infiltration more proximally than X-rays have suggested or of intramural involvement, and these changes may be seen in the main bronchus or even trachea and so influence the decision as to proper treatment.

Lymphatic Spread

Evidence of involvement of lymph nodes should be sought. Occasionally an enlarged paratracheal node indents the trachea; more commonly a subcarinal gland mass, metastatic from a carcinoma in either lung, can be appreciated as a broadening of the carina, sometimes with bulging of the medial wall of the contralateral main bronchus. A metastatic lymph node can invade one or other recurrent laryngeal nerve, causing an abductor paralysis of the affected nerve. At first sometimes intermittent or partial, it becomes complete and persistent. On the right side the node in question is one of the upper paratracheal group, involving the nerve where it hooks around the subclavian artery, and metastatic from a primary tumour in either the right or the left lung. On the left side, and this is more commonly seen, the nerve is usually involved by a metastasis in a subaortic lymph gland (often originating from a carcinoma in the adjacent upper lobe) which invades the nerve as it hooks around the arch of the aorta close to the ligamentum arteriosum. (The primary tumour may itself invade the nerve directly.)

Vocal Cord Paralysis

The bronchoscopist should examine the movements of the vocal cords. (He should of course examine the cords themselves: concurrent laryngeal carcinoma occurs and laryngitis is often seen). Under local anaesthesia the movements can be observed during respiration and more decisively by asking the patient to phonate. The principal evidence of a recurrent laryngeal nerve lesion is a loss of the power of abduction, so that the affected vocal cord will move towards the mid-line from the neutral position but not away from it. With a complete paralysis the cord is virtually inert. Under general anaesthesia it may be more difficult to observe movements, especially if a muscle relaxant is employed; however, it is usually possible to observe movements at the end of the procedure, as the patient resumes spontaneous breathing but before he is fully conscious. The movements can usually be observed adequately through the bronchoscope but sometimes it is better to change to a laryngoscope. Allowance must be made for possible unequal rates of recovery of the muscles of the two cords. If there is any doubt it may be best to repeat laryngoscopy on another occasion, without general anaesthesia.

Distant Metastases

A second carcinoma is sometimes found at bronchoscopy. Especially if this is a mucosal tumour, it may be metastatic to the primary growth and perhaps have arisen by transbronchial embolism. Occasionally there is evidence of parenchymal pulmonary metastases. It is always difficult to be certain that such neoplasms are not separate primary tumours.

A general anaesthetic gives the operator an opportunity to palpate the abdomen under ideal circumstances. Metastases in the liver or occasionally in coeliac glands or retroperitoneal tissues are sometimes disclosed in this way.

Collecting Specimens for the Pathological Laboratory

Histology

With the rigid bronchoscope, generous biopsies can be obtained from the accessible major bronchi.

With the fibrescope mini-biopsies can be taken with flexible forceps passed through the suction channel; oval cupped forceps provide specimens about 1 mm in diameter. It is usually best to take several. These can be taken under direct vision from any accessible lesion, and also from peripheral tumours or diffuse infiltrations (transbronchial biopsy) preferably with radioscopic guidance.

Cytology

Secretions can be collected in a container inserted between the sucker and its tubing. If sparse, flush the sucker through by dipping its tip quickly in saline, or inject up to 50 ml of saline into the appropriate bronchus before suction.

Some cytologists prefer brushings. A small brush, usually passed through the suction channel of the fibrescope, sweeps cells from the lining of the chosen bronchus; these cells are transferred to a microscope slide, immediately immersed in fixative. Using a disposable brush and withdrawing the fibrescope while the brush remains in the projected positions avoids the risk of cross-contamination between patients. Radioscopic guidance may be useful (see p. 70).

Microbiology

Secretion or saline washings can be sent in a sterile container for examination and culture, as concomitant bacterial or (rarely) tuberculous infection may be present; alternatively a small swab may be rubbed on the bronchial wall and dipped in transport medium.

Dangers and Complications

Rigid bronchoscopy, properly conducted in skilled hands, is a safe procedure and complications are negligible. The principal danger is bleeding, which is occasionally severe and on very rare occasions has been fatal. A less frequent danger is that of causing obstruction of an already compromised airway. Less serious complications include damage to teeth and lips, muscle pains and occasionally fever (see p. 150).

Haemorrhage

Haemoptysis is a common symptom with bronchial carcinoma, and it is not surprising that bleeding can occur at bronschoscopy on contact with the instrument or particularly with the sucker. Such bleeding prolongs the examination and may interfere with the view obtained, but is seldom serious. Haemorrhage from a conventional biopsy may, however, be dangerous. Such bleeding may come from the bronchial circulation, with systemic blood pressure, or from the pulmonary circulation, especially if a biopsy is taken inadvertently from a normal bronchus in close contact with a large branch of the pulmonary artery, as is found in the basal segments of the lower lobe. The pressure in the pulmonary arteries is lower, but there is little muscle in the wall and copious blood loss may occur.

Management of Haemorrhage. Most bleeding will cease spontaneously. Minor bleeding can often be controlled by the surface application of adrenaline 1 in 1000, applied by a small swab held in a carrier. The control of more serious haemorrhage may be very difficult. Occasionally an immediate thoracotomy may be indicated, i.e. if bleeding is life threatening and if the carcinoma appears to be one best treated surgically. This possibility is a reason for carrying out rigid bronchoscopy under circumstances that allow a safe thoracotomy. It is also a reason for knowing the haemoglobin level of all patients receiving bronchoscopy. If serious bleeding occurs, whether or not thoracotomy is performed, blood transfusion should be instituted. An intravenous drip should be set up and serum sent to the laboratory for cross matching. To prepare an operation inevitably takes several minutes. Meanwhile the bleeding may have seized spontaneously, but if not an attempt should be made to control it by tamponage. Sometimes it is possible to plug the bleeding bronchus with ribbon gauze, or to occlude it with a bronchus blocker or a balloon catheter.

It is always difficult to control serious bleeding. It is essential to remove fluid blood and clot from the bronchial tree and to avoid airway obstruction. This is done by suction. For this reason a sucker of adequate power and sufficient lumen must be available.

Obstruction of the Airway

Another important but uncommon complication of bronchoscopy is obstruction of the airway. This is seldom an important complication unless the airway is already compromised, as by a tumour obstructing one main bronchus and growing across the carina so that the other is partly obstructed, or by a recurrent tumour following pneumonectomy. In such cases serious effects inevitably follow obstruction of the limited remaining lumen. Blood clot may complete the obstruction. This can be removed by suction.

Minor Complications

Abrasions or contusions of the lips and gums should be avoided. Damage to the teeth sometimes occurs. A preliminary inspection minimises the risk. The patient's consent to the removal of loose teeth should be obtained. Crowns are sometimes dislodged.

Muscle pains following the use of a short-acting relaxant drug by the anaesthetist may be a minor disability.

Subcutaneous emphysema very rarely occurs. A mucosal tear caused by the instrument or biopsy forceps occasionally allows air to escape into the peribronchial sheath and so into the mediastinum and root of the neck. No action is usually necessary and the air is quickly absorbed.

Spread of Tumour

A patient with a bronchial carcinoma sheds malignant cells into his bronchial tree continuously, and pathologists usually accept that spread of bronchial carcinoma by transbronchial embolism sometimes occurs. The bronchoscopist will occasionally find a small mucosal deposit separate from the main tumour which may have arisen in this way. Theoretically it is possible that the manoeuvres of bronchoscopy might encourage such spread, but there is no evidence to support this theory.

Cleaning and Sterilising the Instruments

Proper care of the equipment is very important. Gentle handling and careful cleaning of the fibrescope and its suction channel are essential and will allow many years of good service in continual use. Cleaning is best done by someone with special interest and training in this field.

Practice has shown that there is no need to carry out bronchoscopy with the full sterile precautions demanded for an open operation, but there must always be a risk of carrying infectious organisms from one patient to another and a small possibility of tissue contamination leading to confusion in histology or cytology. The rigid bronchoscope, biopsy forceps and so on may be autoclaved. It is not, however, possible to autoclave either the fibrescope or rigid telescopes; these must be sterilised by immersion, e.g. in chlorhexidine for 20 min.

It is probably best to regard the fibrescope as something that cannot be properly sterilised, and certainly not by a short period of immersion, and to be cautious in its use, especially if tuberculous infection is suspected. Adequate immersion time must be allowed, so if a series of bronchoscopies with the fibrescope is to be carried out at one sitting it is best to have available at least two instruments.

Bronchoscopy After Thoracotomy

A bronchoscopy is occasionally indicated at the completion of a thoractomy, before a patient leaves the operating suite, e.g. if after a lobectomy the remaining part of the lung fails to ventilate fully. It may be wise to confirm this with an X-ray before proceeding to bronchoscopy, which may demonstrate simply obstruction by blood clot or mucus.

During early recovery, bronchoscopy will sometimes be indicated for bronchial toilet or for relief of persistent atelectasis that has failed to respond to physiotherapy. If repeat bronchoscopy is thus demanded, it may be better to establish tracheostomy to allow regular suction.

Recording and Photography

The findings at bronchoscopy must be carefully recorded in the patient's case notes. The operator's account is best accompanied by a sketch diagram.

Many bronchoscopists use a printed form, kept separately in the notes. As well as spaces for patient details, the form has a diagram of the bronchial tree on which to indicate, for example, the position of a polypoid tumour or a broadened carina (Fig. 5).

BRONCHOSCOPY REPORT

Date   27 June 1983

Surgeon   Mr Meredith Brown

Anæsthetist   Dr Stoneham

Anæsthetic   Local (lignocaine)

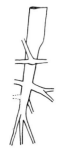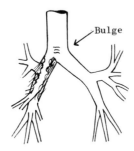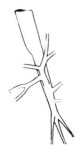

Bulge

Bronchoscopy performed with the fibrescope under local anaesthesia.

The vocal cords appeared normal but the left was paralysed.

The upper trachea was normal. The posterior wall of the lower trachea bulged forwards. The appearances suggested infiltration by a bronchial carcinoma extending from the right bronchial tree.

The carina and left bronchi appeared normal, but a good view was not had.

The right upper lobe bronchus was not seen and may be completely obstructed. The right bronchi were all oedematous with irregular mucosa.

The appearances were very suggestive of a carcinoma perhaps arising in the right upper lobe bronchus but now infiltrating the right bronchial tree and trachea.

A biopsy was taken and brushings sent for cytology.

M Meredith Brown

Fig. 5. A sample bronchoscopy report, with the findings sketched in.

Photography

Excellent photographs of bronchoscopic appearances have been taken through the rigid bronchoscope, and some beautiful examples have been published (Stradling 1981). The photography is time consuming and requires special, expensive equipment; thus it is seldom used for routine recording of findings. On the other hand, photography with the fibrescope is simple and relatively inexpensive. Especially constructed cameras are available which fit on to the eyepiece of the fibrescope. Thirty-five millimetre transparencies provide slides for lectures and demonstrations, and a polaroid camera gives a colour print for the patient's record.

Video-Tape Recording

The appearance at fibreoptic bronchoscopy may be viewed by a second person, using an image splitter attached to the eyepiece. The second image may also be received by a video camera which transmits it to a television screen or to a recorder.

Acknowledgements. I am grateful for assistance received in preparing this chapter from many persons, especially:
The Department of Medical Illustration, South West Surrey Health Authority
Miss Debbie Sutton, Medical Secretary

References

Brock RC (1946) The anatomy of the bronchial tree. Oxford University Press, Oxford
Gellert AR, Rudd RM, Sinha G, Geddes DM (1982) Fibreoptic bronchoscopy: the effect of the experience of the operator on diagnostic yield of bronchial biopsy in bronchial carcinoma. Br J Dis Chest 76(4):397–399
Sanders RD (1967): Two ventilating attachments for bronchoscopes. Del Med J 39:170–173
Stradling P (1981) Diagnostic bronchoscopy, 4th edn. Churchill Livingstone, Edinburgh
Thoracic Society (1950) Report on the nomenclature of broncho-pulmonary anatomy. Thorax 5:222–5

Chapter 5

The Role of Cytology in Diagnosis

Gordon Canti

Historical Background

The historical development of clinical cytology in the diagnosis of chest disease has been fully documented by Grunze (1960). The concept of the cell as a biological unit was established by Schwann (1839) in the early part of the nineteenth century. Müller (1838) published a drawing of mammary cancer cells which is quite remarkable in view of the primitive microscopes available at that time. Illustrations of exfoliated cells including cancer cells from the respiratory tract can be found in monographs by Donné (1845) in Paris and Walshe (1846) in London. A few years later some very accurate illustrations of malignant squamous cells from a cancer of the pharynx were published by Beale (1860), but it was not until 1887 that the first diagnosis of carcinoma of the bronchus was made in spontaneously raised sputum (Hampeln 1887). The first cytological diagnosis of malignancy in serous effusions was recorded by Lücke and Klebs (1867).

The development of the paraffin block section towards the end of the nineteenth century tended to turn the attention of pathologists away from the cytological towards the histological study of disease. Interest in sputum cytology was rekindled in the 1930s in papers by Dudgeon and Wrigley (1935), Gloyne (1937), Barret (1938) and Gowar (1943), using the so-called 'wet film' technique (fixing the smear in alcoholic solutions while still wet) originated by Dudgeon and Patrick (1927). Finally, Wandall (1944) established the value of sputum cytology beyond doubt by the publication of an 84% success rate in 100 cases of lung cancer. Other papers were published at the time and many have been published since, but the application of cytology to the diagnosis of lung cancer has been slow to develop owing to the lack of trained cytopathologists.

Papanicolaou's discovery of the value of cytology in the detection of pre-malignant lesions of the cervix (Papanicolaou and Traut 1943) stimulated interest in exfoliative cytology and was mainly responsible for the establishment of cytology laboratories and the training of technical and qualified staff. From these centres interest and knowledge of pulmonary cytology has developed, but its application is still limited by a shortage of experienced cytopathologists.

Sputum Cytology

Clinical Application

In those medical centres where a cytological service is available, an examination of the sputum is now the preferred method of establishing the diagnosis in a suspected case of lung cancer.

Sputum cytology has obvious advantages over other methods of diagnosis: it is quick, devoid of trauma, and can be performed on the out-patient and repeated as often as necessary; it examines secretions from the whole of the bronchial tree and is therefore capable of making an early diagnosis which may be lifesaving; it is equally practical for establishing the diagnosis in advanced disease before instituting treatment by cytotoxic drugs or radiotherapy; and it is highly specific and usually successful in identifying the histological type of the tumour. The disadvantages are as follows: the investigation is time consuming and requires highly trained technicians and pathologists to achieve acceptable accuracy; a positive result does not indicate the site of the lesion or its operability; not all patients can produce adequate sputum; and not all sputa from patients with lung cancer contain malignant cells. The test is therefore not very sensitive, but it is superior to other methods of investigation in terms of convenience, cost and accuracy (Laurie and Szaloky 1971).

The clinician needs to have some idea of the sensitivity of any investigation that is being employed. This is a particularly difficult question to answer in the case of sputum cytology because of the subjective nature of the test and the reliance that must be placed on the experience of the cytologist. Malignant cells have to be sought among numerous inflammatory and degenerate cells in bronchial secretion; the sensitivity of the test will therefore depend to a considerable extent on the time spent on each case — in other words on the resources of the laboratory. A negative report on sputum is generally considered of little value until at least three specimens have been examined (Oswald et al. 1971). Several slides must be made from each specimen, and each one has to be methodically screened. This may take up to 45 min of the microscopist's time. If those patients who cannot produce a satisfactory specimen of sputum are excluded, the first three specimens should yield 60%-70% positive for malignant cells (Boddington and Spriggs 1965). The yield progressively increases with the number of specimens examined (Farber et al. 1948; Philps 1954). Numerous papers have been published claiming a detection rate of up to 90% (Russell et al. 1963), but these claims are somewhat misleading as they are made by dedicated individuals often working under research conditions, with unlimited time to examine numerous specimens. Some of the high detection rates are achieved at the expense of unacceptably high false-positive rates; others have achieved high figures by including their 'suspicious' reports among the positives — a practice which ignores the reality of the situation as the clinician cannot act on the basis of a 'suspicious' report except in the direction of repeating the test or initiating some other investigation. Nevertheless, it has been shown that a high detection rate can be achieved if a sufficient number of specimens are examined. It must, however, be appreciated that one microscopist cannot effectively screen more than 10–15 specimens a day owing to eye fatigue — a matter which the clinician should bear in mind when ordering the test. Overloading of the department can only result in a loss of efficiency.

The low resectability rate of lung cancers at the time of diagnosis has stimulated some attempts to obtain earlier diagnosis by cytological screening of selected groups of people. These programmes have had little success (Rome and Olson 1961; Taylor et al. 1981).

The group of people most at risk in this country are the heavy smokers. The Royal College of Physicians' Report (Royal College of Physicians of London 1971) showed that the highest incidence of lung cancer is in those smoking more than 25 cigarettes per day in the age group 55–74 years (see p. 16). Bearing in mind that the majority of these tumours would be of the slow-growing squamous cell type, it would be more rewarding to screen heavy smokers in the 45–54 age group. Even then, only 1 in 200 would have lung cancer, and by the time the malignant cells were present in the sputum a high proportion of cases would have fairly advanced disease. Grzybowski and Coy (1970) found malignant cells in 1 of 125 smokers over the age of 40, but these people had been selected because they had, in addition, chronic bronchitis or long-standing radiographic changes.

Sputum cytology is too expensive a test in terms of skilled manpower and too insensitive to hold out any hope of improving the prognosis of lung cancer by screening symptomless persons. However, a case might be made out for screening very high risk groups such as uranium miners (Saccomanno et al. 1965) or those exposed to asbestos (McDonald et al. 1980).

Collection of Specimen

The efficiency of the test depends largely on the quality of the specimen submitted to the laboratory. Many patients are unaware of the difference between sputum and saliva; it is therefore important to explain that the products of a deep cough are required. It may be necessary in some cases to collect the specimen under supervision. Good bronchial secretion is most easily obtained in the early morning before any contamination with food has occurred and when overnight secretions will have accumulated. In order to increase the chances of finding malignant cells, three specimens should be collected on three successive mornings and despatched to the laboratory on the day of collection. Sputum keeps reasonably well for up to 24 hours in temperate climates provided it is in an airtight container and not in a warm place; it is therefore best kept in a refrigerator until despatched.

Most laboratories prefer fresh specimens, but in hot climates or where transport is likely to take more than 24 hours, the specimen should be preserved in 50% alcohol. This will slow down cytolysis and prevent drying, but the consequent increase in the viscosity of the mucus causes problems in smear preparation.

Cytological investigation of naturally produced sputum should be given preference if the service is available. There are occasions, however, when a bronchoscopy is desirable at an early stage in the investigation. If at all possible, a pre-bronchoscopic sputum specimen should be collected, as cytological appearances are difficult to interpret for several days after bronchoscopy owing to the traumatic effect on the bronchial epithelial cells.

Saline washings obtained at bronchoscopy should be despatched to the laboratory without delay as cell morphology deteriorates rapidly in saline.

Laboratory Technique

In the laboratory various portions of the specimen are selected for smearing on to slides, taking the necessary hygenic precautions. A few laboratories still use a wet film technique, in which the cells are stained supravitally with 1% methylene blue. This method is quick and cheap but has the disadvantage that the slides cannot be reviewed as there is no permanent record. Most cytologists prefer fixed preparations. The smears are fixed while still wet in 95% alcohol or an alcohol–ether mixture. the stain used is a matter of personal preference. Haemotoxylin and eosin, as used for histological staining, is quite adequate, but the Pananicolaou method, though basically an H&E stain, has certain advantages. The eosin is combined with other cytoplasmic stains and applied in alcoholic solution; this increases the transparency of the smear and produces a polychromatic effect which, though not specific, improves the visibility of some malignant cells (Plate 1). Some laboratories 'concentrate' the cells by treating the sputum with a mucolytic agent and making smears from the cell suspension. This method may achieve a more comprehensive sample of the whole specimen but the relationship of malignant cells to each other in a cluster or streak of mucus is often as diagnostically significant as the morphology of individual cells and this evidence is destroyed by the mucolysis.

Usually two or three smears are made from each specimen; these are then methodically screened under the low power for atypical cells. In cytology laboratories this screening is done by trained technicians, who mark any suspicious cells for the attention of the pathologist; each slide takes 5–10 min. Some malignant cells are so numerous that the diagnosis is obvious on the first slide, but in some sputa the malignant cells are so few or poorly preserved that it may be necessary to examine many smears before coming to a conclusion.

There is no general agreement on the method of reporting. Some cytologists will report cells as 'consistent with malignancy' and some all too frequently report 'suspicion of malignancy'. It is my opinion that the pathologist should take responsibility for the diagnosis and report unequivocally. When there is only a suspicion of

---

Plate 1. Sputum; malignant squamous cells. With the Papanicolaou stain, the immature cells stain blue-green, the well differentiated cells stain red and the keratinised cells stain orange. (× 225)

Plate 2. Sputum; degenerate malignant squamous cells. (× 225)

Plate 3. Sputum; small celled (oat cell) carcinoma. Note the absence of cytoplasm and the characteristic mutual moulding of the nuclei. (× 225)

Plate 4. Sputum; well differentiated bronchogenic adenocarcinoma cells. When well differentiated, these cells tend to stay in papillary clusters. (× 225)

Plate 5. Sputum; alveolar cell carcinoma. The cells appear relatively benign and are often present in large numbers, singly and in small clusters. (× 225)

Plate 6. Pleural fluid; very active mesothelial cells. Note the pleomorphism and the mitotic figure. (× 225)

Plate 7. Pleural fluid; metastatic adenocarcinoma originating from a primary in the stomach. The cells have been stained with periodic acid – Schiff reagent (PAS) to demonstrate mucus secretion at one pole of the cell (× 225)

Plate 8. Pleural fluid; mesothelioma. The cells have been stained with PAS reagent to demonstrate the glycogen which appears as semi-circular granules around the nucleus. (× 225)

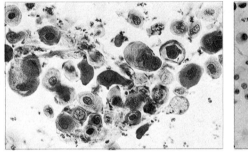

Plate 1

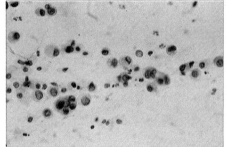

Plate 5

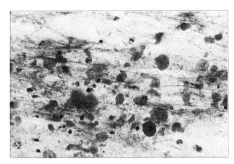

Plate 2

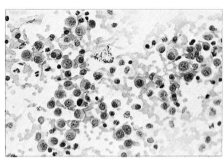

Plate 6

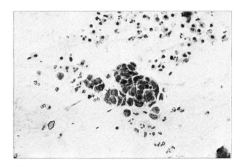

Plate 3

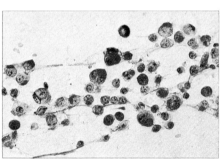

Plate 7

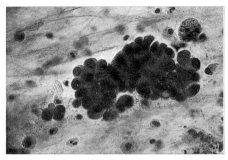

Plate 4

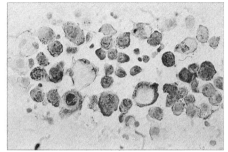

Plate 8

malignancy, no contribution can be made to the diagnosis and the report should be negative. When the cytological diagnosis is 'almost certain' it could be reported as such with a request for further specimens for confirmation. By this means the proportion of 'suspicious' reports can be kept to well below 10% of all positive reports.

Microscopic Appearances

Squamous Cell Carcinomas

Malignant squamous cells are the type most commonly seen. The sputum is usually purulent or mucopurulent and often blood stained. The malignant cells are large and pleomorphic, with abundant cytoplasm which stains polychromatically with the Papanicolaou technique (Plate 1); the keratinised cells stain a bright orange. Even when necrotic, the malignant cells are still identifiable from the bizarre shapes of the ghost cells (Plate 2). The majority of squamous cell carcinomas present no problem in cytological diagnosis but if they are poorly differentiated there may be some difficulty in histological typing. Unfortunately atypical squamous epithelial cells arising in the squamous metaplastic epithelium of the bronchi can closely resemble the malignant cells of a well differentiated carcinoma; these account for most of false-positive reports. The problem is discussed in the section entitled 'False-Positive Reports'. Metastatic squamous cell carcinoma in the lung is so rare that unless there is strong evidence to the contrary, the finding of malignant squamous cells in the sputum is virtual proof of a primary bronchogenic tumour.

Small Cell (Oat Cell) Carcinoma

These cells are not so easily detected in the sputum, as they are little larger than lymphocytes, which they sometimes closely resemble. Fortunately they usually occur in thin or mucoid specimens and, being hyperchromatic, they stand out against the clear background. They often occur in small groups or loose clusters which spread out into streaks when smeared on to a slide. They have little or no cytoplasm so that the nuclei are closely packed and often moulded in such a characteristic way (Plate 3) that they can be identified cytologically with confidence, which is important in practice as the treatment is usually different from that of the other two main histological types. The presence of oat cells in the sputum is proof of a primary bronchogenic carcinoma.

Some of the oat cell carcinomas are composed of rather larger cells which do not exhibit the characteristic moulding and may be difficult to differentiate from the poorly differentiated small cell type of squamous carcinoma. The intermediate type may show some glandular or papillary arrangement of the cells suggestive of a poorly differentiated adenocarcinoma.

Bronchogenic Adenocarcinoma

Adenocarcinoma cells are usually found in mucoid specimens. The cell size and nuclear–cytoplasmic ratio are intermediate between those of the malignant squamous cell and the oat cell. In well differentiated tumours the malignant cells are seen in small groups or clusters showing some organisation suggestive of their epithelial or glandular origin (Plate 4).

A particular variety of adenocarcinoma is the alveolar (or bronchiolar–alveolar) cell carcinoma. Cytologically these tumours are distinguished by the benign appearance of the cells and their presence in very large numbers in the sputum, which is often copious and watery, like saliva. The small round or oval cells resemble alveolar cells and appear singly or in characteristic clusters composed of 10–20 cells (Plate 5). Some of these tumours are composed of cells of more malignant appearance and are then not so easily distinguished from well differentiated bronchial adenocarcinoma.

Large Cell Undifferentiated Bronchial Carcinoma

The frequency with which this histological type is diagnosed in sputum varies considerably among cytologists. It is generally used to describe those undifferentiated malignant cells which appear too large for oat cell carcinoma. It includes those tumours which the histologist classifies as large cell undifferentiated, but will on occasion include a few squamous cell carcinomas and adenocarcinomas which are too poorly differentiated for histological typing in sputum smears (see p. 141).

Metastatic Carcinoma

Metastatic tumours tend to be in the lung parenchyma and only ulcerate at a late stage into the bronchial lumen; the exfoliation of malignant cells into the sputum is likely to occur later in the history of the lesion than is the case with a primary in the bronchus. The yield of positive sputa will therefore be lower at the time of the first investigation. Yields of 50% or less are the usual experience (Koss et al. 1964). When ulceration does eventually occur, the numerous necrotic cells in the sputum may alert the cytologist to the possibility of a metastatic lesion. The majority of metastatic tumours are adenocarcinomas; they are rarely distinguishable morphologically from bronchogenic adenocarcinomas. Although many bronchogenic adenocarcinomas have a fairly distinct morphology which the cytologist recognises by experience, there are no unequivocal features. However, if the laboratory is informed of a clinical suspicion of metastatic tumour, it is often possible for the cytologist to report the malignant cells as 'consistent with metastatic tumour', especially if some rather atypical morphology is encountered.

Other Tumours

Rarely giant cell tumour of the lung, lymphomas and sarcomas of various types can be diagnosed by sputum examination. Adenoid cystic carcinomas, carcinoids and bronchial adenomas do not exfoliate naturally, but have occasionally been diagnosed by brushings or aspirations taken at bronchoscopy. Squamous cell papilloma of the bronchus sheds large numbers of benign squamous cells into the bronchial secretion and can occasionally be diagnosed by cytology.

Non-malignant Conditions

In the course of examining the sputum for malignant cells, the cytologist may find evidence of asbestosis, asthma, pulmonary infarction, and herpetic, cytomegalic and other viral infections; among organisms that can be seen are *Aspergillus, Monilia, Pneumocystis carinii,* and *Strongyloides stercoralis.*

False-Positive Reports

The morphology of atypical benign cells can be deceptive, resulting occasionally in the reporting of malignant cells in the sputum of patients who do not have cancer. These are the true false-positives, but only intensive investigation and the passage of time will establish the fact that a mistake has been made in cytological interpretation.

When a positive report is not corroborated by the clinical evidence, a check should be made to exclude the possibility of errors in identification of the specimen or possible contamination in the laboratory. If necessary, further specimens should be examined.

The cytologist should be advised of the situation and asked to review the slide; a more critical evaluation may result in an amended report. Atypical bronchial epithelial cells under certain inflammatory conditions can resemble well differentiated adenocarcinoma cells; degenerate cells in which only the nuclei remain can be mistaken for small cell carcinoma. Such mistakes are rare compared with the difficulties in interpretation of atypical squamous cells, which come into a different category.

Auerbach et al. (1961) showed that squamous metaplasia, dysplasia and carcinoma in situ were present in the bronchial epithelium of a high proportion of smokers and there is evidence that squamous cell carcinoma develops from these atypical epithelia (Raeburn and Spencer 1953). Fortunately for the cytologist, atypical squamous cells from these lesions are not seen as frequently as the incidence of the epithelial changes might lead one to expect — presumably because there is little exfoliation at this stage in the development of carcinoma. Later, when the lesion becomes invasive, there is a marked increase in cell exfoliation due to a loss of cohesion which is one of the characteristic features of malignancy.

The atypical squamous cells from a pre-invasive lesion are not always distinguishable from malignant cells of a well differentiated carcinoma and account for most of the 'false-positive' reports (Fig. 1).

If after review the presence of malignant cells is confirmed by the cytologist, every effort should be made to locate the lesion; there is a good chance that it will be resectable. If no lesion can be found and the cells are of the squamous type, it must be assumed that a carcinoma in situ is present. Sometimes a blind biopsy will demonstrate this. A regular follow-up of the patient is essential as an invasive lesion may develop several years later (Melamed et al. 1963; Canti 1966).

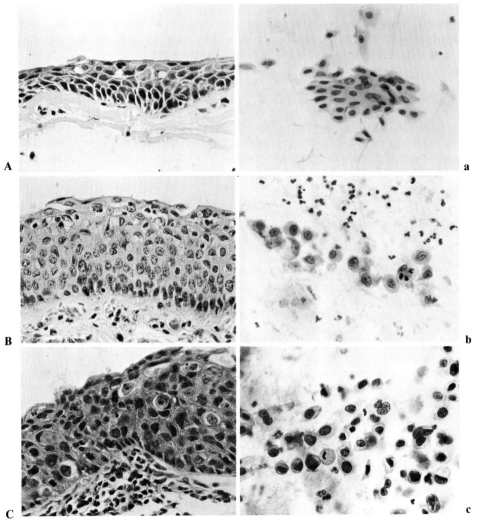

Fig. 1. Stages in the development of squamous cell carcinoma of the bronchus, with corresponding exfoliated cells. (In every case magnification is × 520.)
A Squamous metaplasia of bronchial epithelium. **a** Metaplastic squamous epithelial cells in sputum. Small cells with bland nuclei are seen.
B Dysplasia in metaplastic squamous epithelium. **b** Atypical metaplastic cells, showing a slightly raised nuclear–cytoplasmic ratio and some chromatin clumping. The cells are slightly suggestive of malignancy.
C Carcinoma in situ of the bronchus. **c** Malignant squamous cells showing raised nuclear–cytoplasmic ratio, hyperchromasia and pleomorphism. Morphologically the cells are indistinguishable from those of an invasive tumour.

It follows from this that if sputum cytology is to fulfil its life-saving role in identifying early occult carcinomas, an occasional false-positive report is almost unavoidable but the risk of an unnecessary lobectomy or thoracotomy is minimal as

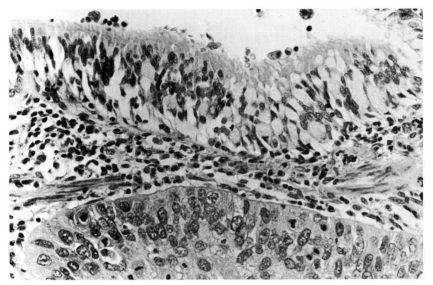

Fig. 2. Invasive squamous cell carcinoma covered by intact bronchial epithelium (× 320). The tumour was visible bronchoscopically, but the sputum was negative.

no operation is likely to be undertaken until the lesion has been located. While every effort must made to pick up the early case, it is desirable to keep the false-positive rate below 1% of positive reports, otherwise confidence in the method will be lost.

The laboratory should be informed of any clinical aspects of the case which might be responsible for the production of atypical cells, e.g. recent bronchoscopy, radiotherapy, cytotoxic drugs, suspect viral infection or chronic inflammatory disease, particularly tuberculosis.

False-Negative Reports

To the cytologist a false-negative implies that malignant cells were present in the sputum, but missed on screening. Experience of re-examining subsequently diagnosed cases suggests that this happens only rarely. The majority of false-negatives are undoubtedly due to failure of the patient to produce an adequate specimen of sputum or lack of laboratory capacity to examine a sufficient number of specimens. As already mentioned, where unlimited facility exists, usually under research conditions, a number of workers have been able to report malignant cells in the sputum in up to 90% of cases of lung cancer. There appears to be a residuum of about 10% of patients with lung cancer whose sputum remains negative however many specimens are examined. This is due in some cases to small peripheral lesions with little or no open connection with the main bronchial tree. In some large central growths the bronchus is occluded either by the tumour or by enlarged peri-bronchial lymph nodes. Even some bronchoscopically visible tumours do not yield a positive sputum, either because the exfoliated cells are too necrotic for identification or because the carcinoma remains covered by intact bronchial epithelium (Fig. 2).

Bronchoscopy

Since the introduction of the fibreoptic bronchoscope (Hattori et al. 1964), it is probably more economic to proceed to bronchoscopy after the first three or four specimens of sputum have failed to produce a diagnosis.

Even if tumour is visible, a biopsy is not always successful either because it does not contain tumour or because it is too small or damaged for interpretation. Cytological preparations may be more successful and should always be taken in addition to biopsy. There is no general agreement as to whether brushings, aspirations or washings give the best yield; it seems to depend much on the site of the lesion and the skill of the operator.

Owing to drying or distortion of the cells or poor display due to interference by blood or fibrin clot, malignant cells are not so easily identified as in sputum and it is also more difficult to differentiate the various histological types.

Fine Needle Aspiration

The presence of an enlarged lymph node in a patient suspected of carcinoma provides an opportunity for a rapid diagnosis by fine needle aspiration; the technique is simple and can be performed at the time of the first consultation. If the result is negative or inconclusive little time and effort will have been wasted; if positive, the patient will have been spared the inconvenience and possibly the discomfort of some more invasive investigation.

Failure to obtain a positive result is rarely due to any difficulty in identifying the malignant cells; it is more likely to be due to failure to extract the cells from a hard fibrous node. Successful aspiration depends very much on using the correct technique.

A 10-ml syringe fitted with a 21 gauge needle (venepuncture size) is all the apparatus required; some 3.8% sodium citrate solution should be at hand for immediate use. A special handle attachment to the syringe has been designed to facilitate the maintenance of negative pressure during aspiration, but this is somewhat cumbersome and may not be available. The position of the withdrawn piston can be maintained by exerting pressure on the flange of the barrel with the thumb, but this is quite a strain on the hand and liable to result in in a rather hurried and inaccurate aspiration. It is better if some form of wedge of the right length can be inserted between the flange of the barrel and the head of the piston so as to prevent retraction. The author uses the thicker half of a needle casing cut across accurately (otherwise it will slide out). This can be placed in position by an assistant or, better still, hinged to the head of the piston with Sellotape; the wedge can then be swung into position with the forefinger.

The correct sequence of manoeuvres is important. The node is first located and steadied between the fingers and transfixed with the point of the needle; no anaesthetic is required. The piston is withdrawn to about 4-ml (giving about 1 atm negative pressure) and wedged as described; this will necessitate having both hands on the syringe for a short while. Then with one hand palpating the tumour and the other hand now grasping the lower end of the syringe, the needle can be accurately relocated. There is no need to hurry at this stage as the patient is unlikely to experience pain once the skin has been pierced. The needle should then be moved back and forth several times as though making punch biopsies. Before withdrawing, the piston must be released. The syringe is then detatched from the needle, recharged with air, and the contents of the needle gently transferred on to slides. Smears should be fixed in alcohol or spray fixed before drying has occurred. Some pathologists may prefer air-dried smears for Romanowski staining and at least one air-dried smear should always be made if lymphoma is suspected. If there is sufficient material for only one smear, it is often possible to obtain enough for a second smear by recharging the syringe with air and forcibly expelling it through the needle. If little or no visible material is obtained, a few millilitres of 3.8% sodium citrate solution should be drawn up and taken to the laboratory in the syringe. In the unfortunate event of blood appearing in the syringe, there will be little time to make smears as clotting will be rapid owing to rupture of platelets and admixture with tissue juice. To give the laboratory the best chance of finding any malignant cells which may be present in the blood, the syringe should be filled with 3.8% sodium citrate solution as quickly as possible and despatched to the laboratory without delay. Sometimes the aspirated material is tightly wedged in the needle and comes out with a splash when forcibly expelled. It is a wise precaution to have several slides laid out in apposition to avoid losing any of the specimen.

In a small proportion of cases, when other methods have failed to obtain a histological diagnosis, it may be necessary to aspirate the lesion directly through the chest wall.

Pleural Effusion

Malignant disease in the chest is frequently accompanied by pleural effusion. This is not necessarily caused directly by metastatic deposits in the pleural membrane; circulatory or lymphatic obstruction or inflammatory disease in the lung distal to a bronchial carcinoma may be the immediate cause of the effusion. When pleural metastases are present, the fluid usually contains malignant cells, but occasionally pleural metastases can be demonstrated histologically by biopsy or at post-mortem in cases in which no malignant cells were found in the fluid. This could be due to the problem of identifying malignant cells, but the possibility of negative fluid with a positive pleural biopsy is supported by the observation that the pleural deposits are often covered by a dense layer of fibrous tissue. Conversely, malignant cells are sometimes seen in the fluid when no pleural metastases can be demonstrated. The absence of pleural involvement is equally difficult to prove owing to the impracticability of sectioning the whole of the pleural membrane.

Only about 50% of cases of malignant disease in the chest contain malignant cells in the fluid. A negative report therefore does not exclude malignant disease, but a positive report establishes the diagnosis of malignancy and may also contribute information regarding the histological type of the tumour and the probable site of the primary. In many cases there is a history of a primary carcinoma outside the chest, most commonly in the breast; it is then usually possible for the cytologist to confirm that the morphology of the cells in the fluid is consistent with the known primary.

Collection of Specimen

A high proportion of pleural fluids will clot within a few hours; it is not possible to predict which fluids will eventually clot, but blood-stained specimens from a traumatic tap usually clot within a few minutes. Reliable cytological preparations cannot be made from the centrifuge deposit of fluids containing clots; it is therefore essential that anticoagulant is added immediately to all specimens on aspiration. About one-third by volume of 3.8% sodium citrate solution will prevent clotting in most cases, but will not arrest clotting once it has started. If the fluid is blood stained or clots are already present, heparin at the rate of 1000 units per 10 ml of fluid will prevent any further clotting. The possibility of clotting can be further reduced by collecting the specimen directly into anticoagulant in the container. The quantities used are not critical.

In many effusions the malignant cells are so abundant that a few millilitres of fluid is sufficient, but some effusions contain only an occasional malignant cell and a larger quantity of fluid is required for their detection. It is also sometimes necessary to make several preparations for special staining techniques. The quantity of fluid sent to the laboratories should therefore be generous: at least 50 ml is preferred.

Immediate despatch to the laboratory is desirable though not as essential as some publications suggest. Provided clotting has not occurred, the majority of fluids do not deteriorate within 24 hours.

Laboratory Technique

The fluid is centrifuged and smears made from the deposit; some are fixed in alcohol for Papanicolaou and other special staining techniques, and some are air dried for Romanowski type staining, especially if a lymphoma is suspected. Very small samples (which are sometimes unavoidable) can be centrifuged directly onto slides in the cytocentrifuge. Clotted samples can be treated with enzymes to extract the cells, but the results are not very satisfactory unless the malignant cells are present in large numbers. Heavily blood-stained specimens can be treated by a variety of methods to reduce the red cell content and concentrate the malignant cells.

Microscopic Appearances

The pleural membrane is normally covered by a single layer of mesothelial cells. These are large flat polygonal cells which are easily identified in scrapings of the pleura owing to their uniform appearance and tendency to remain in monolayered sheets. When an effusion is present these cells desquamate into the fluid and become rounded-up, but their morphology usually remains distinctive. Under certain conditions, however, the mesothelial cells proliferate and the detached cells multiply in the fluid, which is an excellent culture medium. Mitotic activity and clustering may be present and, in addition, many of the cells show degenerative changes due to ageing. The result is a wide variety of morphological features which may be difficult to distinguish from malignancy (Plate 6). Lymphocytes most commonly accompany the mesothelial cells but polymorphs, histiocytes, lympho-plasmacytoid cells and eosinophils may be present according to the degree and nature of the inflammatory reaction.

Malignant cells, like mesothelial cells, can develop an independent existence in the fluid and grow as in tissue culture. Under these conditions morphological features such as, for example, the columnar shape of adenocarcinoma cells, are lost and the more benign looking, well differentiated malignant cells come to resemble mesothelial cells.

Radiotherapy and treatment with cytotoxic drugs can cause morphological changes in mesothelial cells which may be mistaken for malignancy. This most frequently occurs in cases of breast carcinoma which have been treated by radiotherapy; the mesothelium inevitably receives a fairly heavy dose of radiation, which may produce morphological changes for many years after the cessation of treatment. The cytologist should therefore always be informed of any past therapy.

Considerable experience is therefore needed to avoid erroneous diagnosis and to identify some of the less conspicuous malignant cells. However, with adequate specimens and good preparations the majority of fluids present no problem (Spriggs 1972).

Although squamous cell carcinoma is the commonest form of lung cancer, malignant squamous cells are rarely seen in pleural effusions; this must be due either to the behaviour of the tumour or to the inability of malignant squamous cells to survive in serous fluid.

The majority of the positive fluids contain adenocarcinoma cells and the majority of these originate from a primary outside the chest (Plate 7). Only occasionally is the morphology or histochemical staining sufficiently specific to enable the cytologist to identify the primary site.

The one type of malignant cell in pleural effusions which can be confidently identified as of bronchial origin is that of the small cell (oat cell) carcinoma. These small hyperchromatic cells retain their characteristic morphology in fluids; cells from some of the embryonic tumours have a rather similar appearance, but confusion is unlikely to occur owing to the different age group and clinical histories of the patients.

Occasionally patients with a lymphoma present clinically with a pleural effusion. Initially the case may be suspected as being carcinoma of the bronchus, but examination of the pleural fluid will reveal numerous atypical lymphocytes, blast cells or other abnormal cells indicating the presence of a lymphoma.

The cytological diagnosis of mesothelioma is particularly difficult. In some cases, especially when there is a sarcomatous element, there may be no mesothelial cells present in the fluid and cytological investigation therefore cannot contribute to the diagnosis. In the more benign well differentiated mesotheliomas, the fluid contains numerous mesothelial cells, showing perhaps increased activity but no evidence of malignancy. The cytological picture does not differ from that seen in reactive mesothelial proliferation, but the presence of a pure mesothelial cell population and the absence of inflammatory cells may arouse suspicion of neoplasia. Pleural biopsy is not always conclusive, but the persistent recurrence of the effusion showing the same cytological picture over a period of weeks or months may eventually lead to the conclusion that there is no alternative diagnosis. More typically the fluid will contain numerous very active mesothelial cells, some of which show malignant changes; the diagnosis of this type is relatively simple. The poorly differentiated mesotheliomas produce cells of undoubted malignancy, but there may be difficulty in distinguishing them from adenocarcinoma cells. The demonstration of glycogen granules in these cells is fairly conclusive evidence of their mesothelial origin (Plate 8) as these granules are frequently seen in mesothelial cells, but are rarely present in adenocarcinoma cells.

References

Auerbach O, Stout AP, Hammond EC, Garfinkel L (1961) Changes in bronchial epithelium in relation to cigarette smoking and in relation to lung cancer. N Engl J Med 265:253–267

Barret NR (1938) Examination of the sputum for malignant cells and particles of malignant growth. J Thorac Surg 8:169–183

Beale LS (1860) Examination of sputum from a case of cancer of the pharynx and the adjacent parts. Arch Med 2:44

Boddington MM, Spriggs AI (1965) Cytological diagnosis of cancer: its uses and limitations. Br Med J I:1523–1528

Canti G (1966) Carcinoma-in-situ of the bronchus. Some aspects of carcinoma of the bronchus. A symposium. Teare D, Fenning J (eds) 41–50 King Edward VII Hospital, Midhurst, England

Donné A (1845) Cours de microscopie complémentaire des etudes medicales. Bailliére et fils, Paris

Dudgeon LS, Patrick CV (1927) A new method for the rapid microscopical diagnosis of tumours with account of 200 cases so examined. Br J Surg 15:250–261

Dudgeon LS, Wrigley CH (1935) On the demonstration of particles of malignant growth in the sputum by means of the wet film method. J Laryngol Otol 50:752–763

Farber SM, Benioff MA, Frost JK, Rosenthal M, Tobias G (1948) Cytological studies of sputum and bronchial secretions in primary carcinoma of the lung. Dis Chest 14: 633–664

Gloyne SR (1937) The cytology of sputum. Tubercle 18:292–297

Gowar FJS (1943) Carcinoma of the lung: the value of sputum examination in diagnosis. Br J Surg 39:193–200

Grunze H (1960) A critical review and evaluation of cytodiagnosis in chest diseases. Acta Cytol IV:175–198

Grzybowski S, Coy P (1970) Early diagnosis of carcinoma of the lung. Simultaneous screening with chest X-ray and sputum cytology. Cancer 25:113–120

Hampeln P (1887) Über einen Fall von primären Lungen-Pleura-Carcinom. St Petersburger Med Wochenschr 17:137–139

Hattori S, Matsuda M, Nishihara H, Horai T (1964) Early diagnosis of small peripheral lung cancer: brushing method under X-ray television fluoroscopy. Dis Chest 45:129–142

Koss LG, Melamed MR, Goodner JT (1964) Pulmonary cytology — a brief survey of diagnostic results for July 1st 1952 until Dec. 31st 1960. Acta Cytol 8:104–113

Laurie W, Szaloky LG (1971) Sputum cytology in the diagnosis of bronchial carcinoma. Med J Aust 1:247–251

Lücke A, Klebs E (1867) Beitrag zur Ovariotomie und zur Kenntnis der Abdominalgeschwülste. Arch Pathol Anat 41:1–14

McDonald JC, Liddell FDK, Gibbs GW, Eyssen GE, McDonald AD (1980) Dust exposure and mortality in crysotile mining 1910-1975. Br J Ind Med 37:11–24

Melamed MR, Koss LG, Clifton EE (1963) Roentgenologically occult lung cancer diagnosed by cytology: report of 12 cases. Cancer 16:1537–1551

Müller J (1838) Über den feineren Bau und die Formen der krankhaften Geschwülste. Reimers, Berlin

Oswald NC, Hinson KFW, Canti G, Miller AB (1971) The diagnosis of primary lung cancer with special reference to sputum cytology. Thorax 26:623–631

Papanicolaou GN, Traut HF (1943) Diagnosis of uterine cancer by the vaginal smear. Commonwealth Fund, New York

Philps FR (1954) The identification of carcinoma cells in sputum. Br J Cancer 8:67–96

Raeburn C, Spencer H (1953) A study of the origin and development of lung cancer. Thorax 8:1–10

Rome DS, Olson KB (1961) A direct comparison of natural and aerosol produced sputum collected from 776 asymptomatic men. Acta Cytol 5:173–176

Royal College of Physicians of London (1971) Smoking and health now. Pitman Medical, London

Russell WO, Neidhardt HW, Mountain CF, Griffith KM, Chang JP (1963) Cytodiagnosis of lung cancer: a report on a four-year laboratory clinical and statistical study with a review of the literature on lung cancer and pulmonary cytology. Acta Cytol 7:1–44

Saccomanno G, Saunders RP, Archer VE, Auerbach O, Kuschner M, Beckler PA (1965) Cancer of the lung: the cytology of sputum prior to the development of carcinoma. Acta Cytol 9:413–423

Schwann T (1839) Mikroskopische Untersuchungen über die Übereinstimmung in der Struktur und dem Wachstum der Tiere und Pflanzen. GD Reiner, Berlin.

Spriggs AI (1972) The cytology of effusion in the pleural, pericardial and peritoneal cavities, 2nd edn. Heinemann, London

Taylor WF, Fontana RS, Uhlenhopp MA, Davis CS (1981) Some results of screening for early lung cancer. Cancer 47[Suppl]:1114–1120

Walshe WH (1846) On the nature and treatment of cancer. Taylor and Walton, London

Wandall HH (1944) A study on neoplastic cells in sputum. Acta Chir Scand 91[Suppl]:1–143

Chapter 6

Percutaneous Needle Biopsy of Pulmonary Tumours

Robert Dick and Benjamin Timmis

Percutaneous transpleural needle biopsy of the lung (PTNB) is not a new procedure. It has been practised over many years since its introduction in the last century by Leyden, who aspirated organisms causing a pneumonia (Leyden 1883) and then by Menetrier, who 3 years later diagnosed a bronchial carcinoma by needle aspiration (Menetrier 1886). Since that time, several large series have been reported, using either an aspirating or a cutting technique (Lauby et al. 1965; Dahlgren and Lind 1969; Allison and Hemingway 1981; Gallo Curcio et al. 1983). Until recent years, PTNB has not been as popular a procedure in the United Kingdom as in the United States and Scandanavia because of its complications. However, with the advent of aspiration biopsy using relatively narrow gauge needles, the procedure has become safer and now has a secure place in the diagnosis of isolated pulmonary lesions, many of which will be neoplastic.

The discovery of a pulmonary lesion on the chest radiograph demands a precise and rapid diagnosis in view of the ever-present risk of malignancy. Small peripheral asymptomatic bronchial carcinomas (Fig. 1) have the best prognosis (Buell 1971; Steel and Buell 1973) and early diagnosis is clearly important. Two large studies (Good and Wilson 1958; Good 1963) have stated that the incidence of a solitary pulmonary lesion on the chest radiograph is about 0.1%. The nature of such a solitary lesion will vary with ethnic and geographical background, age, industrial exposure and smoking habits of the subjects radiographed. Of all solitary mass lesions seen on a chest radiograph in patients over 50 years of age, 30%–50% will be carcinomas, whilst the risk falls almost to zero in those under 40 years (Trunk et al. 1974; Higgins et al. 1975). Granulomas and localised areas of infection account for the majority of the non-malignant cases (Sinner 1982).

Once the chest radiograph or fluoroscopy has established the presence of a solitary pulmonary lesion, it may be further delineated by tomography, either simple or computed (CT). The diagnostic pathway now includes sputum cytology, bronchoscopy, bronchial lavage, PTNB and thoracotomy. Exfoliative cytology of the sputum is only applicable to those tumours which shed cells and are connected to bronchi (Grubb, personal communication). Since the common location for adeno-carcinomas and metastases is peripheral, they are less likely to shed cells into the bronchi for ultimate retrieval from sputum. Both PTNB and open thoracotomy of such lesions will give a higher diagnostic yield than either exfoliative cytology or bronchoscopy (Sargent et al. 1974; Walls et al. 1974). PTNB is a preferable diagnostic procedure to thoracotomy, since it is quick, performed under local anaesthetic, and relatively simple and safe. Furthermore, the patient need remain in

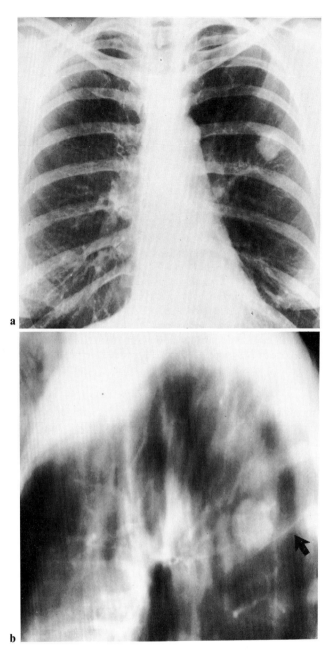

Fig. 1a,b. 64-year-old female, asymptomatic. **a** PA chest X-ray. **b** Lateral tomogram showing lesion of left upper lobe just above the posterior end of the oblique fissure (*arrowed*). Biopsy: squamous carcinoma.

hospital only 6 h after the biopsy, and, barring implications, can sometimes avoid an overnight stay.

Depending upon the site of the isolated pulmonary lesion on the chest radiograph, patients fall broadly into three groups. For those with hilar masses, fibre-optic bronchoscopy and biopsy is preferred (Smiddy et al. 1971). For peripheral masses with negative sputum, PTNB is the initial investigation (Dick et al. 1974). In the third group of those with masses which are adjacent to yet not contiguous with the hilum, we employ a combined approach, starting with fibre-optic bronchoscopy and proceeding to PTNB at the same session if the lesion is not visualised via the bronchoscope (Johnson et al. 1979).

Indications and Contra-indications

There are a number of *indications* for PTNB:

1. The investigation of a mass lesion demonstrated on the chest radiograph, especially where it is peripherally situated and where sputum culture/cytology and bronchoscopy (if indicated) have failed to furnish a diagnosis (Fig. 2).
2. The investigation of a mass lesion demonstrated on the chest radiograph in a patient known to be suffering from malignancy. Biopsy will establish whether or not the new lesion represents a metastasis or other pathology (Fig. 3). Resection of a solitary pulmonary metastasis may significantly improve the patient's prognosis.
3. The investigation of an unresolved pneumonic consolidation, where the nature of the underlying cause (infective or non-infective) remains unknown despite other diagnostic tests (Fig. 4). Sometimes direct retrieval of an offending organism is obtained, allowing specific chemotherapy to be utilised.
4. Any other persistent localised lung lesion that cannot be diagnosed by other methods (Fig. 5).
5. Pleural masses sometimes associated with rib destruction (Fig. 6), though often without (Fig. 7).

Contra-indications to PTNB are few, and include:

1. Bleeding diatheses, including patients on anticoagulant therapy. In practice, a fine gauge (21,22) needle can be safely employed in this group.
2. Suspected vascular lesions, such as an aneurysm or arteriovenous malformation.
3. Suspected echinococcus cyst; dissemination of hydatids may occur following needle puncture, and severe anaphylaxis result.

The following are *theoretical contra-indications*, and provided small gauge needles are used and complications dealt with immediately, many in the following group can safely be biopsied:

4. Severe pulmonary hypertension, which increases the risk of post-biopsy haemorrhage.
5. Previous pneumonectomy on the contralateral side of the chest.
6. Severe pulmonary emphysema where lung function tests indicate that even a small pneumothorax would seriously impair the patient's respiratory reserve.
7. The inability of the patient to co-operate with procedure, or his or her refusal to undergo definitive treatment irrespective of the biopsy result.

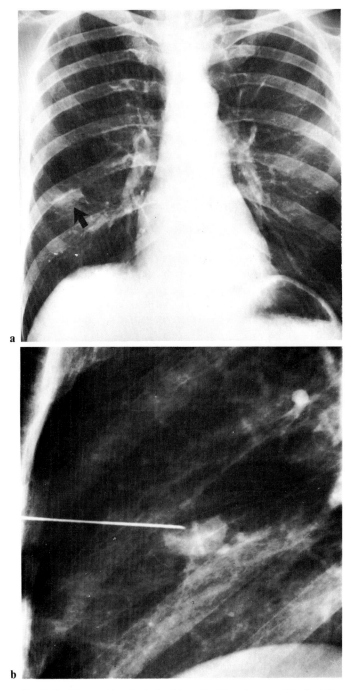

a

b

Fig. 2a,b. 55-year-old male clerk with cerebral lymphoma. **a** PA chest X-ray showing small lesion in the right middle lobe (*arrowed*). **b** Lesion transfixed by aspiration biopsy. Cytology: granuloma.

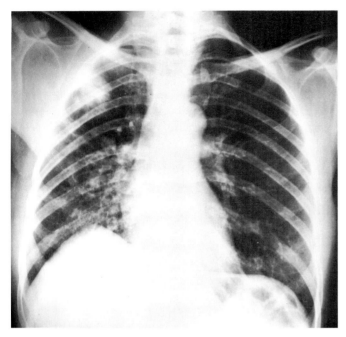

Fig. 3. 52-year-old Iraqi, with right mastectomy followed by radiation. PA chest X-ray showing a discrete shadow in the right upper lobe. Biopsy: radiation pneumonitis; no malignancy.

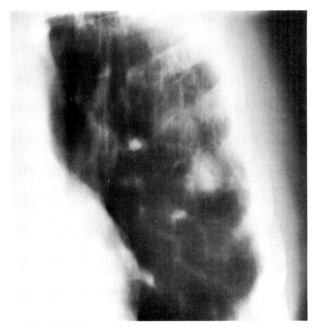

Fig. 4. 57-year-old male with previous radiotherapy of right Pancoast tumour. Shadowing appeared anteriorly in the left lingula. Biopsy: chronic inflammatory tissue.

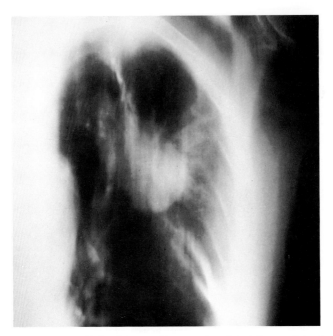

Fig. 5. 72-year-old Greek lawyer. Tomography of the left upper lobe shows an irregular mass and also pleural calcification from known TB pleurisy. Biopsy of mass: squamous cell carcinoma.

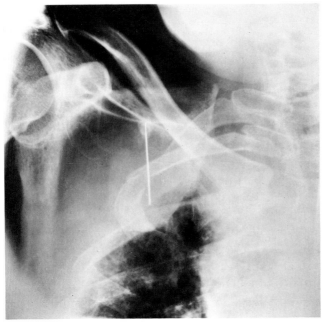

Fig. 6. 50-year-old company director. Peripheral mass destroying right second rib. Biopsy: undifferentiated carcinoma.

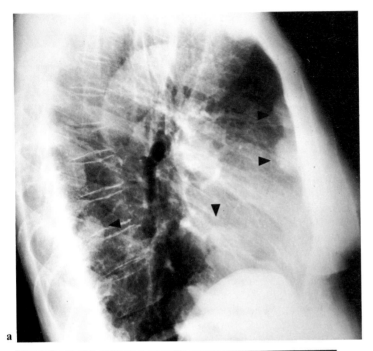

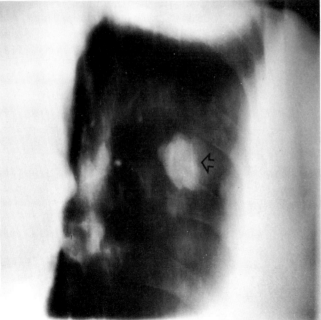

Fig. 7a,b. 58-year-old female with previous removal of malignant mediastinal thymoma. **a** Lateral chest X-ray showing multiple pleural masses over the anterior, posterior and inferior surfaces of both pleural cavities (*arrowheads*). **b** Tomography of right chest anteriorly demonstrating lobulated pleural mass between the anterior ribs (*arrowed*). Biopsy: malignant thymoma.

Technique of Percutaneous Transpleural Needle Biopsy

An explanation of the procedure is given to the patient in the ward or clinic, and informed consent obtained. Even though vomiting is never a complication, it is prudent to have a 4-h fast, and blood coagulation studies are done. If there are doubts about respiratory reserve, formal assessment should be undertaken during the week before the procedure. Certainly the patient requires to be capable of lying flat on an X-ray table for 10–15 min, without distressing dyspnoea.

When the patient has reached the screening table, 10–20 mg Diazemuls (emulsified diazepam; Kabivitrum Ltd, United Kingdom) is given intravenously. During the procedure, small increments of diazepam may be added if the patient remains anxious, though some confident patients will reject all sedation yet find the procedure perfectly acceptable. It is always important to ensure that the patient is able to co-operate with the procedure throughout; thus oversedation is to be avoided.

Examination of the pulmonary lesion on the PA and lateral chest radiograph and during AP and lateral fluoroscopic screening must be undertaken most carefully, for selecting the approach and the subsequent accuracy of the biopsy depend on this. A radiograph should be taken *on the day of the aspiration biopsy* prior to the procedure, to ensure that a lesion has not altered (or cleared) since the X-ray performed days or weeks before. We routinely employ a 'C' arm image intensifier (Fig. 8), finding this more convenient than simultaneous 'bi-plane' screening. Though possible, it is less precise to perform the biopsy with single-plane screening. Under fluoroscopy, the lesion is first located in both the PA and lateral fields. A small lesion in a large patient may be difficult to visualise on lateral screening, and recourse to previously obtained lateral tomograms may be necessary to help find it (Fig. 9). If the lesion cannot be seen at all on lateral screening, the procedure is abandoned, there being no place for a 'blind biopsy' following a calculated guess as to where the lesion may be. Usually, with careful screening, lesions as small as 1.5 cm can be identified.

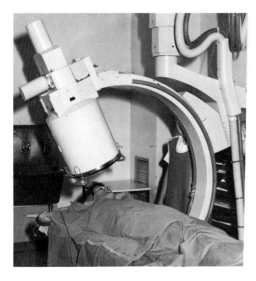

Fig. 8. Patient on table prior to biopsy. The equipment, including the 'C' arm, is demonstrated.

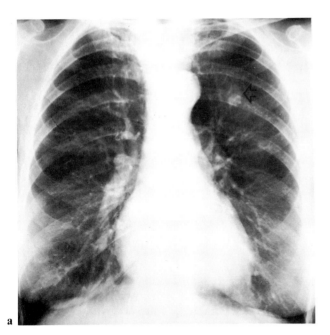

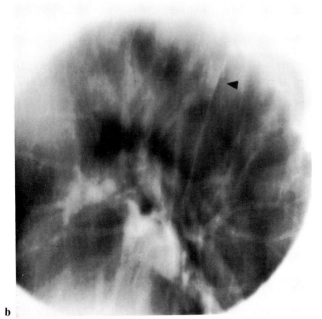

Fig. 9a,b. 68-year-old female admitted for routine operation. **a** PA chest showing small 1.5-cm lesion in the left upper lobe (*arrowed*). **b** Lateral tomogram showing lesion anterior to the oblique fissure (*arrowhead*). The lesion could not be seen on routine lateral chest film. Biopsy: undifferentiated carcinoma.

Once the lesion is seen during screening, an assessment is made as to the most direct approach. One usually chooses the shortest route, placing the patient into a prone, supine or oblique position. For example, if a lesion is situated in the apical segment of the lower lobe, the approach is from the rear, rather than a longer anterior approach which would pass through large vessels in or adjacent to the right hilum. When choosing the skin site, it is important to (a) adjust the image intensifier so that the lesion lies in the middle of the field, otherwise errors of positioning due to parallax will arise, and (b) to position the patient so that an approach will be supracostal, not infracostal, which may injure the neurovascular bundle.

Aspiration biopsy is performed with a strict aseptic technique. A skin marker having been placed on the precisely localised site of entry to the thorax, the marker is pressed into the skin to leave an imprint, quickly removed, and the skin cleaned and draped with sterile towels. The skin at the marker site is infiltrated down to the pleura with 5 ml 1% lignocaine; the position is checked on the screen (Fig. 10) and a 2-mm skin incision made to facilitate insertion of the aspirating needle. We are currently using a 15 cm long 20 s.w. gauge screw biopsy needle (Surgimed, A/S Denmark) (Fig. 11). It is advanced vertically towards the lesion in the AP plane (Fig. 12). The 'C' arm image intensifier is now positioned for lateral screening, and the needle advanced during lateral screening (Fig. 13). During insertion through the pleura, the patient is asked to hold his or her breath temporarily. Apart from this, the biopsy proceeds during quiet respiration. Excessive inspirations and expirations are to be avoided, and no patient can remain apnoeic for the few minutes the actual biopsy requires.

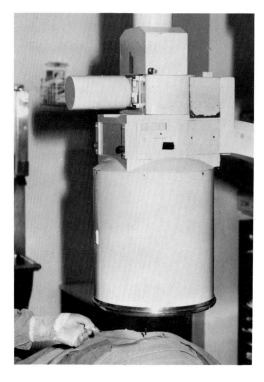

Fig. 10. Local anaesthesia has been injected into the chest wall over the lesion to be biopsied. Accurate position is checked by X-ray screening.

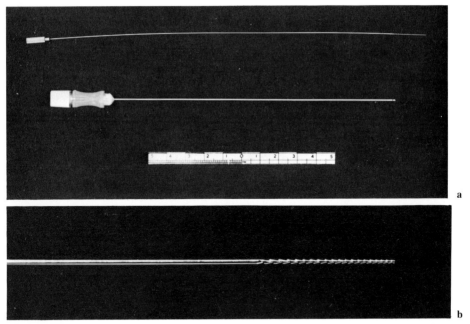

Fig. 11. a The needle and stylet used for aspiration biopsy. **b** Close-up view of spiralled tip of replacement stylet.

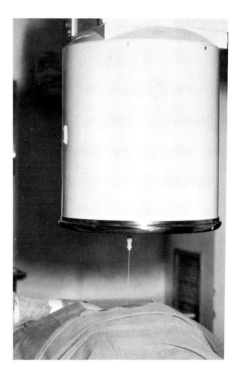

Fig. 12. Biopsy needle inserted; AP screening.

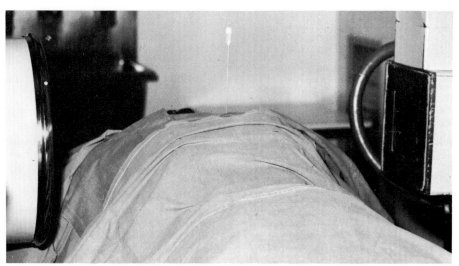

Fig. 13. Biopsy needle inserted; position checked during lateral screening.

Whilst the needle is gently advanced during lateral screening, its hub may be gripped with a pair of horizontally held forceps, so as to minimise radiation exposure to the operator's hands. Usually, however, the radiographer can 'cone' tightly on to the lesion, unless it is very superficial. When the needle tip reaches the pulmonary mass a slight resistance is commonly felt and screening may reveal slight movement of the lesion as it is 'nudged' by the needle tip. A small, firm, well defined lesion may slide to one side when the needle tip reaches its surface. If this occurs a rapid thrust of the needle usually transfixes it. Quiet respiratory movement should now show the lesion and needle tip to be moving together.

The central stylet is now removed, and replaced with a slightly longer one with a spiralled tip which is gently screwed into the lesion to loosen cells. It is withdrawn, and any material trapped in the thread of the 'corkscrew' smeared directly on to a slide. A 20-ml syringe and two-way tap are next attached to the hub of the aspirating needle. Strong aspiration is initiated, and cells already loosened by the screw should enter the aspirating needle and may reach the tap. Excessive aspiration should be avoided, as should further advancement of needle and syringe, since both of these manoeuvres can result in a bloody aspirate entering the syringe, with 'swamping' of vital cells. Before removing the needle, tap and syringe as an entity, the tap is turned off, so that material remains in the syringe: in this way, aspiration of chest wall tissue into the needle during its removal is avoided.

If aspiration is unproductive, a second aspiration is performed and invariably supplies representative material. Should air from a bronchus or blood from a vessel be aspirated, then the needle tip is introduced to an adjacent area and aspiration repeated. Material finally obtained is injected on to a slide (Fig. 14) and then spread over it using the aspirating needle shaft (Fig. 15). It should be fixed immediately to avoid 'air-drying'. The presence of a cytologist in the screening room to advise quickly on the adequacy of the specimen is invaluable, a cellular specimen being quickly recognised (Fig. 16). Occasionally necrotic material or pus is aspirated and sent for microbiology in addition to cytology (see p. 71).

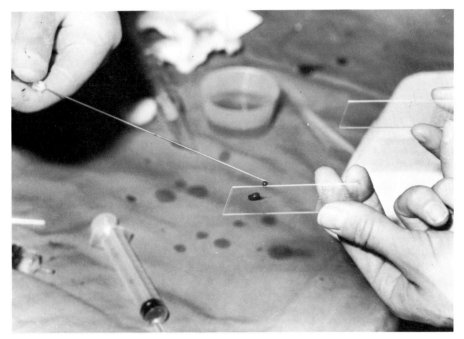

Fig. 14. Drop of aspirated material being injected onto slide.

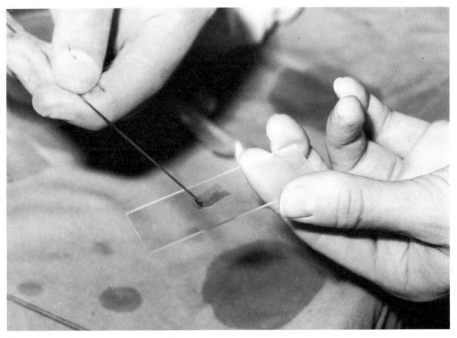

Fig. 15. Smearing of material over slide surface.

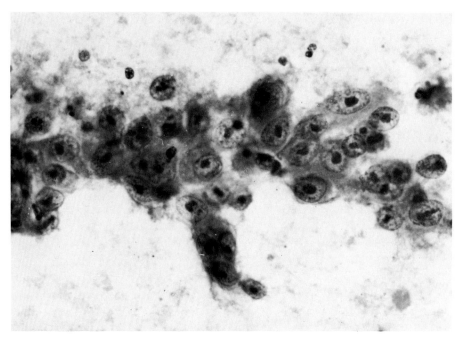

Fig. 16. Aspiration cytology of a lung mass showing a sheet of non-keratinised malignant cells; the nuclei are disproportionately large and have granular chromatin and prominent macronucleoli. Histological investigation of lobectomy specimen showed poorly differentiated squamous carcinoma. Papanicolaou stain, × 254.

We normally puncture a lesion twice to obtain different specimens; however, if a rich aspirate of 'gritty' material results from the first biopsy, it is prudent to complete the procedure immediately, since in the unlikely event of cytology being negative a repeat biopsy can easily be arranged within a day or so. Other workers (Allison and Hemingway 1981) adhere strictly to a single puncture technique, the outer shank being advanced after each biopsy, so obtaining material from different levels of the same lesion. The advantage of this method is that only a single puncture is made of the pleura and lung; thus it may be safer.

After the needle is withdrawn from the chest, a small Elastoplast is placed over the site of entry. Some claim that massaging the skin and subcutaneous tissues over the puncture site may minimise the risk of pneumothorax (Sargent et al. 1974). We have found no evidence that either this or lying the patient down on the puncture site reduces the incidence of pneumothorax.

Prior to leaving the fluoroscopy table, the patient is carefully screened for any evidence of pneumothorax. As well as screening in expiration, a formal expiratory PA chest radiograph is taken. A lesion recently biopsied will sometimes appear larger, and fuzzy-edged, presumably due to local haematoma around the site of biopsy. Before returning to the ward on bed rest, the patient is warned that slight haemoptysis and some chest pain are common sequelae to biopsy, and that should the lung show more than a little collapse, it can be readily re-expanded following percutaneous insertion of a tube attached to an underwater drain. In our experience it is most unusual for a pneumothorax to occur as late as 6 h after the procedure — certainly most patients having a morning biopsy can return home in the early evening and those having one in the afternoon are usually discharged the following morning.

Discussion

A successful diagnostic procedure should have high patient acceptability, be easy, quick and safe to perform, and have a high positive yield with no false-positives. With good imaging, the use of small gauge needles and high-quality cytology, PTNB fulfils these criteria.

Before the advent of image intensifiers, positive rates as low as 40% were published (Lauby et al. 1965). Modern screening facilities allow lesions as small as 1–2 cm to be seen and biopsied, some workers being confident to biopsy those as small as 3 mm (Nordenstrom 1972, personal communication). Clearly the size of the lesions on which attempts are made will modify the percentage yield, though our own results on lesions of a variety of size and shape and totalling 774 biopsies over an 8-year period have a 90% positive yield. This figure is also reported by other workers (Allison and Hemingway 1981; Berquist et al. 1980; Poe and Tobin 1980).

The site and depth of a lesion within the thorax do not influence its suitability for biopsy, since either an anterior, a posterior or a lateral approach may be used. Both long and short bevelled needles have been used without influencing results. A 20 gauge needle with both a plain and then a corkscrew stilette offers the best compromise through which a large enough specimen can be obtained with the least trauma. When a large lesion has invaded the chest wall directly, perhaps with bony destruction, then in addition to aspiration cytology, a formal histological specimen may also be obtained using a Trucut needle.

Diffuse or fibrotic lesions are not suitable for aspiration and may be investigated by the trephine drill technique or by open biopsy. Drill biopsy provides a better histological specimen than an aspiration biopsy, but also has a higher complication rate, presumably due to the larger calibre of needle used (Steel and Winstanley 1969). Open biopsy is the most certain method of obtaining a histological diagnosis; however, it requires a general anaesthetic, and not surprisingly has a higher complication rate than other methods (Zavala and Bedell 1972).

False-positive results do not appear to be a significant problem with aspiration biopsy, and in our centre no patient given a cytological diagnosis of malignancy has subsequently been found to have benign disease. The false-negative rate appears to be 5%–10% depending on the experience of the radiologist and cytologist involved. There are several reasons for failure to obtain representative tissue: The biopsy may be from an inflammatory area distal to a neoplastic bronchial occlusion. Secondly, it may be from the centre of a necrotic mass, be it neoplastic or inflammatory. Thirdly, a small firm lesion may move away from an advancing needle point, or be so hard as to defy puncture. Usually primary and metastatic neoplasms in the lung are softer than benign neoplasms and granulomas, and penetration is not a problem. Once a lesion has cavitated, biopsy should be from the periphery of the lesion, rather than from the unrepresentative necrotic centre.

Several hazards may follow aspiration biopsy. They include pneumothorax, pulmonary haemorrhage, bronchopleural fistula, empyema, air embolism, tumour embolism and tumour implantation in the biopsy track (Meyer et al. 1970; Lauby et al. 1965; Sinner 1976). Apart from pneumothorax, most complications occur rarely. The factors that appear to influence the incidence of post-biopsy pneumothorax include the calibre of the biopsy needle, the number of insertions of needle through pleura and lung, the length of time the needle is left within the lesion, and finally, the confidence and experience of the operator (Allison and Hemingway 1981). Most series report a pneumothorax rate of 20%–25%, though personal experience where CT scans were performed immediately after fine needle PTNB shows that a very shallow asymptomatic pneumothorax is common, this being undetectable on the chest X-ray. The number of patients requiring tube drainage is less than 5% in our hands.

Out of a total of more than 9000 needle biopsies in the literature, there have been six deaths. The association with the use of large bore needles is clear, three dying from haemoptysis, and one each from tension pneumothorax, air embolism and cause unspecified (Meyer and Ferrneci 1970; Adamson and Bates 1967; Woolf 1954). One patient who died from haemoptysis was so heavily sedated that he was unable to clear his airway; this should never occur. A second case of fatal haemoptysis was in the presence of severe pulmonary hypertension, whilst Woolf (1954) reported fatal air embolism whilst the procedure was being performed on a patient with severe dyspnoea. The possibility of tension pneumothorax must be borne in mind whilst performing any percutaneous lung biopsy, and the radiologist must recognise this immediately and have ready access to a chest drain.

Needle track implantation of tumour has been reported by several authors (Oschner et al. 1947; Berger et al. 1972); the result is either secondary deposits along the needle track or malignant effusions. It seems, however, that the risk of needle track seeding is extremely small, Nordenstrom and Bjork (1973) reporting only one definite case in a series of 4000 biopsies.

Percutaneous needle biopsy is a simple, 15-min, low cost (Gobien et al. 1983) procedure which patients tolerate well. Many appear to feel no discomfort whatsoever, when, following instillation of local anaesthetic down to the pleura, the aspirating needle is advanced into the lesion itself, and some express surprise when the procedure is announced to have been completed. We have had one patient with a neurofibroma who experienced severe pain. Whilst considering the various risks of aspiration biopsy, and balancing these against the expected high diagnostic yield, it should be borne in mind that the only practical diagnostic alternative at that particular stage in the patient's work-up is thoracotomy.

Conclusions

Percutaneous transpleural needle biopsy of discrete lung lesions suspected of being malignant tumours is a simple and safe diagnostic procedure involving clinicians, radiologists and cytologists as a team. The method is reliable, the diagnostic yield being greater than that for competing procedures, except thoracotomy. Accurate localisation of a lesion prior to biopsy is of fundamental importance and starts with good quality PA and lateral chest radiographs (Fig. 17), often supplemented by

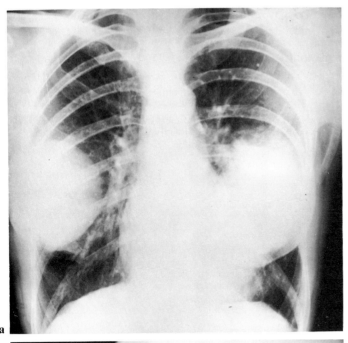

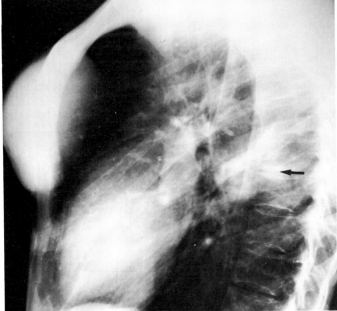

Fig. 17a,b. 40-year-old female with haemoptysis. **a** PA chest X-ray shows bilateral mammoplasties. Between a calcified node at the left hilum and the left mammoplasty there is an area of lung infiltration. **b** Lateral chest X-ray; the lesion lies in the apical segment of the left lower lobe (*arrowed*). Biopsy: final histology, adenocarcinoma.

tomography. With modern screening facilities, virtually all lesions are accessible for biopsy. Should the first biopsy yield material that is inadequate for a certain diagnosis, a repeat biopsy is worthwhile and invariably provides a representative and definitive specimen. Pneumothorax is the only significant hazard, though only 5% of patients will require a pleural drain.

A correct diagnosis is made in over 90% of patients. The procedure now has a secure place in the diagnosis of any lung lesion suspected to be carcinomatous. It should be used earlier and more frequently to allow prompt and definitive therapy for any persistent lung lesion that cannot be diagnosed by non-invasive means.

References

Adamson JS, Bates JH (1967) Percutaneous needle biopsy of the lung. Arch Intern Med 119:164–169

Allison DJ, Hemingway AP (1981) Percutaneous needle biopsy of the lung. Br Med J 282:875–878

Berger RH, Dargan EL, Huang BL (1972) Dissemination of cancer cells by needle biopsy of lung. J Thorac Cardiovasc Surg 63:430–432

Berquist TH, Bailey PB, Cortes DA, Miller WE (1980) Transthoracic needle biopsy. Mayo Clin Proc 55:475–481

Buell PE (1971) The importance of tumor size in prognosis for resected bronchogenic carcinoma. J Surg Oncol 3:539–551

Dahlgren SE, Lind B (1969) Transthoracic needle biopsy or bronchoscopic biopsy? Scand J Resp Dis 50:265–272

Dick R, Heard BE, Hinson KFW, Kerr IH, Pearson MC (1974) Aspiration needle biopsy of thoracic lesions: an assessment of 227 biopsies. Br J Dis Chest 68:86–94

Gallo Curcio C, Rinaldi M, Tonachella R, Donnorso RP (1983) Role of percutaneous fine needle aspiration in the diagnosis of lung cancer: Our experience with 140 patients. Oncology 40:177–180

Gobien RP, Bouchard EA, Gobien BS, Valicenti JF, Vujic IV (1983) Thin needle aspiration biopsy of thoracic lesions. Impact on hospital charges and patterns of patient care. Radiology 148:65–67

Good CA (1963) The solitary pulmonary nodule: a problem of management. Radiol Clin North Am 1:429–438

Good CA, Wilson TW (1958) The solitary circumscribed pulmonary nodule. JAMA 166:210–215

Higgins GA, Shields TW, Keehn RJ (1975) The solitary pulmonary nodule. Arch Surg 110:570–575

Lauby VW, Burnett WE, Rosemund GP, Tyson RR (1965) Value and risk of biopsy pulmonary lesions by needle aspiration. J Thorax Cardiovasc Surg 49:159–172

Leyden H (1883) Über infectiose Pneumonie. Dsch Med Wochenschr 9:52–54

Johnson N Mcl, Dick R, Casselden P, Clarke SW (1979) Fibreoptic bronchoscopy and fluoroscopic percutaneous needle biopsy — a combined approach to the investigation of thoracic lesions. Radiography XLV 540:273–275

Menetrier P (1886) Cancer primitif du Puomon. Bull Soc Anat 11:643

Meyer JE, Ferrneci JF, Janower ML (1970) Fatal complications of percutaneous lung biopsy. Review of the literature and report of a case. Radiology 96:47–48

Nordenstrom B, Björk VO (1973) Dissemination of cancer cells by needle biopsy of the lung. J Thorac Cardiovasc Surg 65:671

Oschner A, Debakey M, Leonard Dixon J (1947) Primary cancer of the lung. JAMA 135:321–326

Poe RH, Tobin RE (1980) Sensititivity and specificity of needle biopsy in lung malignancy. Am Rev Respir Dis 122:725–729

Sargent EN, Turner AF, Gordonson J, Schwinn CP, Pashkyo O (1974) Percutaneous pulmonary needle biopsy. Report of 350 patients. Am J Roentgenol Radium Ther Nucl Med 122:758–768

Sinner WN (1976) Complications of percutaneous transthoracic needle aspiration biopsy. Acta Radiol [Diagn] (Stockh) 17:813–825

Sinner WN (1982) Fine-needle biopsy of hamartomas of the lung. Am J Roentgenol Radium Ther Nucl Med 138:65–69

Smiddy JF, Ruth WE, Kerby GR, Renz LE, Raucher C (1971) Flexible fibreoptic bronchoscope. Ann Intern Med 75:971–972

Steel JD, Buell PE (1973) Asymptomatic solitary pulmonary nodule. J Thorac Cardiovasc Surg 65:140–151
Steel SJ, Winstanley DP (1969) Trephine biopsy of the lung and pleura. Thorax 24:576–584
Trunk G, Gracy DR, Byrd RB (1974) The management and evaluation of the solitary pulmonary nodule. Chest 66:236–239
Walls WJ, Thornbury JR, Naylor B (1974) Pulmonary needle aspiration biopsy in the diagnosis of Pancoast tumours. Radiology 111:99–102
Woolf CR (1954) Applications of lung biopsy with a review of the literature. Dis Chest 25:286–301
Zavala DC, Bedell GN (1972) Percutaneous lung biopsy with a cutting needle: analysis of 140 cases and comparison with other biopsy techniques. Am Rev Respir Dis 106:186–193

Chapter 7

The Role of Computed Tomography in the Management of Bronchial Carcinoma

Stephen J. Golding

One of the principal benefits of the recent developments in imaging techniques has been improvement in the investigation of malignant neoplasms. Computed tomography (CT) has a particularly important place in oncology, being a valuable technique for demonstrating primary tumours and detecting metastases to lymph nodes and other organs (Husband 1981; Husband and Golding 1982). However, CT scanners are expensive and present in only limited numbers in the United Kingdom. CT examinations are also time consuming and it is necessary to select for investigation only those patients in whom useful information will be obtained. In practice this usually means that the technique is carried out when a management decision, for example to submit the patient to surgery, depends upon the result of the examination.

Accurate assessment of patients with carcinoma of the bronchus is valuable because the extent of disease is an important factor in planning treatment (Kirsh et al. 1976; Choi et al. 1980). In this chapter the technique of CT is described and its value in the diagnosis, staging and treatment of this tumour is considered. Situations where CT is indicated in preference to other investigations are discussed and a diagnostic regime for the pre-operative assessment of these patients suggested.

Technique

Computed tomography is a technique which uses X-rays to produce a cross-sectional image of the patient. The system originally described by Sir Godfrey Hounsfield (Hounsfield 1973) could only examine the head but has undergone rapid development and refinement and now may be used to investigate all areas of the body. An account of the technical aspects is given here in outline only and for more information the reader is referred to Pullan (1979) or Parker (1981).

The basis of CT is similar to that of conventional radiography in that the image is obtained by transmission of an X-ray beam through the patient. In CT a thin beam produced by a conventional X-ray tube is passed through the patient and the intensity of the emergent beam is measured by a bank of electronic detectors. This indicates the density to X-rays of the tissues in the beam. The tube and the detectors rotate around the patient and the large number of measurements obtained are analysed by a computer system. The X-ray density, or attenuation value, of all the cross-section is calculated and displayed as a two-dimensional grey-scale image, dense structures being shown as white (Fig. 1a). The image is viewed by television monitor and is usually recorded photographically.

This process is a very sensitive measure of attenuation value and a wide range is recorded. The attenuation values, now called Hounsfield Units (HU), are expressed on a scale in which water has a value of zero units, air a value of -1000 HU and a dense bone a value between $+400$ and $+1000$ HU. A grey-scale image representing the complete scale would contain fine differences in contrast which are not appreciated by the human eye. The viewing system is therefore designed so that a selected range of values or visible 'window' can be chosen from any region of the scale. In Fig. 1a a window of 500 HU at a level of zero Hounsfield units is displayed. This demonstrates bone and soft tissues but the lungs are not seen since the attenuation values of these are below the visible window. Reducing the level of the window to -700 HU shows the pulmonary vessels and lung fields (Fig. 1b).

Computed tomography is therefore comparable to conventional radiography in that the image is based on the density of the patient's tissues to X-rays and the images are readily appreciated by those familiar with chest radiographs. The principal difference between CT and radiography is that cross-sectional images are not subject to the superimposition of structures which occurs in conventional radiography. For example, in Fig. 1a the individual structures of the mediastinum are seen distinct from each other and from the overlying soft tissues, whereas on the chest radiograph they all contribute to the normal mediastinal shadow. Another difference is that the density discrimination of CT is far greater than that of radiography and small differences in attenuation value can be recorded. An advan-

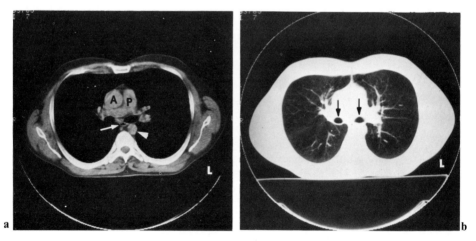

Fig. 1. a Normal CT section of the chest at the level of the right hilum. The ascending aorta (*A*) and main pulmonary artery (*P*) are seen separately. The descending aorta (*arrowhead*) is seen posterior to the left main bronchus and there is air in the oesophagus medial to this (*arrow*). **b** Same CT section. The viewing characteristics have been altered by reducing the window level to -700 HU, showing the pulmonary vessels within the lung fields. Only the air-containing main bronchi (*arrows*) are now seen within the mediastinum.

tage of this is that the density of vessels is increased after an intravenous injection of contrast medium and this technique is useful in distinguishing mediastinal vessels from other tissues.

The examination is usually carried out with the patient supine and a series of CT sections is taken through the area of interest. It is customary for patients to be starved for a few hours before the examination if intravenous contrast medium is to be given but apart from this no specific preparation is required for the investigation of the chest. Since the scanning action takes a significant time (usually between 4 and 10 s), the images are liable to artefact from patient movement. Sections are therefore obtained during suspended respiration but artefact is also produced by cardiac action and pulsation of major vessels. This is minimised by using a short scan time but nevertheless cardiac and arterial pulsation is an important source of image degradation in thoracic CT. Serious artefact is also produced if metal clips have been used in previous surgery.

CT in Diagnosis and Staging

Diagnosis

Bronchial tumours demonstrated by CT usually appear as masses with similar attenuation values to muscle or other soft tissues (Fig. 2). Masses may be spherical or lobulated and are usually well circumscribed but may show evidence of spiculation. Necrosis within the tumour produces areas of lower attenuation value and cavitation is easily detected (Fig. 3). The relationship of tumours to the chest wall or mediastinum (Fig. 4) is readily appreciated on cross-sectional images.

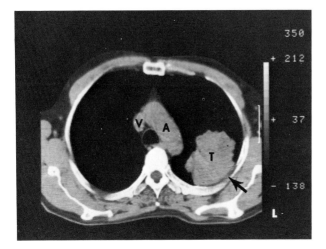

Fig. 2. CT section at the level of the aortic arch showing a large primary tumour (*T*) lying peripherally in the left upper zone. There is a clear soft tissue plane (*arrow*) between the tumour and the chest wall. *A*, aorta; *V*, superior vena cava. No chest wall involvement was found at surgery.

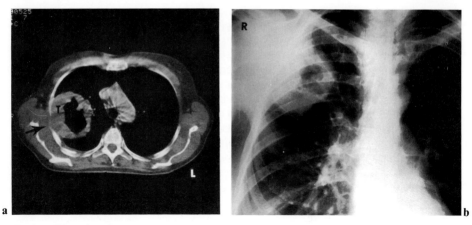

Fig. 3. a CT section showing a large cavitating tumour (*T*) in the right upper zone. The tumour has invaded the chest wall, eroding the adjacent rib (*arrow*). **b** A chest radiograph shows the tumour but does not demonstrate the erosion of the rib.

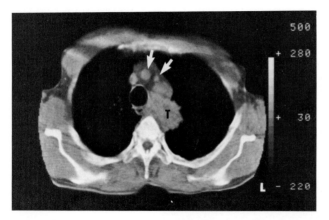

Fig. 4. CT section showing a tumour (*T*) which has infiltrated the left side of the upper mediastinum, displacing the trachea to the right. Anterior to the tumour the innominate and left common carotid arteries are seen (*arrows*); the left subclavian artery is surrounded by the tumour and is not seen separately.

It is well accepted that at present CT is the most accurate method of detecting small nodules in the lung fields. Studies comparing the number of pulmonary metastases demonstrated by CT with those found at radiography or whole lung tomography have shown an increased yield over both techniques (Muhm et al. 1978; Husband et al. 1979). This suggests that CT should be the investigation of choice for the detection of a small pulmonary tumour. However, the majority of patients with bronchial carcinoma have a significant abnormality on the chest radiograph at presentation. In practice, therefore, CT is unlikely to be commonly required for the detection of a primary tumour within the lung fields except when there is strong clinical evidence that such a tumour exists and the conventional studies are normal (McLoud et al. 1979).

Tumours which are adjacent to the mediastinum are more difficult to demonstrate by radiography and conventional tomography. Quite large mediastinal masses can exist without producing alteration in the mediastinal contour. The cross-sectional display provided by CT is very suitable for demonstrating the structure of the mediastinum, and tumours may be detected by CT despite a normal chest radiograph (Crowe et al. 1978). The technique is less reliable in detecting masses in the pulmonary hilum because most tumours have similar attenuation values to adjacent vessels. Artefact from pulsation of the pulmonary artery may also degrade the image of the hilum and although the hilum may appear prominent (Fig. 5) it is not normally possible to distinguish the normal and abnormal components. In this situation CT confers no advantage over conventional radiography or tomography (Mintzer et al. 1979). However, Glazer et al. (1983) have recently shown that by obtaining a rapid series of thin CT sections of the hilum following a bolus injection of contrast medium, masses may be demonstrated which are not seen using the standard technique. The relevance of this work to the detection of small hilar carcinomas has yet to be determined.

There are two major drawbacks to the use of CT in the diagnosis of bronchial carcinoma. Firstly, most tumours have attenuation values similar to other soft tissues and the CT appearances do not usually distinguish between benign and malignant lesions. Work in the United States has suggested that benign pulmonary nodules may be characterised by unusually high attenuation values attributable to microscopic calcification not detectable on conventional tomograms (Siegelman et al. 1980). Unfortunately this has not been confirmed by other workers (MacMahon et al. 1983). In British patients CT is unlikely to provide evidence of calcification if it is not present on conventional tomograms, and a nodule detected by CT should be regarded with the same degree of suspicion as one discovered by chest radiography (Edwards and Fry 1982). The second drawback is that CT, in common with chest radiography, cannot distinguish pulmonary tumours from consolidation in the

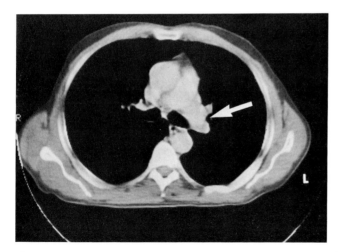

Fig. 5. CT section showing prominence of the left hilum (*arrow*) due to carcinoma. Intravenous contrast medium has been given and the vessels appear dense but it is not possible to distinguish the tumour from the normal structures.

surrounding lung. Occasionally consolidated lung may show an increase in attenuation following intravenous contrast medium and the tumour may be revealed as an area of relatively low density but this is an infrequent finding. If, as commonly occurs, pulmonary collapse or consolidation surround the tumour, it may be impossible either to define the tumour margins or to detect it at all.

CT-Guided Percutaneous Biopsy

In general, imaging techniques alone do not allow a precise diagnosis of neoplasia to be made. Bronchial carcinoma may be diagnosed by sputum cytology or transbronchial biopsy if the tumour is situated centrally. If the tumour lies peripherally or neither technique provides a result, percutaneous needle biopsy (Chap. 6) offers an alternative to open biopsy. Various imaging techniques may be used for percutaneous biopsy, including fluoroscopy, ultrasound and CT.

Computed tomography is an accurate means of needle localisation and the technique is a safe, effective method of obtaining material for cytology or histology (Husband and Golding 1983). However, fluoroscopically guided biopsy is simple, rapid and less costly than CT and is more likely to be used for chest lesions as these are usually visible on fluoroscopy. Nevertheless, there are several situations where CT is the imaging method of choice. The most important of these is a mass within the mediastinum, especially if situated in the thoracic inlet or near major vessels (Adler et al. 1983). The vessels are clearly seen and a needle route avoiding these is chosen (Fig. 6). CT-guided biopsy may also be required for pulmonary and mediastinal lesions which cannot be localised adequately on fluoroscopy. The technique is valuable for biopsy of pleural tumours because puncture of the underlying lung is avoided. In addition, the detection by CT of areas of tumour necrosis may be used to avoid obtaining unrepresentative tissue samples when biopsy is guided by either imaging technique (Pinstein et al. 1983).

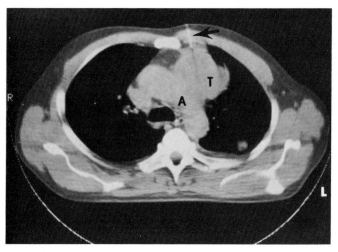

Fig. 6. CT-guided biopsy of tumour (*T*) invading the mediastinum anterior to the aortic arch (*A*). The needle (*arrow*) has been inserted to the left of the sternum and is directed posterolaterally, avoiding the aorta.

Staging

The prognosis of bronchial carcinoma is closely related to the extent of disease at presentation (Little et al. 1983). Treatment policy is influenced both by the histological type and by the stage at presentation (Kirsh et al. 1972; Choi et al. 1980), and it is important that staging investigation is as accurate as possible. When CT is introduced into conventional staging programmes a significant number of patients are found to have more extensive disease than was formerly suspected (Emami et al. 1978; Harper et al. 1981). Staging consists of assessment of the primary tumour and the detection of metastases to lymph nodes and to distant organs (TNM staging) (Mountain et al. 1974) (see p. 180).

Assessment of the Primary Tumour (T-Stage)

The extent of the primary tumour and its relationship to surrounding structures is readily appreciated on cross-sectional images. Tumours which extend to the surface of the lung may be shown to be separated from the chest wall by a soft tissue plane (Fig. 2), or erosion of ribs and extension through the chest wall may be evident (Fig. 3). The absence of a clear soft tissue plane between the tumour and the chest wall does not, however, always indicate that the parietal pleura is involved (Baron et al. 1982). Tumours adjacent to the mediastinum may infiltrate the mediastinal fat and extend between the vessels or around the oesophagus and trachea (Fig. 4). Compression of mediastinal vessels and venous thrombosis may also be detected by CT.

Computed tomography is more accurate than chest radiography in detecting or excluding tumour extension into the chest wall or the mediastinum (Crowe et al. 1978; McLoud et al. 1979; Baron et al. 1982). The objective of assessing the relationship of the primary tumour to the mediastinum and chest wall is that a confident prediction can be made as to whether the tumour is resectable. Infiltration between the mediastinal vessels or other organs indicates inoperability, as may extension into ribs or through the chest wall (Webb et al. 1981a). In a study carried out at the Royal Marsden Hospital a prediction of operability was based on the CT appearances in ten patients who subsequently underwent surgical exploration. Five patients had primary tumours adjacent to the chest wall and in all five the CT prediction of operability was correct (Table 1). Five other patients in this study had tumours related to the pulmonary hilum and the CT prediction was correct in only three of these. The extent of hilar tumour was overestimated in two patients, leading to an incorrect prediction. This emphasises the difficulty in assessing hilar masses.

Table 1. CT prediction of operability (ten patients)

	Prediction	No. of patients	Correct	Incorrect
Peripheral masses	Inoperable	3	3	—
	Operable	2	2	—
Hilar masses	Inoperable	2	—	2
	Operable	3	3	—

Detection of Lymph Node Metastases (N-Stage)

Bronchial carcinoma tends to spread to hilar lymph nodes and then to nodes in the mediastinum (Kirsh et al. 1972; Heitzman et al. 1982). Large hilar and mediastinal lymph node masses are usually detectable by chest radiography and indicate a poor prognosis but it is the presence, not necessarily the extent, of lymph node involvement that determines survival following surgery (Kirsh et al. 1976).

The cross-sectional display and superior density discrimination of CT allow lymph node masses to be demonstrated which are not seen on the chest radiograph (Goldwin et al. 1977; Husband et al. 1979). Enlarged lymph nodes are seen as discrete rounded soft tissue densities in the mediastinal fat between the normal structures (Fig. 7). Their demonstration is facilitated by obtaining CT sections after intravenous administration of contrast medium since the vessels opacify but lymph nodes do not. Larger lymph node masses obliterate the fat planes between the mediastinal structures and also distort the mediastinal contour, but even these may not be identified on the chest radiograph or conventional tomograms (Fig. 8). CT is also very accurate in excluding lymph node involvement in patients who have on the chest radiograph a mediastinal contour which is suspicious or equivocal (Fig. 9) (Baron et al. 1981).

Although CT is capable of demonstrating enlarged lymph nodes at almost all sites in the mediastinum, lymph node masses in the pulmonary hilum are more difficult to detect (Faling et al. 1981). In the same way that conventional tomograms appear to be more valuable when there is a primary hilar mass, tomography in the oblique plane appears to be the technique of choice for detecting hilar lymph node enlargement (Mintzer et al. 1979). However, Webb et al. (1981b) have shown that by using rapid scans and thin sections with intravenous contrast medium the anatomy of the pulmonary hilum can be studied and small lymph node masses demonstrated. The clinical relevance of this to the assessment of the pulmonary hilum is still under evaluation.

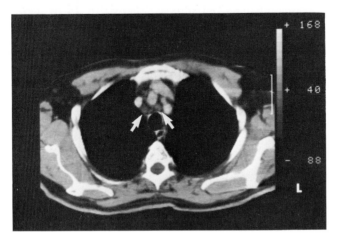

Fig. 7. CT section showing two mildly enlarged lymph nodes (*arrows*) lying posterior to the right brachiocephalic vein and innominate artery. Intravenous contrast medium has been given to opacify the mediastinal vessels, and the lymph nodes are distinguished by the fact that they do not take up contrast medium.

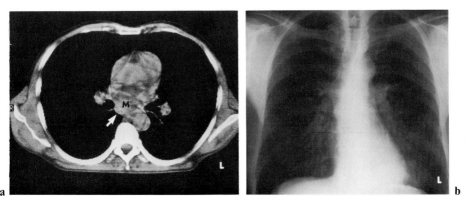

Fig. 8. a CT section showing a large subcarinal lymph node mass (*M*). The mass obliterates the surrounding soft tissue planes and distorts the mediastinal outline posteriorly (*arrow*). Compare this image with the similar area in Fig. 1a. **b** The chest radiograph shows no evidence of lymphadenopathy.

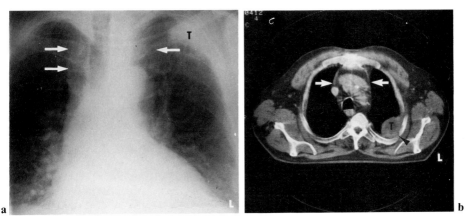

Fig. 9. a Chest radiograph showing a left apical tumour (*T*). The superior mediastinum appears wide (*arrows*), suggesting lymph node metastases. **b** CT section through the superior mediastinum shows that the mediastinal widening is due to excessive fat deposition around the mediastinal vessels (*arrows*). No soft tissue plane is seen between the tumour and the chest wall (*arrowhead*). Intercostal extension of tumour was found at surgery.

It should be stressed that CT does not demonstrate the internal architecture of lymph nodes and enlargement is the only criterion of abnormality. It is therefore not possible to distinguish lymph node enlargement due to neoplastic involvement from inflammatory disease or reactive hypertrophy. Nevertheless, Baron et al. (1982) have shown in a study of 98 patients with carcinoma of the bronchus that lymph nodes with a transverse diameter greater than 2 cm almost always indicate neoplastic involvement. In their study lymph nodes less than 1 cm in diameter were very unlikely to contain tumour. This is borne out by the work of Rea and his colleagues (Rea et al. 1981). Lymph nodes greater than 1.5 cm in diameter are abnormal but enlargement may be due to causes other than malignancy.

Table 2. Number of abnormal mediastinal lymph nodes detected by CT vs mediastinoscopy or thoracotomy in 12 patients

Site of nodes	No. of abnormal nodes	
	CT	Mediastinoscopy/ thoractomy
Anterior mediastinal	2	2
Right paratracheal	3	4
Left paratracheal	1	1
Subcarinal	—	2
Beneath aortic arch	—	1
Right tracheobronchial	3	4
Right hilum	3	3
Left hilum	1	2

The possibility of CT as a non-invasive alternative to mediastinoscopy has attracted much attention. CT has the advantage of being non-invasive but detects lymph node enlargement only and the appearance of enlarged lymph nodes is non-specific. At mediastinoscopy biopsy of normal sized lymph nodes can be carried out but the technique is invasive and not all areas of the mediastinum can be visualised (Trinkle et al. 1969). Several workers have suggested that CT has a high accuracy in excluding mediastinal lymph node disease and have suggested that normal CT appearances obviate staging by surgical means (Rea et al. 1981; Faling et al. 1981). However, the author's experience does not support this view. In a study at the Royal Marsden Hospital 12 patients underwent staging by CT before mediastinoscopy or thoracotomy. CT detected enlarged nodes in only 13 of 19 lymph node sites subsequently shown to contain disease. The overall accuracy of the technique was 94% (Table 2). These figures compare favourably with the false-negative rate reported by Underwood et al. (1979) but they suggest that at present CT cannot completely replace surgical staging of these patients. The author's personal recommendation would be that patients who have no evidence of mediastinal lymph node involvement on the chest radiograph should undergo staging by CT. Lymph nodes greater than 2 cm in diameter may be assumed to represent disease but biopsy should be carried out on smaller degrees of lymph node enlargement and in these circumstances the CT findings are useful in directing mediastinoscopy (Baron et al. 1982). If the mediastinum appears normal at CT it cannot be assumed that disease is absent and direct mediastinal investigation is required. However, the number of patients shown by mediastinoscopy to have abnormal nodes may well be so small that it is preferable to proceed direct to staging at thoracotomy without an additional mediastinal procedure (Goldstraw et al. 1983). Clearly this is an area that requires further study and it is probable that with greater experience, more reliance will be placed on the CT findings.

Detection of Distant Metastases (M-Stage)

The spread of malignant tumours to other organs generally precludes local treatment. The likelihood of this occurring at presentation in bronchial neoplasms depends upon the histology (Little et al. 1983). Carcinoma of the bronchus shows a tendency to early spread to the skeleton, brain, liver and adrenal glands, and a significant number of patients must be assumed to have disseminated disease at presentation (Engelman and McNamara 1954; Matthews et al. 1973).

Skeletal scintigraphy (isotope scanning) is the investigation of choice for the detection of metastases to the skeleton. The technique has a very high sensitivity and demonstrates skeletal deposits that are not detected on conventional radiographs and tomograms (O'Mara 1974; Kirchner and Simon 1981). Multiple areas of radionuclide uptake almost certainly indicate metastases but a single abnormality on the scintigram may represent a benign or malignant lesion (Corcoran et al. 1976). Conventional radiographs of such areas are frequently normal because as much as half the bone may be destroyed before the disease becomes detectable radiographically (Edelstyn et al. 1967). Percutaneous or surgical bone biopsy may be required to exclude disease before radical surgery to the primary tumour. Recently CT has been shown to be more accurate than conventional tomograms in demonstrating abnormalities at areas of abnormal nuclide accumulation and may therefore be a non-invasive alternative to biopsy (Muindi et al. 1983).

Computed tomography is the technique of choice for detecting cerebral metastases. It is less invasive than cerebral angiography and more sensitive than radionuclide studies (Paxton and Ambrose 1974; Deck et al. 1976). However, radionuclide studies are more generally available and provide an acceptable first-line investigation, CT being reserved for those patients in whom scintigraphy fails to demonstrate metastases (Nisbet et al. 1983). Cerebral metastases from carcinoma of the bronchus usually appear on CT as areas of lower attentuation than the surrounding cerebral tissue and may show enhancement following intravenous contrast medium (Deck et al. 1976). Metastases in the liver may be demonstrated by CT, ultrasound or isotope studies. CT is rather more sensitive in detecting metastases than the other two modalities (Snow et al. 1979) but in practice ultrasound and isotope studies are more readily available and are more likely to be carried out first, CT being reserved for difficult diagnostic problems. CT is, however, very definitely the technique of choice for detecting masses in the adrenal gland (Eghrari et al. 1980). When the adrenal glands of patients with carcinoma of the bronchus are examined by CT, a significant number of patients are found to have metastases in one or both adrenal glands (Fig. 10) (Nielsen et al. 1982). This technique is now an

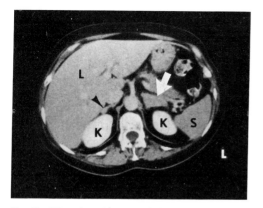

Fig. 10. CT section of the upper abdomen showing enlargement of the left adrenal gland (*arrow*) due to metastatic bronchial carcinoma. *L*, liver; *K*, kidneys; *S*, spleen; *arrowhead*, right adrenal gland.

obligatory part of the pre-operative investigation of these patients because a number of patients who have no evidence of spread elsewhere are found on CT to have adrenal metastases (Sandler et al. 1981). Recently Pagani has reported a study in which patients with carcinoma of the bronchus who had normal CT appearances of their adrenal glands underwent CT-guided biopsy (Pagani 1983). Forty-three biopsies were carried out and five morphologically normal glands were found to contain microscropic deposits of carcinoma. The relevance of this work to staging patients with bronchial carcinoma has yet to be evaluated but the study supports the view that many patients have widespread disease at presentation.

CT in Treatment

CT-Assisted Radiotherapy Planning

The objective of radiotherapy is to deliver a high dose of radiation to a tumour with minimal damage to the surrounding structures. To do this accurately needs a precise plan of the tumour in relation to the surrounding organs and the body contour. An inaccurate plan may mean that part of the tumour receives little radiation and a normal organ is damaged.

The images provided by CT are an excellent basis for radiotherapy planning since they show the tumour, the body outline and the other organs clearly. Software programmes are now available whereby treatment plans can be constructed directly from the CT image. The technique requires that the patient be examined under similar conditions to those of treatment, usually supine using an examination couch with a flat top (Hobday et al. 1979). The technique must also make allowance for inaccuracies arising in the course of treatment. Respiration is an important source of inaccuracy since the tumour may move during breathing and the treatment volume must be increased to allow for this. The sections are therefore repeated during quiet respiration and are compared with the initial sections. The images are then transferred to a computer planning system. The tumour margin and important adjacent organs are outlined on the monitor using a touch-sensitive light pen and the computer produces a treatment plan and isodose curves superimposed on the image (Fig. 11).

Data from CT images may also be used to influence radiotherapy planning quantitatively. Dose calculations have to take into account the density of tissues through which the beam passes before it reaches the tumour. In conventional radiotherapy planning only an approximate allowance can be made for this, but the attenuation values from CT images can be used to make precise inhomogeneity corrections (Hobday et al. 1983). This is particularly important in the thorax, where treatment beams pass through tissues of greatly differing density such as lung and bone.

Several studies have shown that CT-assisted radiotherapy planning is more accurate than conventional methods (Goiten et al. 1979; Hobday et al. 1979; Seydel et al. 1980). When CT is introduced into the conventional regimes more than 30% of treatment plans may be changed, the most common change being to increase treatment volume. Thus it is anticipated that CT-assisted radiotherapy planning will result in more reliable control of local tumour spread.

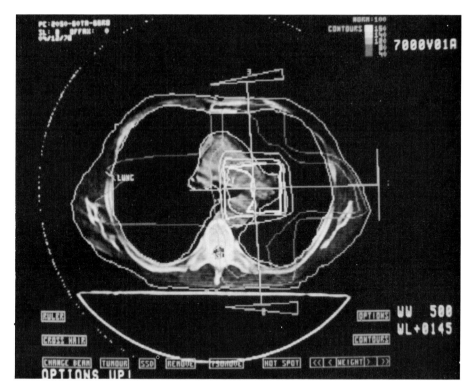

Fig. 11. CT-assisted radiotherapy planning. The left hilum is enlarged by a bronchial carcinoma. Three treatment beams and the isodose distribution are superimposed on the CT image. (Reproduced by courtesy of International General Electric Company of New York Limited)

Monitoring Response to Treatment and Detection of Relapse

Precise measurements of tumour volume can be made from CT examinations and these are valuable for monitoring the response to treatment in some tumours. However, the technique has proved disappointing in the case of carcinoma of the bronchus. In a pilot study carried out at the Royal Marsden Hospital five patients with inoperable small cell carcinoma of the bronchus were examined at monthly intervals during chemotherapy. CT provided more information than the chest radiograph in one patient but this did not alter the patient's treatment. In the remaining four patients CT provided no more information than the chest radiograph and was less informative in one of these. As discussed above, CT assessment of the tumour becomes inaccurate when there is consolidation or collapse of the surrounding lung. This may happen at any time during treatment or alternatively parenchymal changes may resolve. In these circumstances both CT and chest radiographs may be difficult to assess. This affected the radiological assessment of two patients in this pilot study.

Computed tomography does appear to be valuable in the detection of recurrent tumour after pneumonectomy. In only a small number of patients is the pneumonectomy space completely obliterated and in most patients the area shows uniform attenuation values in keeping with fluid. Recurrent tumours in this space are difficult to detect by radiography but CT may reveal a soft tissue mass within the fluid.

Conclusion — The Influence of CT on Patient Management

The clinical value of an investigation depends upon the effect it has on the treatment of the patient. The treatment of choice for carcinoma of the bronchus is surgical resection, if this is feasible. Only a small number of patients presenting with carcinoma of the bronchus are in fact suitable for radical resection. Post-mortem evidence also suggests that many patients who appear to have localised tumours at surgery in fact have disseminated disease (Matthews et al. 1973).

Since introducing CT into staging of bronchial carcinoma usually results in the assessment being changed to a more advanced stage, it is reasonable to suppose that this will lead to fewer patients undergoing unsuccessful thoracotomy. A possible pre-operative investigation protocol is shown in Table 3. Diagnosis is usually made by sputum analysis or biopsy and simple investigations should be carried out first — if the initial chest radiograph shows definite signs of inoperability, other investigations are unnecessary. Skeletal scintigraphy is non-invasive and generally available and may therefore be the next investigation. Patients without skeletal metastases may then proceed to CT. This examination should include the liver and adrenal glands and will also permit examination of the lung fields for occult pulmonary metastases. This regime should identify those patients who may proceed to mediastinoscopy or direct to thoracotomy as preferred.

Table 3. A suggested pre-operative imaging regime

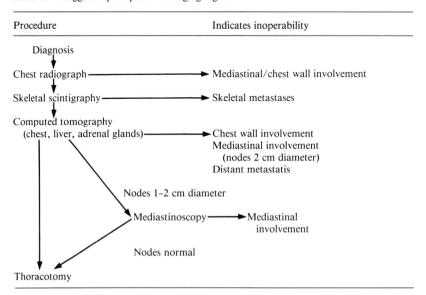

Procedure	Indicates inoperability
Diagnosis	
Chest radiograph	Mediastinal/chest wall involvement
Skeletal scintigraphy	Skeletal metastases
Computed tomography (chest, liver, adrenal glands)	Chest wall involvement Mediastinal involvement (nodes 2 cm diameter) Distant metastatis
Nodes 1–2 cm diameter	
Mediastinoscopy	Mediastinal involvement
Nodes normal	
Thoracotomy	

Table 4. Other uses of CT

Diagnosis:	Detection of occult tumour
	CT-guided percutaneous biopsy
Staging:	Investigation of single scintigraphic abnormality in skeleton
	Detection of cerebral metastases
Treatment:	CT-assisted radiotherapy planning
	Detection of recurrence following pneumonectomy

The other possible uses of CT are shown in Table 4. This is a developing field and imaging techniques are changing all the time, with refinements in existing techniques and development of new ones. Continued study in liaison with clinicians and pathologists will be required to identify the most effective investigation regimes. Nevertheless, our present state of knowledge suggests that as CT becomes more generally available and those involved in the management of thoracic disease become more familiar with CT findings, a greater number of patients with bronchial carcinoma will benefit from the technique.

Acknowledgements. I am grateful to Dr Janet Husband of the Royal Marsden Hospital and Mr Peter Goldstraw of the Brompton Hospital for their help and for permission to quote from studies carried out with them. Miss Janet Edmonds provided expert secretarial assistance.

References

Adler OB, Rosenberger A, Peleg H (1983) Fine-needle aspiration biopsy of mediastinal masses. Am J Roentgenol 140:893–896

Baron RL, Levitt RG, Sagel SS, Stanley RJ (1981) Computed tomography in the evaluation of mediastinal widening. Radiology 138:107–113

Baron RL. Levitt RG, Sagel SS, White MH, Roper CL, Marbarger JP (1982) Computed tomography in the pre-operative evaluation of bronchogenic carcinoma. Radiology 145:727–732

Choi NCH, Grillo HC, Gardiello M, Scannell JG, Wilkins EW (1980) Basis for new strategies in postoperative radiotherapy of bronchogenic carcinoma. Int J Radiat Oncol Biol Phys 6:31–35

Corcoran RJ, Thrall JH, Kyle RW, Kaminski RJ, Johnson MC (1976) Solitary abnormalities in bone scans of patients with extraosseous malignancies. Radiology 121:663–667

Crowe JK, Brown LR, Muhm JR (1978) Computed tomography of the mediastinum. Radiology 128:75–87

Deck MDF, Messina AV, Sackett JF (1976) Computed tomography in metastatic disease of the brain. Radiology 119:115–120

Edelstyn GA, Gillespie GA, Grebbell FS (1967) The radiological demonstration of osseous metastases. Clin Radiol 18:158–162

Edwards SE, Fry IK (1982) Prevalence of lung nodules on computed tomography of patients without known malignant disease. Br J Radiol 55:715–716

Eghrari M, McLoughlin MJ, Rosen IE et al. (1980) The role of computed tomography in assessment of tumoral pathology of the adrenal glands. J Comp Ass Tomogr 4:71–77

Emami B, Melo A, Carter BL, Munzenrider JE, Piro AJ (1978) Value of computed tomography in radiotherapy of lung cancer. Am J Roentgenol 131:63–67

Engelman RM, McNamara WH (1954) Bronchogenic carcinoma — a statistical review of 234 autopsies. J Thorac Surg 27:227–237

Faling LJ, Pugatch RD, Jung-Legg Y et al. (1981) Computed tomographic scanning of the mediastinum in the staging of bronchogenic carcinoma. Am Rev Respir Dis 124:690–695

Glazer GM Francis IR, Gebarski K, Samuels BI, Sorensen KW (1983) Dynamic incremental computed tomography in evaluation of the pulmonary hila. J Comp Ass Tomogr 7:59–64

Goitein M, Wittenberg J, Mendiondo M et al. (1979) The value of CT scanning in radiation therapy treatment planning: a prospective study. Int J Radiat Oncol Biol Phys 5:1787–1798

Goldstraw P, Kurzer M, Edwards D (1983) Preoperative staging of lung cancer: accuracy of computed tomography versus mediastinoscopy. Thorax 38: 10–15

Goldwin RL, Heitzman ER, Proto AV (1977) Computed tomography of the mediastinum. Radiology 124: 235–241

Harper PG, Houang M, Spiro S, Geddes D, Hodson M, Souhami RL (1981) Computerized axial tomography in the pretreatment assessment of small-cell carcinoma of the bronchus. Cancer 47:1775–1780

Heitzman ER, Markarian B, Raasch BN, Carsky EW, Lane EJ, Berlow ME (1982) Pathways of tumor spread through the lung: radiologic correlations with anatomy and pathology. Radiology 144:3–14

Hobday P. Hodson NJ, Husband J, Parker RP, MacDonald JS (1979) Computed tomography applied to radiotherapy treatment planning: techniques and results. Radiology 133:477–482

Hobday P, Cassell K, Parker RP (1983) CT-assisted inhomogeneity corrections. Int J Radiat Oncol Biol Phys (in press)

Hounsfield GN (1973) Computerised transverse axial scanning (tomography): Description of system. Br J Radiol 46:1016–1022

Husband JE (1981) Computed tomography in oncology. In: Husband JE, Fry IK (eds) Computed tomography of the body: a radiological and clinical approach. Macmillan, London Basingstoke, pp 210–217

Husband JE, Golding SJ (1982) Computed tomography of the body: when should it be used? Br Med J 284:4–8

Husband JE, Golding SJ (1983) The role of computed tomography-guided needle biopsy in an oncology service. Clin Radiol 34:255–260

Husband JE, Peckham MJ, Macdonald JS, Hendry WF (1979) The role of computed tomography in the management of testicular teratoma. Clin Radiol 30:243–252

Kirchner PT, Simon MA (1981) Radioisotopic evaluation of skeletal disease. J Bone Joint Surg 63: 673–681

Kirsh MM, Prior M, Gago O et al. (1972) The effect of histological cell type on the prognosis of patients with bronchogenic carcinoma. Ann Thorac Surg 13:303–310

Kirsh MM, Rotman H, Argenta L et al. (1976) Carcinoma of the lung: results of treatment over ten years. Ann Thorac Surg 21:371–377

Little AG, DeMeester TR, MacMahon H (1983) The staging of lung cancer. Semin Oncol 10:56–70

MacMahon H, Courtney JV, Little AG (1983) Diagnostic methods in lung cancer. Semin Oncol 10:20–33

Matthews MJ, Kanhouwa S, Pickren J et al. (1973) Frequency of residual and metastatic tumor in patients undergoing curative surgical resection for lung cancer. Cancer Chemother Rep 4:83–93

McLoud TC, Wittenberg J, Ferrucci JT (1979) Computed tomography of the thorax and standard radiographic evaluation of the chest. J Comp Ass Tomogr 3:170–180

Mintzer RA, Malave SR, Neiman HL, Michaelis LL, Vanecko RM, Sanders JH (1979) Computed vs. conventional tomography in evaluation of primary and secondary pulmonary neoplasms. Radiology 132: 653–659

Mountain CF, Carr DT, Anderson WAD (1974) A system for the clinical staging of lung cancer. Am J Roentgenol 120:130–138

Muhm JR, Brown LR, Crowe JK, Sheedy PF, Hattery RR, Stephens DH (1978) Comparison of whole lung tomography and computed tomography for detecting pulmonary nodules. Am J Roentgenol 131:981–984

Muindi J, Coombes RC, Golding SJ, Powles TJ, Khan O, Husband JE (1983) The role of computed tomography in the detection of bone metastases in breast cancer patients. Br J Radiol 56:233–236

Nielsen ME, Heaston DK, Dunnick NR, Korobkin M (1982) Preoperative CT evaluation of adrenal glands in non-small cell bronchogenic carcinoma. Am J Roentgenol 139:317–320

Nisbet AP, Ratcliffe GE, Ellam SV, Rankin SC, Maisey MN (1983) Clinical indications for optimal use of the radionuclide brain scan. Br J Radiol 56:377–381

O'Mara RE (1974) Bone scanning in osseous metastatic disease. JAMA 229:1915–1917

Pagani JJ (1983) Normal adrenal glands in small cell lung carcinoma: CT-guided biopsy. Am J Roentgenol 140:949–951

Parker R (1981) Basic principles. In: Husband JE, Fry IK (eds) Computed tomography of the body: A radiological and clinical approach. Macmillan, London Basingstoke, pp 1–8

Paxton R, Ambrose J (1974) The EMI scanner. A brief review of the first 650 patients. Br J Radiol 47:530–565

Pinstein ML, Scott RL, Salazar J (1983) Avoidance of negative percutaneous lung biopsy using contrast-enhanced CT. Am J Roentgenol 140:265–267

Pullan BR (1979) The scientific basis of computerised tomography. In: Lodge T, Steiner RE (eds) Recent advances in radiology and medical imaging, No. 6. Churchill Livingstone, Edinburgh, London New York, pp 1–15

Rea HH, Shevland JE, House AJS (1981) Accuracy of computed tomographic scanning in assessment of the mediastinum in bronchial carcinoma. J Cardiovasc Surg 81:825–829

Sandler MA, Pearlberg JL, Madrazo BL, Gitschlag KF, Gross SC (1982) Computed tomographic evaluation of the adrenal gland in the preoperative assessment of bronchogenic carcinoma. Radiology 145:733–736

Seydel HG, Kutcher GJ, Steiner RM, Mohiuddin M, Goldberg B (1980) Computed tomography in planning radiation therapy for bronchogenic carcinoma. Int J Radiat Oncol Biol Phys 6:601–606

Siegelman SS, Zerhouni EA, Leo FP, Khouri NF, Stitik FP (1980) CT of the solitary pulmonary nodule. Am J Roentgenol 135:1–13

Snow JH, Goldstein HM, Wallace S (1979) Comparison of scintigraphy, sonography and computed tomography in the evaluation of hepatic neoplasms. Am J Roentgenol 132:915–918

Trinkle JK, Bryant LR, Hiller AJ, Playforth RH (1969) Mediastinoscopy — experience with 300 consecutive cases. J Thorac Cardiovasc Surg 60:297–300

Underwood GH, Hooper RG, Axelbaum SP, Goodwin DW (1979) Computed tomographic scanning of the thorax in the staging of bronchogenic carcinoma. N Engl J Med 300:777–778

Webb WR, Jeffrey RB, Godwin JD (1981a) Thoracic computed tomography in superior sulcus tumors. J Comp Ass Tomogr 5:361–365

Webb WR, Gamsu G, Glazer G (1981b) Computed tomography of the abnormal pulmonary hilum. J Comp Ass Tomogr 5:485–490

Chapter 8

Pre-operative Assessment of Patients Undergoing Surgery for Bronchial Carcinoma

Peter Drings, Ingolf Vogt-Moykopf

The prognosis and therapeutic approach to surgery, radiotherapy or chemotherapy in cases of bronchial carcinoma (Carr 1973; Carter 1979) are primarily determined by the size and histology of the tumour, and the general condition of the patient. On the neoplastic side the grade of malignancy, the tumour doubling time and evidence of vascular invasion are of importance. On the clinical side the age, sex and race of the patient are of significance, together with such symptoms as loss of weight, psychological disturbance or any other general disorder.

Various suggestions have been made with regard to assessing the general condition of the patient, and the Karnofsky scale (1948) is particularly favoured, finding use in therapeutic studies (Table 1).

Tumour spread is determined in accordance with the UICC's[1] TNM classification prior to treatment. The classification is then supplemented postoperatively in the light of histopathological examination of the resected specimen (p TNM) (see p. 180).

The diagnosis and assessment of bronchial carcinoma requires a wide range of investigative methods, the use of which takes into consideration the stress the patient can withstand and the time they take to perform. This programme should confirm the histological nature of the tumour and enable a decision to be reached on subsequent treatment.

Diagnosis and Staging of the Primary Tumour

In assessing the primary tumour and the regional lymph nodes it has proved of more value to distinguish between a standardised basic programme and various supplementary investigative methods (Table 2). In addition, other diagnostic measures are employed to exclude the existence of distant metastases.

Attention is focussed on the most prominent symptoms such as dry cough, fever (retention pneumonia), night sweats and haemoptysis, all of which accompany other pulmonary diseases, such as tuberculosis. Loss of weight, decline in general per-

[1] Union International Contre le Cancer

Table 1. Performance status (Karnofsky scale)

Able to carry on normal activity; no special care is needed	100 Normal; no complaints; no evidence of disease
	90 'Able to carry on normal activity; minor signs or symptoms of disease
	80 Normal activity with effort; some signs or symptoms of disease
Unable to work; able to live at home and care for most personal needs; a varying amount of assistance is needed	70 Cares for self; unable to carry on normal activity or to do active work
	60 Requires occasional assistance but is able to care for most personal needs
	50 Requires considerable assistance and frequent medical care
Unable to care for self; requires equivalent of institutional or hospital care; disease may be progressing rapidly	40 Disabled; requires special care and assistance
	30 Severely disabled; hospitalisation is indicated although death not imminent
	20 Very sick; hospitalisation and active support treatment are necessary
	10 Moribund, fatal processes progressing rapidly
	0 Dead

Table 2. Diagnosis and staging of the primary tumour and regional lymph nodes

Basic diagnostic procedure:
— Case history
— Clinical investigation and physical findings
— Laboratory investigations
— X-rays of the thoracic organs in two planes – PA and lateral with fluoroscopy and tomography if indicated
— Bronchoscopy (bronchial lavage, biopsy)

Supplementary diagnostic procedure:
— Perfusion scintigraphy of the lungs
— Computer tomography
— Mediastinoscopy and needle biopsy
— Thoracoscopy
— Diagnostic thoracotomy

formance, chest pain, dyspnoea and a paraneoplastic syndrome may also indicate bronchial carcinoma. The presence of pain is suggestive of stage T_3. The symptoms and radiographic appearance of bronchial carcinoma can imitate every other pulmonary disease (Grunze 1962) (Fig. 1). Postero-anterior and lateral chest X-rays are supplemented by hilar tomograms. Using fluoroscopy, paradoxical diaphragmatic movements may serve as an indication of a central growth involving the phrenic nerve (T_3 or N_2).

Bronchoscopy

Bronchoscopy is a very important investigative method which is regarded as obligatory before any lung resection (see p. 41). Bronchoscopy not only confirms the diagnosis in 60%–70% of patients but also provides additional information on the T and N stages and determines the nature and technical extent of surgery.

Computed Tomography

Computed tomography of the thorax has proved to be the most sensitive non-invasive method for assessing malignant extension into the mediastinum and for demonstrating small intrapulmonary or pleural tumours. CT scanning is also the method of choice for the diagnosis of suspected cerebral or hepatic metastases, while isotope scanning is the first method to use when demonstrating skeletal metastases (see p. 107).

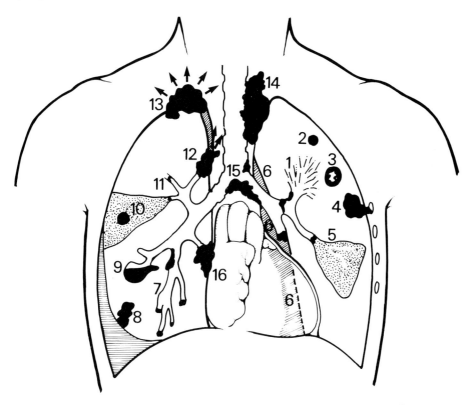

Fig. 1. The most frequent manifestations of bronchial carcinoma (after Grunze): *1*, hilar lung cancer with endobronchial growth (relatively early elicitation of the cough reflex!); *2*, typical round focus; *3*, tumour cavern (note the thick irregular walls!); *4*, subpleural focus infiltrating the chest wall; *5*, obstructive segmental discontinuation with retention in pneumonia, in *10* already with abscess formation; *6*, atelectasis, which is hidden behind the cardiac shadow (lateral X-ray!); *7*, secondary bronchiectasis due to partial stenosis; *8*, focus near to the pleura, with effusion; *9*, necrotising tumour with draining bronchus (abscess symptom!); *11*, obstruction emphysema due to valve occlusion; *12* and *13*, outbreak of carcinoma into the mediastinum, e.g. in the direction of the vena cava (upper inflow congestion!) or as Pancoast tumour; *14*, lymph node involvement in the upper mediastinum and paratracheally, extending to the upper clavicular fossa. Detection by lymph node biopsy according to Daniels or by mediastinoscopy; *15* and *16*, carcinoma spreading to the trachea and pericardium respectively. Caution! A bronchial carcinoma can be masked even in a normal X-ray!

Mediastinoscopy

Mediastinoscopy has been used in many units throughout the western world, but CT scanning is now available as an alternative non-invasive method and is of particular value in those places which cannot be reached at mediastinoscopy, such as the sites of the anterior mediastinal, subaortic and para-oesophageal lymph nodes. However, this method will only detect lymph node enlargement and will not provide evidence of malignancy. A variety of views have been expressed on the indications for mediastinoscopy. Some authors (Goldberg et al. 1974; Maassen 1967; Pearson et al. 1972) use mediastinoscopy in all cases pre-operatively in order to reach a decision as to the further therapeutic strategy. Others, however (Konrad and Schulte 1969), dispute that mediastinoscopy can generally be used to assess the operability of bronchial carcinoma, since even when the lymph nodes are involved, 7%–17% of patients may survive 5 years following successful removal. Vanderhoeft (1979) performs mediastinoscopy only when the tumour is located in the left lung, but the authors consider the following criteria as a reasonable approach to mediastinoscopy:

1. Mediastinoscopy should be employed in cases of central or peripheral carcinoma when there is suspicion of extensive mediastinal involvement, regardless of whether this involvement is ipsilateral or contralateral to the tumour.

Nevertheless, in young patients whose general condition is good, one should perform thoracotomy immediately (foregoing mediastinoscopy), even when the tumour is centrally located, so as not to deny the patient the possibility of resection. In addition, one should take into consideration the secondary changes which may result from mediastinoscopy, making mobilisation of the tracheobronchial tree difficult or even impossible when attempting conservative surgery such as segmental resection.

2. In cases of small cell carcinoma the result of mediastinoscopy determines operability. With our present state of knowledge, involvement of the paratracheal nodes represents a contra-indication to curative resection.

3. In elderly patients, in whom the risks of surgery are greater, a positive result from mediastinoscopy enables thoracotomy to be avoided, regardless of histology.

4. Not only the histological findings, but also palpation during mediastinoscopy is of significance. A pronounced tendency to bleed occasionally rules out the taking of a biopsy. When the operator is able to palpate a fixed hard lymph node, this suffices to indicate inoperability without biopsy.

Mediastinoscopy is the method of choice for exploring the mediastinal lymph nodes, although some authors (Jolly et al. 1973; Deneffe et al. 1983) prefer mediastinotomy. The latter technique is usually undertaken on the right side, but when the primary tumour is located in the left upper lobe an approach from the left is preferred, in correspondence with the assumed path of lymph node metastasis. In the presence of such metastases, mediastinotomy is said to be more informative than mediastinoscopy (Deneffe et al. 1983), but this claim requires confirmation.

Thoracoscopy

In instances of proven effusion in the pleural space one must distinguish between serous and haemorrhagic forms, and thoracoscopy is the only suitable method for this purpose. In our own experience (Vogt-Moykopf and Luellig 1976), pleural metastasis is to be expected in the vast majority of cases of haemorrhagic effusion, while on the other hand serous effusion does not rule out metastasis. In addition to a discrete metastasis, the accumulation of lymph in the presence of central involvement of hilar lymph nodes can result in a serous effusion, and retention pneumonia with inflammatory pleural involvement is a further possible cause.

Laparoscopy

Laparoscopy is indicated for the detection of hepatic metastases where CT scanning does not provide evidence. This technique has been used successfully by various groups (Dombernowsky et al. 1978; Margolis et al. 1974; Muggia and Chervu 1974) to search for metastases in cases of small cell carcinoma. Laparoscopy can detect smaller foci than the previously described methods, as long as the foci are situated on the surface of the liver and are within view. The advantages of laparoscopy are that it makes possible histological confirmation of the diagnosis and assessment of neighbouring structures. As a staging procedure, the use of laparoscopy can be considered in small cell carcinoma when all other methods have produced a negative result, and in non-small cell carcinoma in the presence of a lesion in the liver which cannot be explained by other methods.

Careful palpation of the epigastrium through the diaphragm should always be performed after opening the thorax. In cases of doubt on the right side, the abdomen is opened through the diaphragm in order to obtain precise information, and, if necessary, to perform a hepatic biopsy.

Summary

In considering which diagnostic investigations to undertake, time taken and the subjective stress experienced by the patient must be taken into consideration. In cases of doubt, thoracotomy provides the most reliable information on the site, extension and histological classification of bronchial carcinoma.

Assessment of Operative Risk

General Risk Factors

Assessment of the general condition of the patient with bronchial carcinoma is of decisive significance in the pre-operative review, insofar as most elderly people suffer from accompanying disorders that may increase the risk of the surgical procedure. In this respect the biological reserves of the patient are of considerably more importance than his or her age. In our opinion it is incorrect to lay down an upper age limit, e.g. 70 years, above which all surgical measures for the treatment of bronchial carcinoma are no longer indicated or even contra-indicated: of far more significance are the biological capabilities in relation to the risk factors present (see p. 163). Apart from disturbances in lung function, a series of extrapulmonary risk factors must be considered: disturbances in circulatory function through myocardial and coronary insufficiency, arrhythmia, hypertension, hepatic and renal diseases, metabolic disorders, obesity or undernutrition, alcohol and nicotine abuse, and severe cerebral arteriosclerosis. This list can be extended at will. Nevertheless, the above risk factors in no way represent a contra-indication in the final decision on whether to employ operative measures; rather it is necessary to weigh up the risk in each individual case, bearing in mind also the tumour stage, the presence of any complaints, and complications that could be expected as a result of tumour growth. Patients of advanced biological age and subject to high individual risk constitute the main candidates for organ-sparing operations. In the individual case this means avoiding pneumonectomy by means of plastic techniques on the bronchus itself and/or on the pulmonary artery, or avoiding lobectomy through anatomical or a typical segmental resection. These methods, which should belong to the standard repertoire of every thoracic surgeon, will be discussed later in this chapter.

Functional Risk Factors

In order to make a practicable pre-operative forecast of operative risks, it is advisable to record the relevant data and findings systematically, the importance of each factor being considered in accordance with the frequency of complications which result from it.

In one study (Peter et al. 1980), serious or lethal postoperative complications in the form of renal failure, cardiovascular insufficiency and pulmonary insufficiency occurred in a ratio of 1:3:4.5. Less common complications were hepatic failure, septic shock and pulmonary embolism.

The difficulty in assessing the risks systematically consists in the fact that from the vast quantity of available data one must select a limited number of factors which will make possible a reliable determination of the operative risks. On the one hand there is the danger of considering too many data, on the other, of considering too few data in an effort to produce a simple and easily surveyable system. In the risk evaluation prior to pulmonary surgery, disturbances in lung function play a domi-nant role (so-called functional operability). The risk values of preoperative lung function for spirometry (VC, FEV_1, FEV_1/VC, MVV and RV/TLC), for body plethysmography (R_{aw}), for blood gas analysis (PaO_{2ex} and $PaCO_{2ex}$) and for measurement of pulmonary arterial pressure (PAP_{ex}) are listed in Table 3 (Kristers-son 1974; Matthys and Ruehle 1976).

The flowchart shown in Fig. 2 can be used to evaluate functional operability and to plan pre-operative therapy (Brindley et al. 1982; Fabel 1983; Loddenkemper 1983; Olsen et al. 1975). In this chart the areas of risk are differentiated into various grades of risk, up to inoperability.

Screening or Basic Investigations

1. Besides alterations in the acid-base balance, analysis of blood gases permits an appraisal of the presence of hypoxia or hypercapnia at rest or on exercise. This is

Table 3. Risk values for pre-operative lung function

Vital capacity	VC	under	3.0 l
Forced expired volume in one second	FEV_1	under	2.0 l
Ratio	FEV_1/VC	under	50%
Maximal voluntary ventilation	MVV	under	60 l min^{-1}
Residual volume/total lung capacity	RV/TLC	over	50%
Resistance after bronchodilators	R_{aw}	over	0.5 kPa l^{-1}s
			5.0 cmH$_2$0/l/s
Arterial O$_2$ pressure on exercise	P_aO_{2ex}	under	7.3 kPa
			55 mmHg
Arterial CO$_2$ pressure on exercise	P_aCO_{2ex}	over	6.0 kPa
			45 mmHg
Mean pulmonary arterial pressure on exercise	PAP_{ex}	over	4.7 kPa
			35 mmHg

important as a pre-operative investigation for comparison of the intra-operative and postoperative alterations in blood gases.

2. Spirometry with determination of VC, FEV_1, FEV_1/VC and MVV serves for evaluation of ventilatory reserve.

Normal ventilation is distinguished from restriction or obstruction by means of the measured vital capacity in relation to the normal value and the ratio of forced expired volume in one second to the vital capacity measured. If the basic investigations of spirometry and analysis of blood gases show restriction or obstruction with or without alteration of blood gases, then prior bronchodilator therapy lasting as a rule from 3 to 4 days is carried out, in addition to absolute prohibition of smoking. Besides the effect of a possible improvement, especially of the ventilatory values, the patients can learn the breathing exercises which are necessary after lung resection. The result of therapy is checked by repeat lung function tests.

Inoperability is present in those cases in which the analysis of blood gases on exercise reveals on the one hand arterial hypoxia under 7.3 kPa or on the other hand arterial hypoxia in combination with hypercapnia of more than 6.0 kPa.

Split Function Studies or Supplementary Investigations

On occasion pulmonary function tests such as those described above may be insufficient to assess accurately high-risk patients for surgery. Since the total ventilatory capacity is related to the total perfusion of the pulmonary parenchyma, lung resection will cause a reduction in ventilatory capacity, which, with limitations, corresponds to the amount of functional pulmonary parenchyma removed. The latter can be assessed beforehand by perfusion scintigraphy, which is carried out if the FEV_1 is less than 2.0 litres for a planned pneumonectomy/bilobectomy and less than 1.7 litres for a lobectomy.

By multiplication of the pre-operative FEV_1 with the perfusion of the residual lung (as predicted for after resection) expressed as a percentage of the total perfusion, the postoperative ventilatory capacity can be pre-calculated according to the formula of Kristersson (1974):

$$FEV_1 \text{ (postop)} = \frac{FEV_1 \text{ (preop)} \times \text{perfusion of the residual lung}}{\% \text{ total perfusion}}$$

100

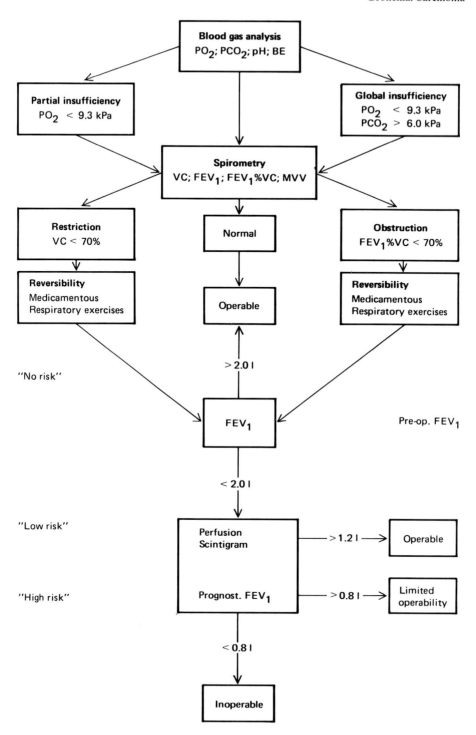

Fig. 2. Pre-operative lung function testing: a flow chart.

This postoperative ventilatory capacity determined semi-quantitatively before operation (expressed by the prognostic FEV_1) is the major functional parameter for evaluation of surgery in risk patients: for pneumonectomy/bilobectomy a pre-operative FEV_1 in excess of 2.0 litres or for lobectomy a pre-operative FEV_1 in excess of 1.7 litres means that surgery involves no functional risk. If, however, pre-operative FEV_1 is less than these guide values, then the prognostic FEV_1 is calculated with the formula according to Kristersson. If the prognostic FEV_1 is more than 1.2 litres, there is operability with low risk. If the prognostic FEV_1 is less than 1.0 litres prior to an intended pneumonectomy or less than 0.8 litres prior to a lobectomy, then there is inoperability. With FEV_1 values between 0.8 and 1.2 litres, the pulmonary arterial pressure on exercise (PAP_{ex}) and/or the airway resistance (R_{aw}) can be measured before and after bronchodilators as a further supplementary investigation of pulmonary function.

In the presence of high risk, there is a limited operability when the pulmonary arterial pressure remains over 4.7 kPa or R_{aw} is over 0.5 kPa 1^{-1}s after bronchodilators.

In the presence of borderline values, it must not be overlooked that the causation of postoperative complications or mortality is multifactorial. Every prediction which is based on only one cardiopulmonary function is necessarily incomplete (Grabor and Ehehalt 1971; Wassner and Timm 1977).

Whether the surgeon removes tissue which is functioning, tissue which is not involved in gas exchange or even tissue which impairs pulmonary function (shunt tissue) is also important for postoperative function (Lockwood 1973). Figure 3 shows the dependence of 30-day mortality on the kind of operation and on the function risk according to Loddenkemper (1983). The high 30-day mortality in extended pneumonectomies or bilobectomies when existing function is poor should be noted; this is an additional indication of the necessity of using types of operation which preserve parenchyma.

Besides the functional state of all vital organs, the general clinical condition of the patient and his readiness to undergo surgery also play a major role in the result.

Despite borderline lung function, a pulmonary operation may be tolerated in the individual case when adequate peri-operative treatment is ensured. This is illustrated by the following example: In a 66-year-old male patient, a wedge incision for bronchial carcinoma ($T_1N_0M_0$), extirpation of a large cyst and decortication were carried out without severe postoperative complications despite multiple functional risk values. The pre-operative FEV_1 was 0.85 litres, the ratio of FEV_1/VC was 29%, the MVV was 30 litres/min, the ratio RV/TLC was 54%, the airway resistance (R_{aw}) was 0.92 kPa 1^{-1}s before and 0.5 kPa 1^{-1}s after bronchodilators, and the 60-Watt exercise P_aO_2 and P_aCO_2 were 9.04 and 7.86 kPa respectively. The warning must be sounded, however, that under extreme risk conditions such an operation is justified only when carried out by an experienced group which has complete mastery of the peri-operative treatment and only when there is opitmal co-operation from the patient.

In every risk patient, there is on the one hand the possibility of not undertaking an operation which might be feasible because of inadequate registration of pre-operative risks, and on the other hand of making a "respiratory cripple" out of the patient by carrying out pulmonary resection on the basis of a false estimation of the existing risk factors.

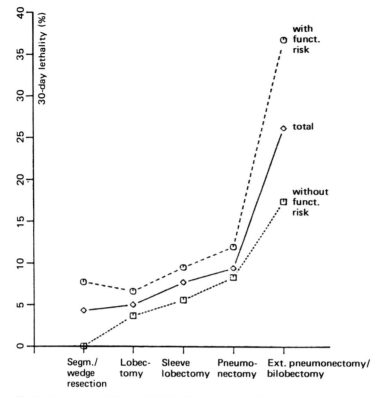

Fig. 3. Dependence of 30-day lethality (%) on the kind of operation and the functional risk according to Loddenkemper.

Preparation for Surgery

Better evaluation of the risk of surgery in terms of lung function is to be expected after carrying out adequate short-term therapy.

The major complications after lung operations include pulmonary atelectasis; the development of postoperative lung failure should be mentioned in this connection. The pre-operative measures against the danger of postoperative pulmonary atelectasis comprise:

1. Improvement of general state of health
2. Absolute abstention from smoking and reduction in alcohol intake
3. Active bronchial clearance with chest physiotherapy, bronchodilators and possibly steroids
4. If indicated, antibiotic treatment

Improvement of General State of Health

Special attention is paid to clearance of the teeth, to good serum albumin values and to a reduction in obesity.

Abstention from Smoking

The patients must be routinely informed of the adverse effect of smoking on the bronchial mucosa and their capacity to expectorate sputum. Nicotine paralyses the cilia of the bronchial mucosa. Even a few days of abstinence from smoking leads to an improvement in ciliary activity.

Bronchial Clearance

Patients frequently have chronic bronchitis in addition to their lung disease requiring surgery. This bronchitis must be improved with (a) breathing exercises; (b) inhalation therapy with bronchodilators, broncholytics and expectorants; and (c) adequate, specific drug therapy.

After pre-treatment for 8 days, pulmonary function is repeated to check the degree of improvement.

Breathing Exercises

The breathing exercises are carried out with the goal of (a) imparting a correct technique of expiration for training and retraining of the respiratory musculature, (b) mobilising the thorax and diaphragm, and (c) improving bronchial clearance. In "wet" lungs (sputum volume more than 20–30 cm³ daily), with bronchitis, bronchiectasis and infected cysts, directed coughing is carried out with changes in the patient's posture. Operations should only be carried out when the amount of sputum declines to below 20 cm³, if possible.

Inhalation Therapy

In inhalation therapy, the following distinctions are made, depending on the method used:

1. Active aerosol inhalation with an ultrasonic or jet nebuliser (driven either by compressed air or a compressor).
2. Passive or tidal inhalation with intermittent positive pressure ventilation (IPPV) via a mouthpiece. Pre-operative inhalation should render the patients familiar with the instruments and methods for postoperative continuation of the treatment.

All patients are subjected to physiotherapy before operation, and this is continued postoperatively. The physiotherapy exercises are a proven means of mobilising the patient for the impending operation. As preparation for surgery, the patient is also given an information sheet. He is instructed to train his breathing and his circulation before and after the operation. This information sheet should also enable him to understand better the unpleasant features associated with the operation.

The pre-operative and postoperative breathing exercises should, if possible, be carried out by the same personnel, since the patients and the personnel know each other. In this way, the efficiency of this important treatment measure is clearly improved.

Inadequate preparation is manifested in an increased rate of postoperative complications. The poorer the preparation, the more frequently is mechanical (bronchoscopic) bronchial clearance necessary postoperatively.

The pre-operative breathing exercises are carried out in patient groups for at least 1 week for half an hour a day. There is concentration on the following: breathing against resistance, e.g. by means of a belt, and exercises in the standing position for general mobilisation and expanding the thorax. Depending on the strength of the patient, exercise with a bicycle ergometer in the sitting position may be instituted.

Drug Therapy

Prior therapy with drugs includes:

Cardiac Glycosides. Pre-operative digitalisation is indicated only in patients with manifest or latent myocardial insufficiency, after prior myocardial infarction, in hypertensives and in patients with atrial fibrillation or atrial flutter. The risks involved in digitalisation due to increased sensitivity of the myocardium to digitalis or to existing overdigitalisation with the danger of ventricular systoles are reduced by monitoring the patient's ECG and determining the digitalis levels.

Antibiotics. Antibiotic prophylaxis is very problematic because of the development of resistance. For this reason, antibiotics are only administered in accordance with the sputum culture and sensitivities in clinically manifest bronchopulmonary infections. If prophylactic administration is decided on, sufficiently high antibiotic levels must be present in the blood and tissue at the time of surgery in order to kill bacteria which have reached the wound and to inhibit their growth. The first dose should hence be applied just before the operation, the optimal time being during the induction of anaesthesia. In the choice of the drug, one must take into account the pathogenic bacteria prevalent in the hospital. Peri-operative antibiotic prophylaxis should not be carried out for more than 24 hours. These measures are controversial at present.

Antidiabetic Agents: Diabetes mellitus invariably increases the surgical risk. Besides the alterations in the vessel wall to be expected and the raised risk of infection, metabolic adjustment of the diabetic can give rise to appreciable difficulties in the postoperative phase. There is a danger of hyperglycaemia as well as of hypoglycaemia caused by overdosage of insulin; in addition, there is the danger of unstable diabetes in the postoperative phase. For this reason, virtually every diabetic is switched to insulin before planned pulmonary resection; the blood and urine sugar is checked regularly and the urine for ketones once a day.

Alcohol abuse constitutes a high risk because of the danger of alcohol withdrawal and delirium tremens occurring postoperatively. In cases of known or suspected alcohol abuse (after questioning of the family and observation on the ward), an adequate period of abstinence with surveillance must be maintained at least during the preparation period.

β-Blockers. Abrupt discontinuation of any long-term hypotensive therapy may be dangerous. Although β-blockers may have a prolonged effect, nevertheless this may be insufficient to prevent dysrhythmias during operation for example. Furthermore, during operation the blood pressure may be labile, particularly with loss of circulating blood volume, the correction of which may require transfusion which itself may precipitate heart failure, especially in patients who have undergone pneumo-nectomy.

As a matter of principle, patients receiving anticoagulant treatment are trans-ferred to heparin, since in potentially fatal haemorrhage the effect of heparin can be abolished very much more rapidly than that of coumarin preparations or acetylsali-cylic acid. With the latter, normal clotting function does not return for 4-6 days after complete replacement of the thrombocytes in the circulation owing to the alteration of their surface properties. In the switch to heparin, a dosage of 3×5000 IU/day can be recommended. Pre-operative or intra-operative administration of partial prothrombin complexes is indicated only in emergency operations and in the presence of Quick values below 30%.

In patients receiving cytotoxic treatment, a treatment interval of at least 2 weeks is observed before operation. After long-term administration of cytotoxics, latent side-effects may persist. Frequently, the functional range of the bone marrow may thus be markedly restricted over a very long period. This applies above all to alkylating agents. After treatment with vincristine, ileus, after adriamycin cardio-toxic side-effects and after bleomycin disorders of lung function due to pulmonary fibrosis may be observed.

Conclusion

The more carefully the pre-operative risks are delimited (i.e. by determination of the risk factors, their prophylactic treatment and the general preparation of the patient), the less severe are the postoperative complications. According to our experience, these measures render prophylactic elective tracheotomy superfluous.

References

Brindley Valter G Jr, Walsh RE, Schnarr WT, Allen GW, Mendenhall MK, Ahlgren EW (1982) Pulmonary resection in patients with impaired pulmonary function. Surg Clin North Am 62:207-210

Carr DT (1973) Diagnosis, staging and criteria of response to therapy for lung cancer. Cancer Chemother Rep 3, 4:303-305

Carter StK (1979) Introduction – what has happened in the last five years. In: Muggia F, Rozencweig M (eds) Lung cancer: Progress in therapeutic research. Raven, New York, pp 1-12

Deneffe G, Lacquet LM, Gyselen A (1983) Cervical mediastinoscopy and anterior mediastinotomy in patients with lung cancer and radiologically normal mediastinum. Eur J Respir Dis 64:613-619

Dombernowsky P, Hirsch F, Hansen HH, Hainau B (1978) Peritoneoscopy in the staging of 190 patients with small-cell anaplastic carcinoma of the lung with special reference to subtyping. Cancer 41:2008-2012

Fabel H (1973) Funktionsstörungen des Lungenkrieslaufes und des Gasaustausches und ihre Bedeutung für die Lungenresektion. Thoraxchirurgie 21:258-262

Goldberg EM, Shapiro CM, Glicksman AS (1974) Mediastinoscopy for assessing mediastinal spread in clinical staging of lung carcinoma. Semin Oncol 1:205-215

Grabow L, Ehehalt V (1971) Die Zuverlässigkeit der präoperativen Funktionsprüfung für endothorakale Eingriffe. Pneumonologie 147:167-170

Grunze H (1962) Tumoren der Thoraxorgane. In: Bartelheimer H, Maurer HJ (eds) Diagnostik der Geschwulstkrankheiten. Thieme, Stuttgart

Jolly PC, Hill LD, Lawless PA, West TL (1973) Parasternal mediastinotomy and mediastinoscopy. Adjuncts in the diagnosis of chest disease. J Thorac Cardiovasc Surg 4:549–556

Karnofsky D, Abelmann WH, Craver LF et al. (1948) The use of nitrogen mustards in the palliative treatment of carcinoma with particular reference to bronchogenic carcinoma. Cancer 1:634–656

Konrad RM, Schulte HD (1969) Die Aussagefahigkeit der Mediastinoskopie zur Beurteilung der Operabilität des Bronchuskarzinoms. Dtsch Med Wochenschr 94:368–372

Kristersson S (1974) Pre-operative evaluation of differential lung function (133_{xe}-radiospirometry) in bronchial carcinoma. Scand J Respir Dis (Suppl) 85:110–117

Lockwood P (1973) Lung function test results and the risk of post-thoracotomy complications. Respiration 30:529–542

Loddenkemper R (1983) Funktionelle Operabilität beim Bronchialkarzinom (prospektive Studie zur Einschaetzung des Operationsrisikos und der postoperativen Lungenfunktion). Habilitationsschrift, Klinikum Charlottenburg der Freien Universitat Berlin

Maassen W (1967) Ergebnisse und Bedeutung der Mediastinoskopie und anderer thoraxbioptischer Verfahren. Springer, Berlin Heidelberg New York

Margolis R, Hansen HH, Muggia FM, Kanhouwa S (1974) Diagnosis of liver metastases in bronchogenic carcinoma. A comparative study of liver scans, function tests, and peritoneoscopy with liver biopsy in 111 patients. Cancer 34:1825–1928

Matthys H, Rühle KH (1976) Lungenfunktionsdiagnostik zur Erfassung des Risikopatienten in der Anaesthesiologie. In: Klin Anasthesiol Intensivther 12:8–13

Muggia FM, Chervu LR (1974) Lung cancer: diagnosis in metastases sites. Semin Oncol 1:217–228

Olsen GN, Black AJ, Swenson EW, Castle JR, Wynne JW (1975) Pulmonary function evaluation of the lung resection candidate. Am Rev Respir Dis 111:379–387

Pearson FG, Nelems JM, Henderson RD, Delarue NC (1972) The role of mediastinoscopy in the selection of treatment for bronchial carcinoma with involvement of superior mediastinal lymph nodes. J Thorac Cardiovasc Surg 64:382–340

Peter K, Unertl K, Heinrich G, Mai N, Brunner F (1980) Das Anaesthesierisiko. Anaesthesiol Intensivmed 9: 240–248

Vanderhoeft P (1979) Regional pre-operative staging of cancer of the left lung. EORTC Symposium on Progress and Perspectives in Lung Cancer Treatment, Brussels

Vogt-Moykopf I, Lullig H (1976) Resultats de biopsie dans le epanchements pleuraux suspects de malignite. Broncho-Pneumologie 26:515–520

Wassner UJ, Timm J (1977) Über die kardioplumonale Insuffizienz nach Lungenresektion und ihre Vermeidung. Zentralbl Chir 102:598–601

Chapter 9

The Histological Varieties of Bronchial Carcinoma

Allen R. Gibbs and Roger M. E. Seal

Introduction

It is important to realise that lung cancer is not a homogeneous entity but instead comprises a number of different histopathological groups and subgroups. A knowledge of the histopathology of lung tumours is not just of academic interest but provides a better framework for ascertaining the aetiology of a given tumour, predicting outcome and determining treatment. For example, small cell carcinoma behaves in a very different way from other types of lung cancer; it metastasises very early and is very often surgically inoperable by the time of diagnosis. On the other hand squamous cell carcinoma, if localised to the lung at operative resection, has a relatively good prognosis. The incidence of squamous cell carcinoma and small cell carcinoma is greatly increased in smokers whereas adenocarcinoma does not show as great an increase.

In this chapter we shall concentrate mainly on the four major groups of lung cancer, viz. squamous cell, small cell, adeno- and large cell carcinoma. We utilise the second edition of the WHO classification of lung tumours for the major groups of lung carcinoma (Table 1). The second WHO classification (World Health Organisation 1981) is reasonably comprehensive and reproducible for the major groups of lung carcinoma, with surprisingly good correlation between small endoscopic

Table 1. Second WHO classification of major groups of lung carcinoma

1. Squamous cell carcinoma (epidermoid carcinoma)
   Variant:
   a) Spindle cell (squamous) carcinoma
2. Small cell carcinoma
   a) Oat cell carcinoma
   b) Intermediate cell type
   c) Combined oat cell carcinoma
3. Adenocarcinoma
   a) Acinar adenocarcinoma
   b) Papillary adenocarcinoma
   c) Bronchiolo-alveolar carcinoma
   d) Solid carcinoma with mucus formation
4 Large cell carcinoma
   Variants:
   a) Giant cell carcinoma
   b) Clear cell carcinoma
5. Adenosquamous carcinoma

biopsy, cytological material and more adequate resection material. However, occasionally a tumour may prove more or less differentiated than the endoscopy biopsy indicated. The histopathological classification of lung tumours is based upon cytological, architectural and histochemical criteria.

Pulmonary tumours can be divided into central (arising from a main, lobar or segmental bronchus) or peripheral (arising distal to a segmental bronchus) (Figs. 1 and 2). Central lesions tend to produce obstructive effects clinically, such as obstructive pneumonitis, bronchiectasis, mucocele, suppuration and rarely obstructive emphysema (Gibbs and Seal 1982a). Peripheral tumours tend to produce symptoms when they become large and/or necrotic, or by involvement of the overlying pleura to produce pain and/or pleural effusions. Apart from local effects, tumours may produce distant effects (a) without evident metastasis (by ill-understood means, e.g. subacute cerebellar degeneration or peripheral neuropathy, or by inappropriate hormone production) or (b) with metastatic spread. The histopathology of the tumour often gives an indication of its behaviour, e.g. small cell carcinoma may produce ACTH and cause Cushing's syndrome; squamous cell carcinoma may produce parathormone and result in hypercalcaemia (see p. 27).

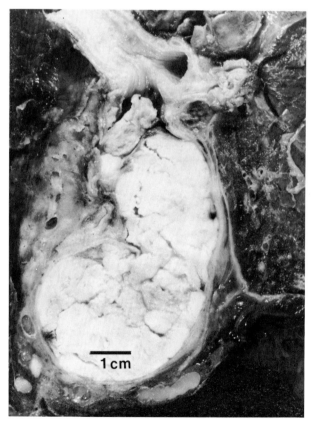

Fig. 1. A central tumour expanding a segmental bronchus. The mucoceles, which are a consequence of the bronchial obstruction, can be seen surrounding the tumour.

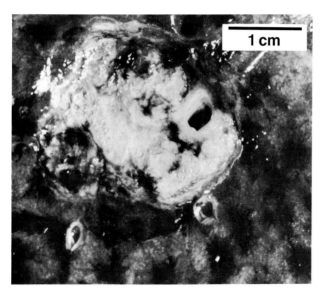

Fig. 2. A peripheral adenocarcinoma occurring in the lung of an ex-miner. Anthracotic foci can be seen in the background lung.

Pathologists and Staging

One of the major problems affecting clinical staging is that the radiological opacities in central tumours are produced partly by the tumour and often largely by secondary inflammatory and mechanical consequences of obstruction. The pathologist's contribution to clinical staging of the tumour includes recognition of pleural involvement by examining pleural biopsies and the demonstration of lymph node involvement after mediastinoscopy. After surgical resection the pathologist should provide a detailed account of the size and extent of the tumour, the involvement or otherwise of visceral and/or parietal pleura, the resected edge of bronchus and regional lymph nodes.

Squamous Cell (Epidermoid) Carcinoma

This type of lung carcinoma appears to be the most common in most series reported from Great Britain and the United States. However, this observation may be apparent rather than real. Melamed and Zaman (1982) have found the prevalence of squamous cell carcinoma to be higher that that of adenocarcinoma but the incidence to be lower, indicating that squamous carcinomas have a slower growth rate than adenocarcinomas. Therefore squamous cell carcinomas appear to be longer clinically occult.

More than two-thirds of squamous cell carcinomas arise from segmental or larger bronchi and thus tend to produce obstructive effects. They are more common in the upper lobes.

Macroscopically, they appear as white or grey, firm, well defined tumours frequently showing necrosis and cavitation. In the rare cases of in situ carcinoma the bronchial mucosa can appear normal or thickened and pale, with loss of ridges and bronchial gland orifices (Melamed and Zaman 1982).

The histological diagnosis of squamous cell carcinoma requires the demonstration of either keratin or intercellular bridges (Fig. 3). It is not sufficient to show stratification without keratin or intercellular bridges. The tumour cells possess hyperchromatic, angulated, pleomorphic nuclei and dense, eosinophilic cytoplasm. Intercellular bridges, cytoplasmic keratin and epithelial pearls are frequent and easily seen in well differentiated tumours but are less frequent and may have to be diligently searched for in poorly differentiated tumours. This tumour often elicits a marked desmoplastic reaction and inflammatory cell response (Fig. 4). The adjacent mucosa may appear normal or show combinations of squamous metaplasia, dysplasia and in situ carcinoma (Fig. 5). With regard to the latter, the surgeon and pathologist must realise that most small flexible endoscopic fragments, though sufficient to diagnose squamous cell carcinoma, often fail to indicate invasion of submucosa, though in almost all instances an invasive intrabronchial growth has been biopsied.

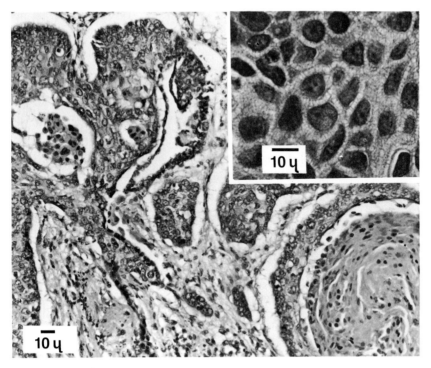

Fig. 3. A well differentiated squamous carcinoma showing stratifications and abundant keratin. *Inset*: Intercellular bridges.

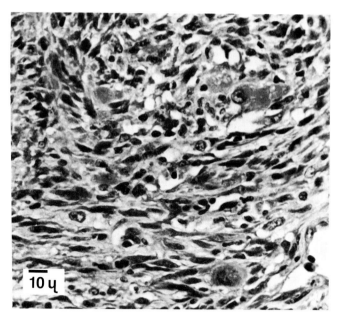

Fig. 4. A moderately differentiated squamous carcinoma showing a florid fibrous stromal reaction (desmoplasia).

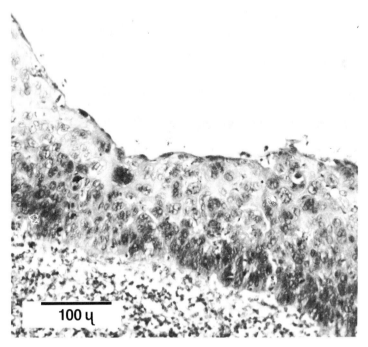

Fig. 5. A bronchial biopsy revealed in situ squamous carcinoma but no invasion. The later resection specimen manifested obvious invasive carcinoma.

We routinely stain all resected lung carcinomas for mucin and we have observed foci of mucin-containing cells in about 10% of otherwise typical squamous cell carcinomas without evidence of glandular formation. This presumably reflects the fact that by electron microscopic examination lung tumours frequently show evidence of more than one type of differentiation (McDowell et al. 1978). We still type these tumours as squamous cell carcinomas but there is room for a study of the relationship of this finding to prognosis.

On rare occasions squamous cell carcinoma may have a pronounced spindle celled component. This has to be differentiated from carcinosarcoma (Litchtiger et al. 1970). Evidence for it being a spindled squamous cell carcinoma is the appearance of merging between obvious squamous cells and spindle cells (Fig. 6). These tumours are usually central polypoid lesions.

The prognosis of squamous cell carcinoma is dependent upon clinical stage. There is almost 100% 5-year survival for in situ carcinoma; 70% 5-year survival for stage I; but less than 10% 5-year survival for stages II and III (Melamed and Zaman 1982). Prognosis also varies with the histological grade, being better in well differentiated than in poorly differentiated squamous cell carcinomas (Goldman 1965; Katlic and Carter 1979).

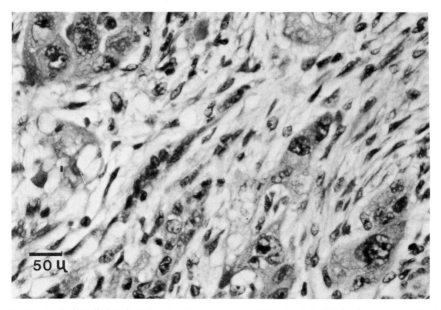

Fig. 6. A spindle celled variant showing three plump keratinised cells indicating its squamous origin.

Small Cell Carcinoma

There is considerable evidence to indicate that small cell carcinoma is derived from endocrine cells. These tumours may contain areas resembling carcinoid tumours;

their cells contain neurosecretory granules ultrastructurally, and they are frequently associated with 'ectopic' hormone production (Bensch et al. 1968).

Small cell carcinomas account for about a quarter of lung cancers. Two-thirds are centrally located and approximately three-quarters are situated in the upper lobes. Macroscopically, the tumours appear as grey-white bulky, soft, fleshy, friable lesions often with areas of necrosis. Involvement of the bronchial mucosa by the tumour leads to thickening and narrowing of the lumen.

The second edition of the WHO classification (World Health Organisation 1981) subdivides small cell carcinoma into:

1. Oat cell carcinoma
2. Intermediate cell type
3. Combined oat cell carcinoma

The oat cell (lymphocyte-like) carcinoma is composed of relatively uniform small cells, about twice the size of a lymphocyte, containing round, oval or carrot-shaped nuclei and scanty basophilic cytoplasm (Fig. 7).

The cells of the intermediate cell type are about half as big again as the oat cell type, and they have round, oval, fusiform or polygonal nuclei with a more open chromatin pattern. Their cytoplasm is sparse but more easily recognised than the oat cell type. Mitoses are readily identified (Fig. 8).

The combined oat cell carcinoma contains foci of squamous or glandular differentiation in addition to the usual oat cell pattern.

All the subtypes of small cell carcinoma may show an arrangement of the cells into sheets, cords, ribbons or pseudorosettes. There is little collagen and inflammatory infiltrate within the tumour. Areas of necrosis are usually conspicuous and in relation to this necrosis, marked basophilic staining of blood vessels and connective tissue by DNA is often seen (Azzopardi 1959) (Fig. 7). A problem facing the pathologist is that small cell carcinomas have a marked tendency to distort by 'crushing' during the biopsy procedure, sometimes so much so that doubt exists regarding the true nature of the lesion.

Small cell carcinoma of the lung has a very poor prognosis, dissemination via the bloodstream and lymphatics occurring very early in the disease. Widespread metastases may be evident when there is only a small primary tumour present within the lung. No clear-cut differences in clinical behaviour have emerged between the various subtypes.

Adenocarcinoma

Adenocarcinomas are characterised by their ability to form glandular structures or mucin within the tumour cells. They may be graded into well, moderately or poorly differentiated tumours according to the prevalence of glandular structures.

More than 90% of these tumours are peripherally located within the lung and they are more common in the upper lobes. They are often subpleural. They are firm, grey and circumscribed with well defined borders or soft, slimy and necrotic. Varying amounts of anthracotic pigment are seen. Rarely an adenocarcinoma may infiltrate the pleura and grow to encase the lung, thus simulating a malignant mesothelioma

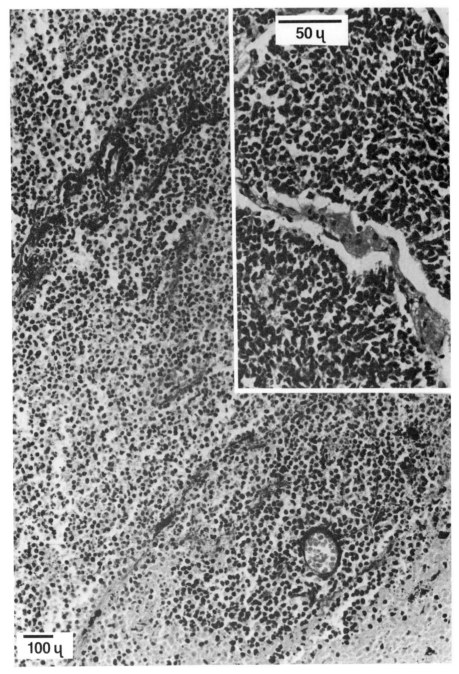

Fig. 7. Oat cell carcinoma showing haematoxyphilic staining of vessel walls. *Inset* shows cells contain dark nuclei with sparse ill-defined cytoplasm.

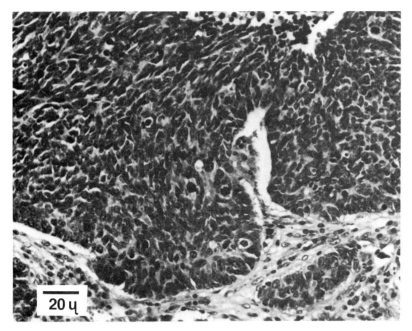

Fig. 8. Small cell intermediate carcinoma showing fusiform and polygonal cells.

(Harwood et al. 1976). Regional lymph node involvement is frequently present, even when the tumour is small.

Adenocarcinoma frequently occurs in patients with pre-existing lung fibrosis. Sometimes adenocarcinoma 'haloes' a localised scar — so-called scar cancer (Raeburn and Spencer 1953). Another recognised combination is cryptogenic fibrosing alveolitis and adenocarcinoma (Meyer and Liebow 1965), and of increasing importance and recognition is the association between lung cancer and asbestos-induced pulmonary fibrosis (Gibbs and Seal 1981b) (Fig. 9). There is no doubt as to the causative role of heavy asbestos exposure sufficient to cause overt 'asbestosis', but there is conflicting evidence of the importance of lesser exposure with mural fibrosis, and the presence of only a few asbestos bodies in the lung parenchyma of lung cancer patients.

The second WHO classification subdivides adenocarcinoma into four subtypes:

1. Acinar adenocarcinoma
2. Papillary adenocarcinoma
3. Bronchiolo-alveolar carcinoma
4. Solid carcinoma with mucus formation

Acinar Adenocarcinoma

Acinar adenocarcinomas usually develop in segmental or subsegmental bronchi. They may appear as sessile endobronchial polyps or circumscribed peribronchial

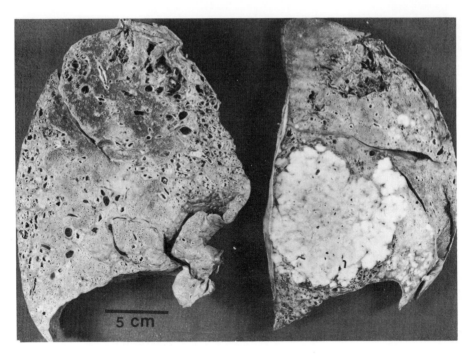

Fig. 9. Bilateral pleural plaques in an asbestos worker. Extensive interstitial fibrosis with honeycombing can be seen in the upper and lower lobes of both lungs. There is also a large peripheral carcinoma in the lower lobe. This tumour was not attributed to asbestos exposure, however, since several asbestos counts were taken and varied between 5000 and 60 000/g of dried lung tissue.

growths. They are characterised by a predominance of acinar and tubular structures (Fig. 10). In addition, papillary or solid areas may be present. Signet ring cells or psammoma bodies may be present on occasion. They often produce considerable mucin. Ultrastructural studies indicate an origin from bronchial mucous glands or bronchial surface epithelium (Kodama et al. 1982).

Papillary Adenocarcinoma

Papillary adenocarcinomas are usually peripheral tumours. They are characterised by a predominance of papillary structures (Fig. 11). In addition, small foci of acini and tubules may be seen. If, as occurs occasionally, the acinar and papillary components appear approximately equal, it should be designated acinar and papillary adenocarcinoma. The papillae have connective tissue cores and are lined by either tall, columnar, non-mucus secreting cells or low columnar peg-shaped cells. Distinction from bronchiolo-alveolar carcinoma may be difficult but papillary adenocarcinomas possess a greater amount of fibrous tissue in their cores. Ultrastructural studies have shown the epithelial cells of some of the papillary adenocarcinomas to possess features of non-mucus secreting bronchial surface epithelial cells, whilst others have features of Clara cells or rarely type II pneumocytes (Shimosato et al. 1982).

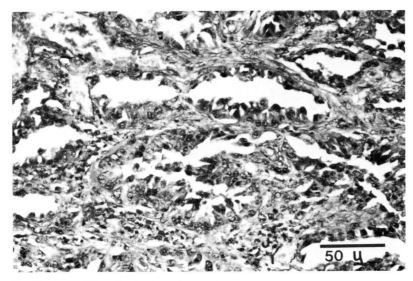

Fig. 10. A well differentiated acinar adenocarcinoma.

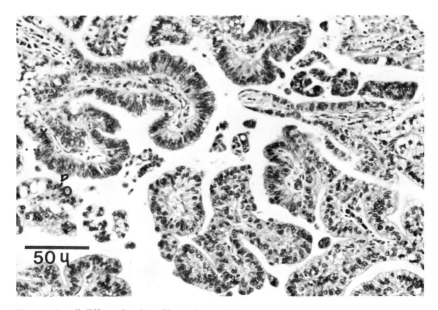

Fig. 11. A well differentiated papillary adenocarcinoma.

Bronchiolo-alveolar Carcinoma (alveolar cell carcinoma, pulmonary adenomatosis)

Bronchiolo-alveolar carcinomas comprise 1%–8% of primary lung malignancies. The tumour first grows as a solitary mass, often in association with a scar, but later forms multiple masses, often affecting both lungs. Sometimes the tumour grows diffusely to look macroscopically like type III pneumococcal pneumonia. Bronchiolo-alveolar carcinomas are often associated with a distinct clinical picture of voluminous bronchorrhea, increasing dyspnoea and cyanosis.

The tumour cells characteristically grow upon and along an intact bronchioloalveolar framework (Fig. 12). Two main cell patterns are seen (Greenberg et al. 1975):

1. Tall columnar cells with bland basal nuclei, forming single rows along delicate alveolar septae and focal papillary infoldings; they may or may not secrete mucin.

2. Low columnar, pleomorphic cells with thickened alveolar septae; the cells contain little or no mucin.

Ultrastructural studies have revealed the cells of some of the tumours to have characteristics similar to bronchiolar mucus cells, whilst others possess features of Clara cells or type II pneumonocytes (Greenberg et al. 1975; Adamson et al. 1968; Kuhn 1972).

Stage I bronchiolo-alveolar carcinoma treated by lobectomy has been reported to have a 5-year survival rate of approximately 50% (Too et al. 1978).

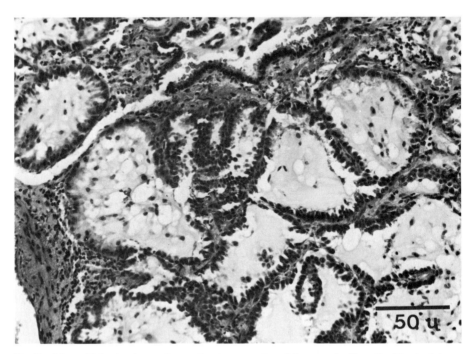

Fig. 12. A bronchiolo-alveolar carcinoma showing parenchymal framework of lung lined by single layer of columnar cells with basal nuclei and with overt mucin secretion.

Solid Carcinoma with Mucus Formation

Solid carcinoma with mucus formation appears to be identical to large cell carcinoma on conventional haematoxylin and eosin sections. However, histochemical stains for mucin reveal the presence of intracellular mucin. The tumour cells have large nuclei, prominent nucleoli, abundant cytoplasm and grow in sheets without the formation of acini or tubules.

Large Cell Carcinoma

This tumour consists of large cells with large vesicular nuclei, prominent nucleoli and copious homogeneous cytoplasm growing in sheets without any evidence of squamous, glandular or small cell differentiation (Fig. 13). The more material is available for examination of a given tumour, the less common is the diagnosis of large cell carcinoma; this is because one is more likely to find a focus of glandular, small cell or squamous differentiation.

Large cell carcinomas are usually bulky, ovoid, soft, grey fleshy masses. They may show foci of necrosis but do not generally cavitate. Approximately 50% are peripheral and 50% central in location. The central tumours do not manifest adjacent in situ carcinomatous change.

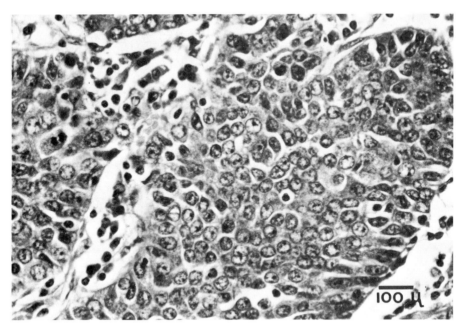

Fig. 13. Large cell carcinoma showing sheets of pleomorphic cells with copious cytoplasm. In spite of the stratified appearance, the absence of keratin and intercellular bridge designates this a large cell carcinoma.

The tumours usually have a delicate stroma. Mitoses are frequently observed. Electron microscopic studies have revealed a variety of features, including squamous, glandular, undifferentiated, endocrine and Clara cells (Bolen and Thorning 1982; Churg 1978; Sidhu 1982).

Large cell carcinoma is treated similarly to squamous cell and adenocarcinoma. Prognosis depends upon stage. Rubinstein et al. (1979) found that of those operated upon, the 5-year survival rate for large cell carconoma without nodal involvement was 52%, whereas with lymph node metastases it was only 10%.

The second WHO classification included two variants of large cell carcinoma: (a) giant cell carcinoma and (b) clear cell carcinoma.

Giant Cell Carcinoma

Giant cell carcinoma is characterised by numerous bizarre giant cells which show cannibalism of leukocytes. Although, in the WHO classification, this tumour is included in the large cell carcinoma group, these tumours may evince foci of glandular or squamous differentiaton. It is a peripheral tumour, frequently large with areas of necrosis. It has often invaded the chest wall by the time of diagnosis.

Microscopically, the striking feature is the presence of bizarre multinucleated cells with abundant eosinophilic cytoplasm containing leukocytes and lymphocytes. The background cells are polygonal or spindled and tend to lack cohesion. The tumour cells are admixed with white blood cells (Fig. 14).

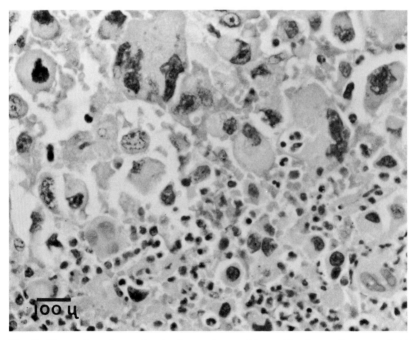

Fig. 14. Giant cell carcinoma showing large, pleomorphic, multinucleate cells, some of which contain white blood cells. A prominent leukocytic infiltrate is a feature of this type.

The incidence of the neoplasm has been variously estimated at between 1% and 10% of lung carcinomas (Carter and Eggleston 1980). Clinically, it usually presents at a younger age than the majority of lung cancers and has a rapidly fatal course (Flanagan and Roeckel 1964).

Clear Cell Carcinoma

The second WHO classification restricts this term to a tumour composed of large cells and lacking evidence of glandular or squamous differentiation (Fig. 15). Tumours complying with these criteria are rare. Katzenstein et al. (1980) found only one such tumour out of 348 cases of lung carcinoma whereas they found a further 14 tumours with a content of more than 50% clear cells but which evinced foci of squamous or glandular differentiation. There appeared to be no significant difference in the behaviour between the tumours with a large content of clear cells and the common lung cancer groups.

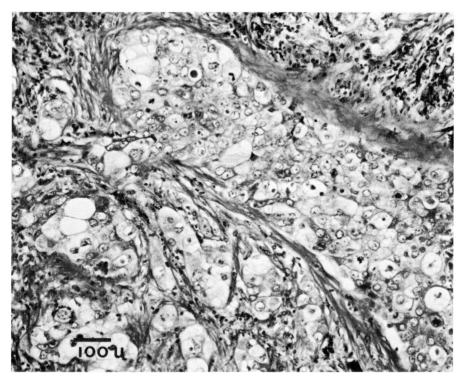

Fig. 15. Clear cell carcinoma composed of sheets of polygonal, large, clear cells which were mucin-negative.

Adenosquamous Carcinoma

These tumours show microscopical features of both squamous and adenocarcinoma in various degrees of differentiation (Fig. 16). The incidence is usually stated to be about 1% of lung carcinomas (Larsson and Zettergren 1976) but in fact careful examination of lung carcinomas will reveal a much higher incidence. To some extent this is borne out by ultrastructural studies, which demonstrate that adeno- and squamous features are commonly present together in lung carcinomas (McDowell et al. 1978). These tumours are said to behave like adenocarcinomas but this requires further study.

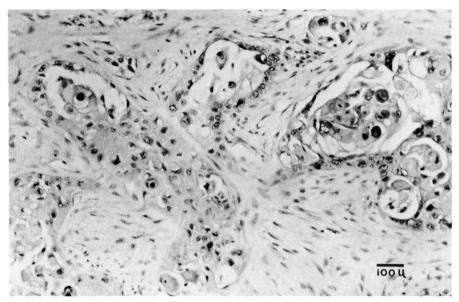

Fig. 16. A well differentiated adenosquamous carcinoma showing both glandular and stromal structures. The fibroblastic stroma is non-neoplastic.

Acknowledgements. We wish to thank Mr. Peter Langham and Mr D. Llewellyn for photographic assistance, and Miss Jayne Stitfall for typing the manuscript.

References

Adamson JS, Senior RM, Merill T (1968) Alveolar cell carcinoma: An electron microscopic study. Am Rev Respir Dis 100:550–557.
Azzopardi JG (1959) Oat cell carcinoma of the bronchus. J Pathol Bacteriol 78:513–519

Bensch KG, Corrin B, Pariente R, Spencer H (1968) Oat cell carcinoma of the lungs: its origin and relationship to bronchial carcinoid. Cancer 22:1163–1172

Bolen JW, Thorning D (1982) Histogenetic classification of pulmonary carcinomas. Pathol Annu 1:77–100

Carter D, Eggleston JC (1980) Giant cell carcinoma. In: Tumours of the lower respiratory tract. Second Series Fascicle, AFIP, Washington 17:155–160

Churg A (1978) The fine structure of large cell undifferentiated carcinoma of the lung. Human Pathol 2:143–156

Flanagan CP, Roeckel IE (1964) Giant cell carcinoma of the lung. Anatomical and clinical correlations. Am J Med 36:214–221

Gibbs AR, Seal RME (1982a) Lung carcinomas. In: Gresham GA (ed) Atlas of pulmonary pathology. MTP Press, Lancaster, pp 103–110

Gibbs AR, Seal RME (1982b) Occupational lung disorders II. Silicate pneumoconioses. In: Gresham GA (ed) Atlas of pulmonary pathology. MTP Press, Lancaster, pp 91–95

Goldman KP (1965) Histology of lung cancer in relation to prognosis. Thorax 20:298–302

Greenberg SD, Smith MN, Spjut HJ (1975) Bronchiolo-alveolar carcinoma — cell of origin. Am J Clin Pathol 63:153–167

Harwood TR, Gracey DR, Yakoo H (1976) Pseudomesotheliomatous carcinoma of the lung. A variant of peripheral lung cancer. Am J Clin Pathol 65:159–167

Katlic M, Carter D (1979) Prognostic implications of histology, size and location of primary tumours. In: Rozencweig M (ed) Treatment of lung cancer. Raven Press, New York, pp 143–150

Katzenstein A-A, Prioleau PG, Askin FB (1980) The histologic spectrum and significance of clear cell change in lung carcinoma. Cancer 45:943–947

Kodama T, Shimosoto Y, Kameya T (1982) Histology and ultrastructure of bronchogenic and bronchial gland adenocarcinomas (including adenoid cystic and mucoepidermoid carcinomas) in relation to histogenesis. In: Shimosato Y, Melamed MR, Nettesheim P (eds) Morphogenesis of lung cancer, vol 1. CRC Press, Boca Raton, vol 1, pp 147–166

Kuhn C (1972) Fine structure of bronchiolo-alveolar carcinoma. Cancer 30: 1107–1118

Larsson S, Zettergren L (1976) Histological typing of lung cancer. Acta Pathol Microbiol Scand A] 84:529–537

Lichtiger B, Mackay B, Tessmer CF (1970) Spindle cell variant of squamous carcinoma. A light and electron microscopic study of 13 cases. Cancer 26:1311–1320

McDowell EM, McLaughlin JS, Mereny DK, Kieffer RF, Harris CC, Trump B (1978) The respiratory epithelium V. Histogenesis of lung carcinomas in the human. J Natl Cancer Inst 61:587–606

Melamed MR, Zaman MB (1982) Pathogenesis of epidermoid carcinoma of lung. In: Shimosato Y, Melamed MR, Nettesheim P (eds) Morphogenesis of lung cancer, vol 1. CRC Press, Boca Raton, pp 37–64

Meyer EC, Liebow AA (1965) Relationship of interstitial pneumonia, honeycombing and atypical epithelial proliferation to cancer of the lung. Cancer 18:322–351

Raeburn C, Spencer H (1953) A study of origin and development of lung cancer. Thorax 8:1–10

Rubinstein I, Baum GL, Kalter Y, Pauzner Y, Lieberman Y, Bubis JJ (1979) The influence of cell type and lymph node metastases on survival of patients with carcinoma of the lung undergoing thoracotomy. Am Rev Respir Dis 119:253–262

Shimosato Y, Kodama T, Kameya T (1982) Morphogenesis of peripheral type adenocarcinoma of the lung. In: Shimosato Y, Melamed MR, Nettesheim P (eds) Morphogenesis of lung cancer, vol 1. CRC Press, Boca Raton, pp 65–90

Sidhu GS (1982) The ultrastructure of malignant epithelial neoplasms of the lung. Pathol Annu 1:235–266

Too LC, Delarue NC, Sanders D, Weisbrod G (1978) Bronchiolo-alveolar carcinoma: a correlative clinical and cytologic study. Cancer 42: 2759–2767

World Health Organisation (1981) Histological typing of lung tumours, 2nd edn. Geneva

Chapter 10

Anaesthesia in the Management of Bronchial Carcinoma

Hilary Howells and Brian Porter

Introduction

The practice of anaesthesia within the management of bronchial carcinoma has developed in parallel with advances in other specialities. The most important change has been the adoption and increasing sophistication of controlled ventilation. Improvements in the fields of drugs, notably neuromuscular blocking agents, and pain relief have also contributed.

Anaesthesia may be required for diagnostic procedures, e.g. bronchoscopy and mediastinoscopy, or for thoracotomy (for resection). This chapter will discuss the principles and current practice of anaesthesia in each of these applications, with reference to the problems met in patients with bronchial carcinoma.

Pain relief is discussed in Chap. 13. Fuller accounts of anaesthesia for thoracic surgery are available in texts on the subject.

Pre-operative Assessment

The condition of the patient should be optimal with respect to the presenting and co-existing diseases and the proposed operative procedure. Measurement of haemoglobin concentrations and basic urine analysis should be performed for all cases; other blood tests should be carried out when appropriate. Routine electrocardiography is probably unnecessary below the age of 40 years unless there is evidence of cardiovascular disease.

Patients with carcinoma of the lung often have widespread pulmonary disease by association with tobacco smoking and chronic bronchitis. Respiratory function tests are commonly carried out during investigation of lung disease but are often surprisingly unhelpful in selecting patients who are able to withstand pulmonary resection. Some measurements associated with a poor prognosis are listed in Table 1.

Malignant disease, especially bronchial carcinoma, is sometimes associated with weakness and lassitude and occasionally also with muscle wasting. The absence of fade after low frequency tetanic stimulation distinguishes this myasthenic syndrome from myasthenia gravis. Patients with myasthenic syndrome display an unpredic-

Table 1. Some measurements associated with a poor prognosis after pulmonary resection (Didolkar et al. 1974; Olsen et al. 1975; Tisi 1979)

Age over 70 years
FVC $< 50\%$ predicted
$FEV_1 < 50\%$ of FVC or < 2.0 l
MBC $< 50\%$ predicted
RV/TLC $< 50\%$
$P_aCO_2 > 6$ kPa
Abnormal ECG

---

table response to neuromuscular blocking drugs, which should only be used with caution: subsequent respiratory support may be required.

The pre-operative visit gives the anaesthetist the opportunity to assess the patient clinically for anaesthesia and to discuss the proposed procedure and subsequent management with the patient. Such discussion involves explanation of the conduct of anaesthesia and postoperative care, including pain relief, physiotherapy and chest drains.

Premedication

Conventional premedication involves the administration of drugs with sedative and antisialagogue activity. The need for premedication in a specific case depends upon the patient, the anaesthetist and the proposed operation.

Inhibiting secretions in the upper airway is especially useful before procedures that involve airway instrumentation, as this provides a potent stimulus to secretion. Atropine is an effective antisialagogue and also protects against bradycardia following incremental administration of suxamethonium if it is given immediately prior to the induction of anaesthesia. The use of atropine avoids the sedative effects of hyoscine, though this and the concomitant provision of mild amnesia may be considered an advantage. Glycopyrrolate may provide a more stable cardiovascular system than either of these two drugs (Mirakhur et al. 1978).

Pre-operative sedation is commonly achieved by use of opioid drugs or benzodiazepines and serves to calm the anxious patient as well as to make the induction of anaesthesia more acceptable to both patient and anaesthetist. Oral lorazepam (2–4 mg) provides suitable sedation with some amnesia. It is best given about 2 hours before operation although timing is not critical owing to the long duration of action. Other benzodiazepines commonly used for premedication include diazepam, nitrazepam and temazepam.

Opioid sedation is associated with analgesia, suppression of the cough reflex and sime respiratory depression. Although intra-operative analgesia may be useful, there is unlikely to be a significant influence on postoperative analgesia requirements or on coughing or respiration unless excessive doses are given. Morphine (0.15–0.2 mg/kg body weight), papaveretum (0.2–0.3 mg/kg) and pethidine (1–2 mg/kg) are the drugs most commonly employed. In general, smaller sedative doses are given for the shorter, diagnostic procedures than for thoracotomy;

patients scheduled for the latter are often given additional benzodiazepine sedation from the pre-operative night.

Anaesthesia for Diagnostic Procedures

Bronchoscopy

Bronchoscopy may be by rigid or flexible, fibre-optic instruments. The rigid bronchoscope is used for assessment of carinal and bronchial rigidity and tumour location in the immediate pre-operative period, or as the instrument of choice for operative procedures, e.g. foreign body removal. Flexible instruments are smaller and can be used for exploration and biopsy down to the third generation of subsegmental bronchus.

Rigid Bronchoscopy

Rigid bronchoscopy is usually performed, for patient and operator preference, under general anaesthesia. The anaesthetic requirements are analgesia, sufficient relaxation to allow easy, atraumatic instrumentation, good oxygenation with effective carbon dioxide elimination, and, if under general anaesthesia, unconsciousness.

Conduct of Anaesthesia. Suitable operating conditions can be achieved by the use of volatile anaesthetic agents, but currently intravenous anaesthesia is the most practised and the most convenient. After suitable premedication, induction is commonly with sodium thiopentone and muscle relaxation obtained by the administration of suxamethonium chloride. Unless the patient was pre-oxygenated, ventilation with 100% oxygen must precede both the spraying of the larynx and upper trachea with lignocaine solution and the introduction of the bronchoscope. Topical anaesthesia applied in this manner reduces the incidence of laryngospasm after short procedures, but may reduce the clearance of debris.

Incremental doses of thiopentone and suxamethonium may be used to prolong the appropriate operating conditions and oxygenation maintained by one of the methods described below. It is important to remember that thiopentone is cumulative and that over-generous administration of suxamethonium may result in a mixed depolarising/non-depolarising neuromuscular block, due to breakdown products, which may prolong the recovery from anaesthesia.

Techniques of Oxygenation. There are four common techniques for maintaining oxygenation during bronchoscopy; all involve sharing the airway with the bronchoscopist.

1. *Apnoeic oxygenation:* Oxygen is insufflated through an endotracheal suction catheter. Blood oxygenation is well maintained but carbon dioxide elimination is poor and the P_aCO_2 rises at approximately 0.4 kPa per minute. This technique is therefore suitable only for short procedures.

2. *Ventilating bronchoscope:* A side arm is available for the supply of fresh gas, the proximal end of the bronchoscope being sealed with a glass window which must be

removed for suction or biopsy. A conventional bronchoscope can be used in a similar manner by the intermittent insertion of a shortened endotracheal tube into the proximal end of the bronchoscope. This technique of oxygenation is often unsatisfactory due to leaks and the mutual interference between anaesthetist and bronchoscopist (Safar 1958).

3. *Venturi jet:* The use of a jet injector attached to the bronchoscope to generate intermittent positive pressure breathing was first described by Sanders in 1967; use of the system has since become widespread. The technique is applicable to children as well as adults for whom the jet needle (16 s.w.g.) is connected to a hand-trigger controlled pressurised oxygen supply (414 kPa). Oxygen is injected intermittently into the proximal end of the bronchoscope. Entrained air allows tidal exchange with oxygen-enriched air sufficient to give effective carbon dioxide elimination and good oxygenation with modest airway pressures (2.5–3.0 kPa). Ventilation is time cycled and pressure limited; smaller jet needles can limit further the peak airway pressure.

4. *High frequency positive pressure ventilation (HFPPV):* This technique allows adequate alveolar ventilation with minimal tidal gas flow and low mean intrathoracic gas pressures. The ventilating gas is delivered through a jet at frequencies of 1–2 Hz, using volumes of 2–3 ml/kg body weight, the inspiratory time being approximately 20% of the respiratory cycle (Borg et al. 1980).

Complications of Rigid Bronchoscopy. If bronchoscopy alone is to be performed, it is desirable that the patient awakes immediately after the end of the procedure and with good airway control. Airway obstruction, drug-induced respiratory depression, debris or blood following biopsy may occasionally contribute to respiratory embarrassment requiring temporary endotracheal intubation and intermittent positive pressure ventilation (IPPV).

The intravenous technique of anaesthesia commonly used for rigid bronchoscopy invites a high incidence of awareness during the procedure. A worthwhile preoperative warning of possible awareness during the removal of the bronchoscope does not excuse inadequate anaesthesia.

Cardiac dysrhythmias are least common when the jet injector oxygenation system is used; this probably reflects the efficiency of the technique. Inadequate anaesthesia and laryngotracheal stimulation are remediable contributors to the occurrence of dysrhythmias; repeated administration of suxamethonium is associated with bradycardia which responds to intravenous atropine and can be prevented by prior administration. Suxamethonium is also associated with muscle pains in the postoperative period. Pretreatment of the patient with a small dose of a non-depolarising neuromuscular blocking drug may reduce the incidence and severity of the problem but also may reduce the effectiveness of the relaxation achieved with suxamethonium.

Fibre-optic Bronchoscopy

Fibre-optic bronchoscopy is acceptable to most patients using topical analgesia and sedation, a method which can also be used for rigid bronchoscopy (see p. 49).

Sedation. Intravenous diazepam has become the most widely used drug for this purpose. Marked respiratory depression sometimes occurs, and unusual pharmacokinetics, ascribed to recirculation from the gastric mucosa, may give a prolonged recovery time. Midazolam is a shorter acting benzodiazepine and may be a more appropriate drug in this clinical context (Brown et al. 1979).

During the bronchoscopy the patient is allowed to breathe spontaneously; mild hypoxia is common.

General Anaesthesia. It may be desirable to perform fibre-optic bronchoscopy under general anaesthesia. In adults the instrument can be conveniently passed through a plastic endotracheal tube, allowing ventilation to be controlled if a self-sealing connector is used (Fig. 1). Anaesthesia may be conducted as for rigid bronchoscopy (q.v.), the difference being the insertion of an endotracheal tube (minimum size 8.0 mm) after neuromuscular blockade. The tube allows maintenance of anaesthesia with gaseous agents if preferred to intravenous anaesthesia. Care should be taken to protect the bronchoscope from damage by clenching of the patient's teeth in the event of inadequate neuromuscular blockade or reflex suppression.

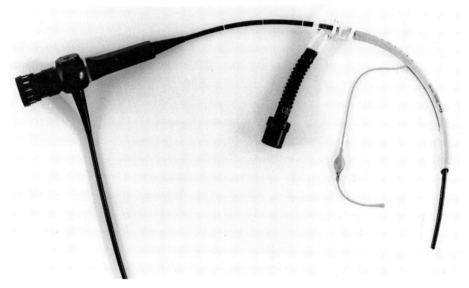

Fig. 1. The fibrescope can be passed through a cuffed endotracheal tube. An airtight adaptor at the proximal end allows the anaesthetist to inflate the patient's lungs through the side tube.

Mediastinoscopy

Mediastinoscopy is carried out under general anaesthesia, commonly in conjunction with bronchoscopy. The procedure is hazardous if there is pre-existing obstruction of the airway or superior vena cava. The effects of such obstruction will be exacerbated by anaesthesia with its concomitant reduction in muscle tone. Anaesthesia will be further complicated by haemorrhage, haemothorax, pneumothorax or air embolism, any of which may result from mediastinoscopy.

Anaesthesia for Mediastinoscopy

Pre-operative sedation need be limited only when there is evidence of airway or superior vena caval obstruction, in which event it is also advisable to pre-oxygenate the patient. Inhalation induction is, in theory, the most appropriate in this situation but in practice it can be more difficult than intravenous induction. Induction is followed by neuromuscular blockade and endotracheal intubation with, for preference, a non-kinking tube. This type of tube is recommended both for its resistance to compression and because the procedure involves turning and extending the head to allow insertion of the mediastinoscope through a suprasternal incision. After intubation, controlled ventilation is continued using nitrous oxide in oxygen, supplemented as necessary, and facilitated by short-acting neuromuscular blocking drugs, for this can be a quick operation. Suxamethonium increments or infusion can be used; the newer non-depolarising drug atracurium is particularly suitable (Payne and Hughes 1981).

Mediastinoscopy Combined with Bronchoscopy

Fibre-optic bronchoscopy can conveniently be carried out in conjunction with mediastinoscopy by passage of the bronchoscope through the endotracheal tube. The use of a self-sealing tube connector allows the continuance of IPPV.

If bronchoscopy is performed at the start of the combined procedure, haemorrhage or debris may necessitate postponement of the mediastinoscopy. Now that short-acting non-depolarising neuromuscular blocking drugs are available (e.g. atracurium), there need be no difficulty in prolonging adequate neuromuscular blockade for rigid bronchoscopy after mediastinoscopy.

Mediastinotomy

The anaesthetic technique described for mediastinoscopy is suitable.

Anaesthesia for Thoracotomy

Physiology of One-Lung Anaesthesia

Mechanical Effect of an Open Hemithorax

An isolated normal lung will collapse due to elastic recoil. Within a closed hemithorax the tendency to collapse is balanced by the outward recoil of the chest wall. Lung expansion then is maintained by virtue of the low negative intrapleural pressure resulting (2–5 kPa). During spontaneous respiration, small fluctuations in this pressure, induced by muscle activity, are responsible for tidal gas flow.

If a hemithorax is opened this equilibrium is lost and the lung will tend to collapse to a degree dependent on the health of the lung. In consequence the mechanical function of the other, closed, hemithorax is deranged because of the mobility of the mediastinum. The result is paradoxical respiration (internal paradox), the mediastinum swinging to the intact side from the partially collapsed lung during inspiration, to return to it on expiration — a pendulum air movement *(pendelluft)*. The problems of the collapsed lung, paradoxical respiration and pendulum air movement can be overcome by controlled ventilation. Occasionally patients can be trained to ventilate preferentially their dependent hemithorax and hemidiaphragm while thoracotomy is performed on the upper hemithorax under local anaesthesia (and acupuncture). This explains how paradoxical respiration is averted in patients undergoing thoracic surgery under acupuncture alone in China. Mediastinal rigidity additionally limits paradox.

Ventilation/Perfusion Relationships

In a subject breathing spontaneously, both ventilation and perfusion are preferentially distributed to the dependent parts of the lungs. During controlled ventilation in the lateral position the upper lung is more compliant, because of the weight pressing on the lower, and so it is ventilated more effectively. The major part of the cardiac output, however, still goes to the lower lung. The result is a worsened overall ventilation/perfusion ratio (V/Q ratio) and so reduced arterial blood oxygenation. This effect may be increased by lung disease or mechanical disruption of cardiac or pulmonary function.

The wasted ventilation of the upper lung can be eliminated by the use of endobronchial intubation and the controlled ventilation of the lower lung. Although this may improve the operating conditions in the upper lung, the remaining blood flow through it is unoxygenated.

Hypoxaemia

The most important effect of the changes in pulmonary physiology during one-lung anaesthesia is hypoxaemia. The severity of it depends upon the amount of blood flowing through the unventilated lung, the V/Q mismatch in the lower lung and the oxygen content of the mixed venous blood. The P_aCO_2 acceptable during anaesthesia for thoracic surgery is an individual requirement but in principle it should be maintained so as to reduce to a minimum any risk associated with hypoxia. It is common practice to use an inspired oxygen concentration of at least 50% during one-lung anaesthesia. Hypoxaemia can be minimised by:

1. Limiting perfusion of unventilated lung by surgical restriction of blood flow and keeping intrapulmonary gas pressures in the ventilated lung as low as possible
2. Selecting a respiratory pattern and inspired oxygen concentration to compensate for the V/Q mismatch in the dependent lung
3. Maintenance of appropriate cardiac output and metabolic state by adequate fluid replacement, correction of dysrhythmias, careful anaesthesia and avoidance of mechanical interference with cardiorespiratory function
4. Insufflation of oxygen at low pressures (10 kPa) to the collapsed lung; this can improve arterial oxygenation, but is of more benefit in non-pulmonary operations because of surgical interference during lung dissection.

Neither manual ventilation nor positive end-expiratory pressure is of proven benefit to oxygenation in this situation.

The elimination of carbon dioxide should present no problem during one-lung anaesthesia, for P_aCO_2 is dependent largely upon alveolar minute ventilation, which should be maintained.

Endobronchial Apparatus

The effects of an open hemithorax have been described above. As referred to earlier, some trained awake individuals can breathe adequately in this situation, but in western medical practice general anaesthesia is preferred for most major surgery, and controlled ventilation then becomes necessary. The management of endobronchial secretions can be improved by the use of endobronchial tubes and bronchial blockers. Double lumen endobronchial tubes allow the independent control of ventilation in the two lungs.

The full range of endobronchial apparatus is extensive and is described fully in texts on thoracic anaesthesia, together with details of the methods of insertion and positioning. For thoracotomy for carcinoma of the lung, the choice of endobronchial apparatus lies most commonly between single and double lumen tubes. Although plastic tubes are becoming available, red rubber tubes are still the most satisfactory.

Single Lumen Endobronchial Tubes

These tubes have a bevel cut to face the side that the tube will enter, and have bronchial and tracheal cuffs. Suitable tubes in current use are briefly described below.

Green–Gordon Right Endobronchial Tube. Four sizes are available. The endobronchial section is offset at an angle of 15°, and the bronchial cuff inflates around a slit in the side wall that allows ventilation of the right upper lobe. The larger two sizes can be introduced under direct vision using an intubating bronchoscope, when it is preferable to remove the carinal hook (Gordon and Green 1955).

Macintosh–Leatherdale Left Endobronchial Tube. Four sizes are available (7–10 mm), and the tubes are curved to fit the oropharynx and the left main bronchus. A third pilot tube permits suction of right lung secretions or the insufflation of oxygen to the right lung. Perforations in the tube wall near the tip allow ventilation should the bevel lie against the bronchial wall. The tube is inserted and positioned blind (Macintosh and Leatherdale 1955).

Brompton–Pallister Left Endobronchial Tube. This tube has three cuffs, the third being a reserve bronchial cuff in case the first is damaged during sleeve resection of the right upper lobe. Two sizes are available (8 and 9 mm), and the tubes are positioned with the aid of an intubating bronchoscope (Pallister 1959).

Double Lumen Endobronchial Tubes

Double lumen tubes have bronchial and tracheal cuffs between which lies the opening of the second lumen. The tubes are angled according to which bronchus they are designed to enter, and are curved to fit the oropharynx. Right-sided tubes have side openings designed to lie opposite the right upper lobe bronchus. Suitable tubes in current use are described below.

Robertshaw Double Lumen Tubes. Right- and left-sided tubes are available, both in three sizes — small, medium and large (corresponding to Magill sizes 8, 10 and 12). The endobronchial segments are angled, 45° for the left side and 20° for the right side. The lumina lie side by side (Robertshaw 1952).

Bryce-Smith Left-Sided and Bryce-Smith-Salt Right-Sided Tubes. Four sizes are available. The lumina lie anterior/posterior so that the long axis of the oval cross-section lies in the long axis of the glottis. These tubes are considered to be less traumatic than the Robertshaw or Carlens tubes (Bryce-Smith 1959; Bryce-Smith and Salt 1960).

Carlens and White Double Lumen Tubes. The Carlens tube was designed for differential broncho-spirometry and is shaped to enter the left main bronchus. The passage of suction catheters through it may be difficult, and there is significant resistance to spontaneous respiration. The carinal hook can make the tube difficult to pass through the larynx. The White tube is similar except that it is shaped to enter the right main bronchus and so has an orifice for the right upper lobe (Björk and Carlens 1950; White 1960).

Selection and Use of Endobronchial Tubes

The use of an intubating bronchoscope to position single lumen tubes under direct vision can be an advantage if there is distortion of the bronchial tree or if rapid, correct positioning of the tubes is important, e.g. bronchopleural fistula.

It may be necessary to withdraw a single lumen tube into the trachea to achieve full expansion of the operated lung after temporary collapse, or to test the integrity of bronchial suture lines. Double lumen tubes allow independent control of the ventilation and suction access to the two lungs. Although their position, when correct, is more stable than that of single lumen tubes, double lumen tubes are more difficult and traumatic to pass because of their size.

The bronchial cuff of single lumen tubes is sometimes left deflated until one-lung anaesthesia is required, so as to maintain the better oxygenation of two-lung anaesthesia for as long as possible. It must be inflated to establish one-lung anaesthesia. For one-lung anaesthesia using double lumen tubes, the catheter mount connection to the operated side is clamped and the suction port in the tube connector opened to allow lung deflation. Secretions should be cleared from the operated lung before re-expansion.

If it proves impossible to position endobronchial apparatus, an endotracheal tube should be used. This is most likely to occur at a second operation involving pulmonary resection, because of distortion of the bronchial anatomy.

Anaesthetic Technique

Pre-operative Preparation

Pre-operative assessment and premedication have been discussed above. It is the practice of some workers to digitalise patients before major thoracic surgery in order to reduce the incidence and cardiovascular disturbance of dysrhythmias in the peri-operative period.

Induction

Intravenous induction is followed by suitable doses of a non-depolarising neuromuscular blocking drug, e.g. pancuronium 0.12 mg/kg, which allows a generous time for bronchoscopy and accurate endobronchial tube placement. If airway or intubation difficulties are expected then suxamethonium may be more appropriate. The endobronchial tube should be secured and for convenience any intravascular cannulae inserted before the patient is positioned for the operation. The operation will usually be done with the patient in the lateral position. After turning the patient the correct function of the endobronchial tube should be confirmed.

Extradural analgesia can be used both for postoperative pain relief and as an adjunct to anaesthesia and this can be a stage at which to insert the catheter. Intercostal nerve blocks are best performed at the end of the operation.

Maintenance

Maintenance of anaesthesia is usually by IPPV using nitrous oxide in oxygen, supplemented as necessary. Opioid drugs, e.g. fentanyl, are commonly given for intra-operative analgesia but generous administration carries a risk of post-operative respiratory depression. Consequently nitrous oxide is frequently supplemented with a volatile anaesthetic agent, e.g. halothane, which also serves to reduce the incidence of awareness, increased when using the high inspired oxygen concentrations administered during one-lung anaesthesia.

Recently there has been increasing use of total intravenous anaesthesia, e.g. combined etomidate and fentanyl infusions (Carli et al. 1983). This avoids the use of volatile agents potentially toxic both to patients and operating theatre staff and of nitrous oxide, which may be deleterious to patients with air-filled cavities. Intravenous anaesthesia is also eminently suitable for use with HFPPV, when the reduction in tidal gas exchange reduces the uptake of volatile agents.

The normal alveolar minute ventilation should be maintained during one-lung anaesthesia, keeping the mean intrathoracic pressure as low as possible. This can be achieved by use of a faster respiratory rate with smaller tidal volumes than for two-lung anaesthesia. Although a high inspiratory/expiratory time (I/E) ratio will improve gas distribution within the ventilated lung, the benefit is offset by the mean pressure increase, and it is preferable to use an I/E ratio of 1:2 or less.

Mechanical ventilation gives a consistent pattern of mediastinal movement, contributing better operating conditions than manual ventilation. The extra versatility of manual ventilation is, however, required to re-expand collapsed lung segments and to test the integrity of bronchial suture lines with controlled inflation at pressures of 3.0–4.0 kPa.

Some thoracic surgery units use HFPPV for thoracotomy. Respiratory rates of 1–2 Hz with gas volumes of 2–3 ml/kg and inspiratory times of 20% of the respiratory cycle are used. The system allows good oxygenation and effective carbon dioxide elimination. The mean intrathoracic pressure is lower than with conventional IPPV and the operating conditions are good owing to the reduced mediastinal displacement (Malina et al. 1981).

Adequate time must be allowed towards the end of the operation for recovery from the anaesthetic drugs, and residual neuromuscular blockade must be effectively antagonised by neostigmine.

Bronchoscopy After Thoracotomy

Occasionally it is desirable to perform bronchoscopy after thoracotomy, at which time the effects of most anaesthetic drugs will be declining. Bronchoscopy may be necessary if there is difficulty in re-expanding collapsed lung segments due to the presence of mucous plugs or blood clot.

Suitable conditions for bronchoscopy at the end of a thoracotomy can be achieved by a small dose of a short-acting neuromuscular blocking drug, e.g. atracurium, without compromising excessively the reversal of the block with neostigmine.

Postoperative Respiratory Care

At the end of the operation an early return to spontaneous respiration avoids positive pressure leaks from bronchial suture lines and reduces the risk of respiratory tract infection from prolonged intubation. Prompt recovery from anaesthesia is also important because pain, secretion retention, intrapleural fluid and the after-effects of lung manipulation all predispose to postoperative respiratory failure. Humidified oxygen and physiotherapy should be given as necessary in the postoperative period.

Sputum retention postoperatively will be likely in those patients with a weak cough who have had tracheobronchial tree anastomoses or who have been heavy smokers. It may be necessary to provide respiratory support for some of these patients in the postoperative period. The endotracheal tube then provides access for fibre-optic bronchoscopy if this is needed. It may be preferable to establish a tracheostomy electively in a patient particularly at risk.

Chest Drains

After lobectomy it is usual to insert an apical and a basal chest drain. Both are connected to underwater seals once the pleura is closed. Manual ventilation expands the residual lung after their insertion and controls lung inflation while the ribs are approximated. Practice differs with respect to the use of low pressure suction on chest drains — although it encourages lung expansion, it may occasionally predispose to haemorrhage and leakage from lung surfaces. Pressures of 1–5 kPa are appropriate.

Drains are not often inserted after pneumonectomy.

Operative Procedures on the Lung

Lobectomy. Lobectomy may be performed with or without sleeve resection, which is carried out if the neoplasm involves the lobar bronchus too close to the main bronchus. In general, anaesthetists and surgeons like the flexibility of differential lung control which double lumen tubes offer both for lobectomy and pneumonectomy. A single lumen endobronchial tube may be preferable if sleeve resection is to be undertaken as less distortion is then caused to the anatomy around the carina. Since the tube is exposed in the operative field, appropriate care must be taken during its insertion to reduce the risk of infection. If a second thoracotomy is performed at a time significantly later than the first, it may be necessary to use an endotracheal tube because of bronchial tree distortion.

Pneumonectomy. Pneumonectomy is associated with a higher hospital mortality than lobectomy. There is also a higher incidence of intra-operative dysrhythmias than during lobectomy, due to the increased mediastinal irritation. A single lumen tube is sometimes preferred for pneumonectomy, as there is less carinal distortion and there is no need for the second lumen of a double lumen tube once the procedure is under way. Postoperative control of pressure within the pneumonectomy space may be required as described above.

Bronchopleural Fistula. The formation of a bronchopleural fistula is a serious complication of pulmonary resection. Although rare, it is more likely after pneumonectomy than lobectomy. It may be associated with infection and it is important to prevent the intrapleural fluid from flooding the bronchial tree. The patient should therefore be nursed in the sitting position, and a chest drain inserted to drain the fluid. If thoracotomy is indicated for surgical closure of the fistula, traditional teaching recommends an inhalation induction of anaesthesia with the patient sitting or intubation of the patient under topical analgesia. In practice it is usually more satisfactory, after pre-oxygenation, and again with the patient in a sitting position, to induce anaesthesia intravenously, e.g. with thiopentone, and to locate an endobronchial tube with the aid of suxamethonium. This method is satisfactory provided that the tube can be positioned quickly and accurately. It is preferable to use a single lumen endobronchial tube, which may be positioned if necessary under direct vision with an intubating bronchoscope. If an endobronchial tube cannot be positioned, an endotracheal tube should be used with gentle IPPV. Under ideal circumstances IPPV is not instituted until the fistula has been isolated. HFPPV, with the associated low airway pressures, would be an advantage in the management of bronchopleural fistula.

Monitoring

Cardiovascular disturbances may be marked during anaesthesia both for diagnostic procedures and thoracotomy. Continuous electrocardiogram display is useful in all cases, especially if used in conjunction with a pulse detector.

Blood pressure can be measured conveniently by the non-invasive sphygmomanometer or oscillotonometer in most cases. For poor-risk patients or major operations, direct intra-arterial pressure measurement allows not only instant and continuous observation of arterial blood pressure, but also ready access to arterial blood for gas analysis and assessment of acid-base status.

Venous access must be available in all cases during anaesthesia, and a good peripheral intravenous infusion is adequate for mediastinoscopy and most thoracotomy cases. A large central venous cannula more reliably allows rapid fluid replacement and also central venous pressure measurement if necessary.

References

Björk VO, Carlens E (1950) The prevention of spread during pulmonary resection by the use of a double lumen catheter. Thorac Surg 20:151–157

Borg U, Eriksson I, Sjörstrand U (1980) High-frequency positive-pressure ventilation (HFPPV): a review based upon its use during bronchoscopy and for laryngoscopy and microlaryngeal surgery under general anaesthesia. Anesth Analg 59:594–603

Brown CR, Sarnquist FH, Canup CA, Pedley TA (1979) Clinical, electroencephalographic and pharmacokinetic studies of a water soluble benzodiazepine, midazolam maleate. Anesthesiology 50:467–470

Bryce-Smith R (1959) A double lumen endobronchial tube. Br J Anaesth 31:274–275

Bryce-Smith R, Salt R (1960) A right sided double lumen tube. Br J Anaesth 32:230–231

Carli F. Stribley GC, Clark MM (1983) Etomidate infusion in thoracic surgery. Anaesthesia 38:784–788

Didolkar MS, Moore RH, Takita H (1974) Evaluation of the risk in pulmonary resection for bronchogenic carcinoma. Am J Surg 127:700–703

Gordon W, Green RA (1955) A new right endobronchial tube. Lancet I:185

Macintosh R, Leatherdale RAL (1955) Bronchus tube and bronchus blocker. Br J Anaesth 27:556–557

Malina JR, Nordström SG, Sjörstrand UH, Wattwil CM (1981) Clinical evaluation of high-frequency positive-pressure ventilation (HFPPV) in patients scheduled for open chest surgery. Anesth Analg 60:324–330

Mirakhur RK, Clarke RSJ, Elliot J, Dundee JW (1978) Atropine and glycopyrrhonium premediation. Anaesthesia 33:906–912

Olsen GN, Block AJ, Swenson EW et al. (1975) Pulmonary function evaluation of the lung resection candidate: a prospective study. Am Rev Respir Dis 111:379–386

Pallister WK (1959) A new endobronchial tube for left lung surgery with specific reference to reconstructive pulmonary surgery. Thorax 14:55–57

Payne JP, Hughes R (1981) Evaluation of atracurium in anaesthetised man. Br J Anaesth 53:45–54

Robertshaw FL (1962) Low resistance double lumen endobronchial tubes. Br J Anaesth 34:576–579

Safar P (1958) Ventilatory bronchoscope. Anesthesiology 19:406–407

Sanders RD (1967) Two ventilating attachments for bronchoscopes. Del Med J 39:170

Tisi GM (1979) Pre-operative evaluation of pulmonary function. Validity, indication and benefits. Am Rev Respir Dis 119:293–310

White GMJ (1960) A new double lumen tube. Br J Anaesth 32-232-234

Chapter 11

Surgical Treatment

Michael Bates

Including:

Pre-operative Radiotherapy for Small Cell Carcinoma

Maurice Sutton

Introduction

This chapter is a personal review of surgical treatment carried out for bronchial carcinoma, which accounted for 41% of the operations performed during 33 years of thoracic surgical practice. The results have been analysed to show the changes which have occurred in the age and sex distribution and in the variety of operations performed. It is interesting to note, comparing other large surgical series reported over the same period, the remarkable similarity in the long-term results irrespective of the country or surgical unit concerned.

Between June 1950 and May 1983, 2800 patients suffering from cancers of the lung were operated on, and of these, 241 had an exploratory thoracotomy only, giving a resectability rate of 91.4%. Up-to-date information has been obtained on all but 17 of the 2559 patients who underwent lung resection. These patients have been considered in three equal periods of 11 years, the first being between June 1950 and May 1961. During most of this period radical pneumonectomy was considered to be the treatment of choice, even when lobectomy would have been possible. There were 195 radical pneumonectomies performed, with 32 hospital deaths: a mortality of 16.4%. During the same period 161 extrapericardial pneumonectomies were performed with 25 hospital deaths: a mortality of 15.5%. While there is little difference between these two mortality rates, they are the reverse of those given by Brock and Whytehead (1955), who quoted 11% mortality for radical pneumonectomy and 18% for extrapericardial pneumonectomy.

By 1959 I had been converted to the principle of lobectomy whenever technically feasible, and subsequently radical pneumonectomy has been performed only when extensive disease was encountered. Although radical pneumonectomy was discontinued as a routine procedure, intrapericardial ligation of vessels is still required together with removal of involved mediastinal and para-oesophageal nodes, but without the removal of the superior mediastinal pleura, the vagus nerve on the right side, paratracheal lymphatics and nodes, and the azygos vein.

During these years the major incidence of bronchial carcinoma for both male and female patients occurred in the 50–59 age group (Table 1). The historical distribution (Table 2) is similar to that in other reported series of the same period. Table 3 demonstrates the high incidence of not only radical pneumonectomy, but also total pneumonectomy compared with lobectomy. It does show the introduction of some conservative surgery, with eight of the lobectomies being of the sleeve variety, but no segmental resection was performed.

Table 1. The age and sex of patients in the first series (1950–1961)

Age	20–29	30–39	40–49	50–59	60–69	70 +	
Males	0	12	80	223	188	29	= 532
Females	0	4	9	9	7	1	= 30

Table 2. Histological findings in the first series (1950–1961)

Variety	Number
Squamous	371
Adenocarcinoma	34
Undifferentiated	100
Small Cell	56
Other	1

Table 3. Operations performed on patients in the first series (1950–1961)[a]

Operation	No. of patients
Pneumonectomy	356
Radical	195
Extrapericardial	161
Lobectomy	214 (8 sleeves)
Segmentectomy	0

[a]Eight patients had two operations.

The second and third series of 11 years show some interesting changes, both in the age and sex groupings (Tables 4 and 5) and in the histological distribution (see Table 6). The considerable increase in the number of patients in the second series was due to additional referral sources as well as an increase from pre-existing sources. The second and third series are of particular interest in that the number of patients in each is so similar that they are strictly comparable, and show that the number of patients requiring surgical treatment did not decline during the last 11 years. A further comparison between Tables 4 and 5 shows that while there were fewer male patients in the third series, more of them were in the older age groups; however, there was an overall increase in female patients in all age groups.

Table 4. The age and sex of patients in the second series (1961–1972)

Age	20–29	30–39	40–49	50–59	60–69	70 +	
Male	1	8	60	361	401	80	= 911
Female	0	3	12	36	37	8	= 96

Table 5. The age and sex of patients in the third series (1972–1983)

Age	20–29	30–39	40–49	50–59	60–69	70 +	
Male	0	7	50	210	420	133	= 820
Female	1	1	18	56	73	21	= 170

Table 6. Histological findings in the second and third series

Variety	Second series (1961–1972)	Third series (1972–1983)
Squamous	647	677
Adenocarcinoma	80	132
Undifferentiated	174	52
Small Cell	102	111
Other	4	9

Age and Sex

Malignant disease in young patients inevitably has a poor prognosis, and with lung cancer one might have anticipated no long-term survivors in the groups under the age of 40. However, in the total series 5 of 36 such patients have survived for 10 years or more (Table 7): the longest survivor is a female who is alive and well today, 24 years after a right upper lobectomy performed when she was 39 for squamous cell carcinoma with a large involved paratracheal node (Bates 1981).

A personal report in 1970 (Bates 1970) gave the results in 100 patients aged 70 and over, operated on for bronchial carcinoma between 1950 and 1968, and anticipated that in the future an increasing number of patients of this age group would require surgery (Bates 1970). Since then a further 183 patients of this group have had resections, of whom 157 were males and 26 females (Table 8). The importance of conservative surgery for this age group was appreciated in 1970, and subsequently

Table 7. Results in patients[a] below 40 years of age (1950–1983))

Years	1	1–2	2–3	3–5	10 +
Deaths	13	9	5	1	1
Survivors					4

[a] Total = 36: 26 males and 10 females

Table 8. Operations performed on patients[a] aged 70 and over (1968–1983)

Operation	Number
Pneumonectomy	56
Lobectomy	111
Segmentectomy	15
Wedge	1

[a] Total = 183: 157 males and 26 females

more than twice the number of patients were treated by lobectomy or segmental resection than by pneumonectomy.

When deciding to perform thoracotomy in a patient in this age group, a policy of resection when technically feasible was adhered to. In a patient of borderline respiratory function who needed pneumonectomy, an elective tracheostomy was performed at the time of surgery and maintained for the first postoperative week.

In two respects the results, shown in Tables 9 and 10, constitute an improvement over those reported in 1970, when 40 of the 100 patients died within a year of operation. First, in the later group, only 43 of 183 patients died in the first year. Secondly, in the earlier group 16 patients had survived for 4 or more years, while 34 survived for this length of time in the later group.

Table 9. Hospital deaths in the 70+ age group (1968–1983)

Operation	Number
Pneumonectomy	12
Lobectomy	17
Segmentectomy	1

Table 10. Survivors and late deaths in the 70+ age group (1968–1983)

Years	1	1–2	2–3	3–4	4–5	5+	10+
Deaths	43	26	16	9	9	10	1
Survivors	5	8	6	6	4	10	0

The quality of life was satisfactory following lobectomy, but pneumonectomy did result in dyspnoea in most patients. The longest survivor was a male patient who had a squamous cell carcinoma removed by lobectomy in 1959 when aged 75. He died at the age of 98 from a cerebral vascular accident.

Tumours in patients of this age group grow just as rapidly as in younger patients, an observation emphasised by Belcher and Anderson (1965) when reviewing a large series of patients treated at the London Chest Hospital. Patients of this age group are extremely co-operative and are appreciative when their lives are extended by even 3 or 4 years. Provided emphasis is placed on conservative surgery, then resection is justified, a policy supported by Sensenig et al. (1966) and by Thompson Evans (1973).

Small Cell Carcinoma

At the end of 1966 a personal review was made of all the cases of small cell carcinoma on whom surgery had been performed.

The results from pneumonectomy were unacceptable (Table 11) and there was only a slight improvement when lobectomy could be performed for peripheral tumours and less advanced disease (Table 12). In the light of these results, it was decided to try the effect of low dose pre-operative radiotherapy.

Table 11. Results of 75 pneumonectomies for small cell carcinoma, 1951-1966

1 A/W at 19 years	7 died between 1 and 2 years
	67 died after average 6 months
	___
	74

Table 12. Results of 18 lobectomies for small cell carcinoma, 1951-1966

1 A/W at 17 years	1 died after 12 years
1 A/W at 15 years	1 died after 6 years
	1 died after 5 years
	1 died after 4 years
	4 died after 1-2 years
	8 died after average $5\frac{1}{2}$ months
	___
	16

Pre-operative Radiotherapy for Small Cell Carcinoma
Maurice Sutton

The use of pre-operative radiotherapy has been explored in many forms of operable malignant disease. The rationale is:

1. It may reduce the number of viable cancer cells so that implantation as a result of the surgical procedure is less likely.
2. It may eradicate malignant cells which, undetected clinically, may lie beyond the margins of the surgical resection.

Surgical procedures do increase the number of malignant cells circultating in the blood and pre-operative radiotherapy should, in theory, reduce these. However, as yet little correlation has been shown between the number of circulating cancer cells in the blood and the incidence of distant metastases.

The drawbacks of pre-operative radiotherapy are:

1. A long course of radiotherapy could significantly delay the operation. This would be undesirable in a treatment schedule in which the operation is the principal therapeutic measure.
2. Pre-operative radiotherapy, if the dose is high, could add difficulties to the actual operation. Early radiation effects include endarteritis affecting capillaries and arterioles and can cause problems with haemostasis. Radiation fibrosis may appear 1 month after radiotherapy has been completed, making dissection difficult and impairing healing of wounds.
3. If host immunity plays a part in the natural history of a particular malignant tumour, then radiation could adversely affect that immunity.

Early trials with pre-operative radiotherapy in bronchial carcinoma were disappointing. They were beset with an unacceptably high incidence of complications.

The first trial was instituted by Bromley and Szur (1955). Pre-operative radiotherapy was given to 65 patients in a dose varying between 3700 cGy and 6000 cGy with an average of 4700 cGy in 5–6 weeks using orthovoltage. This was followed in 4 weeks by surgical resection. Five of the 65 patients developed an empyema not associated with a fistula and 13 developed a bronchopleural fistula — a complication rate of 27%. In this series pre-operative radiotherapy did not appear to influence the overall survival, even though 44% of the irradiated patients had no tumour histologically in the surgical specimen. It was this latter finding that stimulated further trials with pre-operative radiotherapy.

Bloedorn (1973) investigated the use of even higher radiation doses as a pre-operative procedure. His patients received 4500 cGy to an initially large volume of tissue followed by an additional boost of 1000–1500 cGy to fields localised to the tumour site. In this trial the overall survival rate was not improved by the pre-operative radiotherapy and there was a 29% mortality, the most common complications being bronchopleural fistula and empyema.

Other large scale randomised studies (Shields et al. 1970) using similar radiation doses as a pre-operative measure showed no statistically significant difference in survival between those who had had pre-operative radiotherapy and those who had not. In fact, in the pre-operative radiotherapy group, the survival rate decreased as the radiation dose increased. Further advances with this technique were to await the use of low dose pre-operative radiotherapy.

Since 1966 all operable small cell carcinoma of bronchus patients at the North Middlesex Hospital in London have been treated by a combination of pre-operative radiotherapy and pneumonectomy (Bates et al. 1974; Bates 1979; Levison 1980b). The term 'operable' encompassed those tumours that were seen at bronchoscopy to be in the main or intermediate bronchus or at the origin of a lobar bronchus, and from which a positive bronchoscopic biopsy specimen of small cell carcinoma was obtained. Small cell carcinoma, with its particularly malignant propensity and tendency to metastasise, was considered to be the type of tumour that would benefit from this approach.

All patients were treated on a cobalt 60 unit using an opposed pair of fields to cover the tumour and the adjacent mediastinal lymph nodes, the usual field size being 15×10 or 15×12 cm. In the original group of patents 250 cGy minimum tumour dose (MTD) was given daily for seven treatments, usually in 8 days overall time, to a total MTD of 1750 cGy. This dose was arbitrary, but deliberately low as it was considered essential that operation should not be delayed unduly by either the radiotherapy or having to wait for the reaction to treatment to subside.

The subsequent history and X-rays illustrate the response to this treatment. Figure 1 shows a collapsed left upper lobe in a man aged 53 who had a haemoptysis in 1966. Bronchial biopsy revealed a small cell carcinoma in the mouth of the left upper lobe bronchus. There was a marked improvement in this patient following 10 days' treatment with 1750 cGy (Fig. 2), at which time pneumonectomy was performed. Figure 3 shows the situation in December 1983, 17 years later, during which time the patient has remained well and free of symptoms.

Because of the initial favourable results in 17 patients (Fig. 4) and the expectation that increasing the radiation dose might give further improvement, the MTD was raised in 1970 to 2500 cGy administered in ten treatments in 11 days overall time. The results of treatment for this second radiotherapy series of 16 patients were worse with the raising of the MTD, and all died within 5 years (Fig. 5). No explanation was apparent, but perhaps in this instance host resistance was adversely affected by the

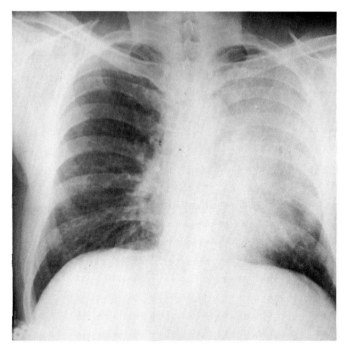

Fig. 1. Collapsed left upper lobe in a male patient ages 53 with small cell carcinoma.

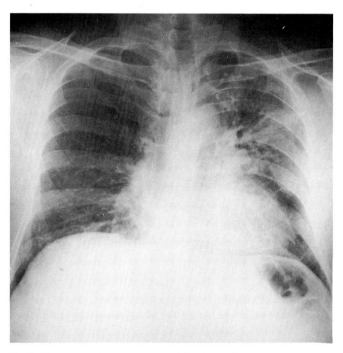

Fig. 2. The same patient as in Fig. 1, following 1750 cGy.

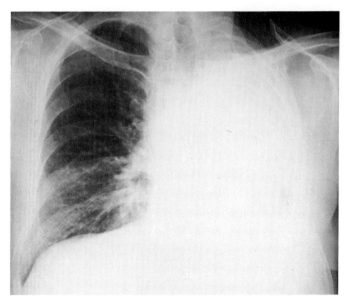

Fig. 3. The same patient as in Figs. 1 and 2 in December 1983, 17 years after pneumonectomy.

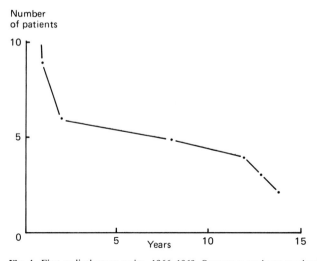

Fig. 4. First radiotherapy series, 1966–1969. Seventeen patients received 1750 cGy pre-operatively.

increased radiation dose (see p. 219). It is interesting to note that in this second radiotherapy series, nearly a third of the operation specimens showed a squamoid appearance. This high proportion of histological difference between the broncho-scopic biopsy and the operation specimen suggests that pre-operative radiation might be responsible (Bates 1975) (Figs 6 and 7).

In 1974 the original MTD of 1750 cGy was reverted to for the third radiotherapy series of 35 patients and it remains the standard pre-operative technique for small cell carcinoma at the North Middlesex Hospital. In this third group of patients, bone, brain and liver scans were performed routinely to aid the decision regarding operability. There is no adverse reaction to this course of radiotherapy and thoracotomy is carried out as soon as possible after its completion.

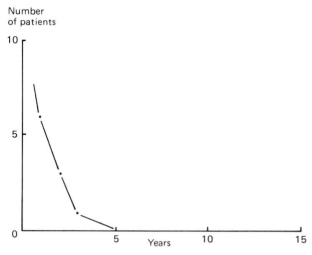

Fig. 5. Second radiotherapy series, 1970–1973. Sixteen patients received 2500 cGy pre-operatively.

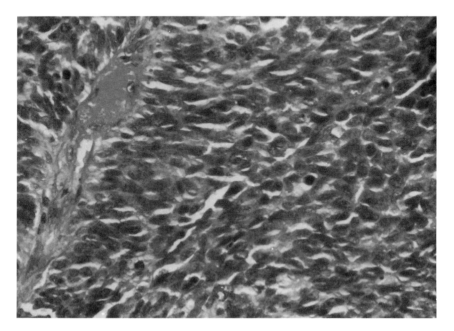

Fig. 6. Small cell carcinoma. H & E, × 70.

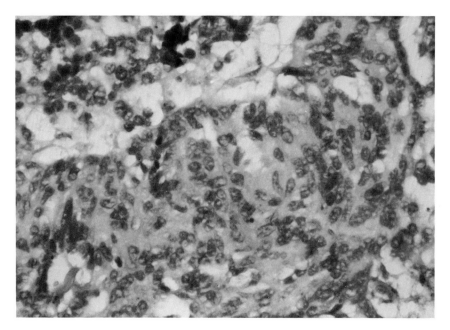

Fig. 7. Irradiated small cell carcinoma showing squamoid change. H & E, × 70.

In all, 68 patients underwent thoracotomy (Bates) and morbidity was low, with bronchopleural fistula causing death in one patient who was given 2500 cGy MTD. The results of the third radiotherapy series of patients are given in Fig. 8. Overall there were 41 patients who were treated with 1750 cGy MTD pre-operatively and were available for 5-year follow-up analysis. Of these, six (15%) were alive at 5 years. Monk and Woods (1975) also showed the beneficial effect of pre-operative radiotherapy in a series of 43 patients with operable small cell carcinoma. They administered pre-operative radiotherapy to a dose varying between 2000 and 4000 cGy MTD followed by pulmonary resection. Ten patients (23%) were alive at 5 years.

While the results in our third radiotherapy series are an improvement on the second radiotherapy series, it is clear that many patients develop widespread metastases within 3 months of surgery. Almost certainly those patients had micrometastases at the time of operation. This cannot be so in all patients or there would be no long-term survivors from surgery alone, of whom many are recorded (Shore and Paneth 1980). Figure 9 demonstrates the reason for the vascular spread of neoplastic cells, both before and during surgery, showing nodules of growth presenting in the left atrium having grown down the lumen of the inferior pulmonary vein.

In 1969 a Medical Research Council (Miller et al. 1969) report said that patients with operable small cell carcinoma '. . . should be advised to submit to radiotherapy rather than surgery'. However, in the light of the North Middlesex Hospital experience it would now seem reasonable to treat patients who present with operable small cell carcinoma with low dose pre-operative radiotherapy followed by pneumonectomy, and perhaps also provide cover with a suitable cytotoxic drug during surgery and the postoperative period (see p. 179).

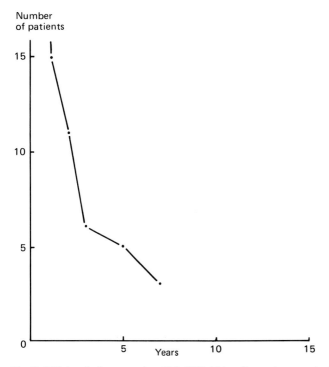

Fig. 8. Third radiotherapy series, 1974–1982. Thirty-five patients received 1750 cGy pre-operatively.

Histology

The incidence of squamous cell growths and small growths has remained constant during the span of 22 years, but there has been a change in the incidence of adenocarcinoma and undifferentiated growths, with a large increase in the number of adenocarcinomas in the last 11 years, and a diminution in the number of undifferentiated tumours (Table 6).

Types of Operation

The tendency towards conservative surgery is shown by the increasing number of sleeve lobectomies and segmentectomies (Table 13).

Sleeve Lobectomy

Of the 46 patients in whom sleeve lobectomies were performed, 18 are still alive and well; the longest survival time is 21 years, and 14 have lived for 5 or more years.

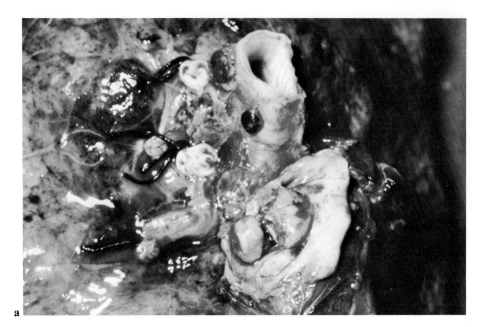

a

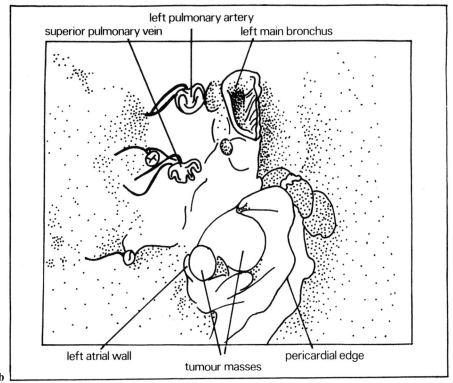

b

Fig. 9. a Mediastinal aspect of left pneumonectomy specimen showing nodules of growth protruding into the left atrial cavity. **b** Diagrammatic representation of **a**.

Table 13. Types of operation ($n = 2589$)[a]

Operation	First series (1950–1961)	Second series (1961–1972)	Third series (1972–1983)	Total
Pneumonectomy	356	532	501	1389
Lobectomy	214	469	459	1142
Sleeve	8	12	26	46
Segmentectomy	0	23	30	53
Wedge	0	1	4	5

[a]Thirty patients had two operations

Even these small numbers give an impression that sleeve lobectomy patients live longer than patients who have undergone a routine lobectomy. It may be that the removal of part of the main bronchus and associated lymphatics is of considerable significance and that more sleeve lobectomies should be performed for upper lobe growths, and not only for those in which the growth is at the origin of the upper lobe orifice.

Segmentectomy

Following the publication by Le Roux in 1972 of satisfactory results obtained from segmentectomy for small peripheral growths, the operation was performed more frequently during the period 1972–1983. Le Roux (1972) reported the results of 17 segmentectomies in a series of 1464 resections, and in 1974 Shields and Higgins reported on 15 segmentectomies in a series of over 3000 resections for bronchial carcinoma. In this personal series of 2559 patients who had resections, 53 were treated by segmentectomy.

Complete anatomical fissures are rare, but are most likely to be found in the lingular and apical lower segments. In this group, although there were only four such complete fissures, the majority of resections were of these two segments.

Indications. Provided there is no peribronchial nodal involvement, segmentectomy is indicated in patients with emphysema, or where previous resection has been performed, in order to conserve lung tissue. Two segments can be removed if a peripheral growth lies across a fissure, such as between the posterior upper and apical lower segments. Segmentectomy should also be considered for the removal of an undiagnosed small peripheral mass which could be tuberculous in nature.

Results (Table 14). Thirty-two per cent of patients survived 5 or more years. Of the 16 patients who survived this long, ten had squamous cell growths, four had adenocarcinoma and two had large cell undifferentiated growths. There was one

Table 14. Results of segmentectomy (1950–1983)[a]

Years	1–5	5–10	10–15	15–20
Deaths	34	9	1	0
Survivors	3	3	1	2

[a]Total no. of patients = 53 (including 23 apical lower segmentectomies and 8 lingulectomies)

hospital death. These figures confirm that limited surgery should be chosen for small localised lesions where there is no segmental bronchial node involvement. This view was shared by Overholt et al. in 1975, in a review of 1848 patients treated by resection for bronchial carcinoma between 1932 and 1974.

Bronchial Closure

Until June 1979 all main bronchi and the majority of lobar bronchi were closed using the Brock technique with figure-of-eight stainless steel wire sutures. This method resulted in a 5% incidence of bronchopleural fistula following pneumonectomy. Since July 1979, all bronchi have been closed with the American TA 30 stapler. In addition, bronchial mucosal healing has been encouraged by the use of a fine running suture along the cut edge of the bronchus. Since using this method, only one bronchopleural fistula has occurred in the last 105 pneumonectomies.

Survival

The 20-year survival figures given in Table 15 show the importance of cell type in determining long term survival: a squamous cell growth with negative node involvement gave the best prognosis, and until now the poor long-term prognosis of adenocarcinoma may not have been realised. In contrast to these results, in 1975 Shields et al., with a comparable number of resections (2349), considered that mediastinal node involvement was of greater significance than cell histology.

Table 15. Twenty-year survivors[a]

	+ ve mediastinal nodes	− ve mediastinal nodes
Squamous	8	19
Adenocarcinoma	0	1
Undifferentiated	3	6
Small	1	1

[a]Of the 39 survivors, 36 were males and 3, females

In the total series there were 39 patients of a possible 769 who survived 20 years (5.1%), while 226 of 1659 survived 10 years (13.6%) and 517 of 2127 survived 5 years (24.3%). These percentages include the hospital mortality, since this gives a realistic estimate of survival rate when advising a patient to accept surgery.

Causes of Death

Hospital Deaths. (Table 16). Although the number of patients in the second series was almost doubled, the hospital mortality was actually reduced by one. Undoubtedly this was due to the introduction of routine antibiotic cover and the

Table 16. Hospital deaths

	1950–1961	1961–1972	1972–1983
Patients	562	1007	990
Deaths	79	78	92

availability of assisted respiration in intensive care units. The increase in the third series was due to the increased age of patients being treated.

Late Deaths. (Table 17). The figures in Table 17 show the remorseless nature of this disease, with 74% of late deaths being due to bronchial carcinoma. Although the figures are depressing, it must be remembered that they take no account of the number of patients who survived 10 or more years before developing a recurrence.

Table 17. Late deaths

Cause of death	Number
Mediastinal recurrence or metastasis	1584
New extrathoracic carcinoma	44
Cerebral or cardiovascular accident	278
Bronchopulmonary or pleural infection	217

Conclusion

It is generally accepted that untreated bronchial carcinoma causes death after an average time of 9 months. In one-third of patients diagnosed, the first symptom is due to a metastasis, and in a further third poor general health precludes surgical treatment, leaving only one-third who are fit for radical therapy.

In the largest collection of patients treated for bronchial carcinoma by different surgeons, Belcher (1983) has shown that survival rates quoted both in England and in America show little variation around a 15% 10-year rate and a 26% 5-year rate (excluding hospital mortality), regardless of the surgeon or hospital concerned. It is therefore clear that surgical technique alone cannot improve on present results.

Squamous cell growths form 60% of bronchial carcinomas, and in spite of trials combining radiotherapy and chemotherapy with surgery, surgical resection remains the most successful form of treatment for this histological variety. For the three other cell types, however, improved results must depend on further research into combination therapy.

References

Bates M (1970) Results of surgery for bronchial carcinoma in patients aged 70 and over. Thorax 25:77–78
Bates M (1975) Treatment of oat cell carcinoma of the lung. Am Heart J 89:675–677

Bates M (1979) Combined radiotherapy and surgery for oat cell carcinoma. Rev Fr Mal Respir 7:740–741

Bates M (1981) Surgical treatment of bronchial carcinoma. Ann R Coll Surg Engl 63: 164–167

Bates M, Hurt RL, Levison V, Sutton M (1974) Treatment of oat cell carcinoma of bronchus by pre-operative radiotherapy and surgery. Lancet I:1134–1135

Belcher JR (1983) Thirty years of surgery for carcinoma of the bronchus. Thorax 38:428–432

Belcher JR, Anderson R (1965) Surgical treatment of carcinoma of the bronchus. Br Med J I:948–956

Bloedorn FG (1973) In: Fletcher GH (ed) Textbook of radiotherapy. Lea and Febiger, Philadelphia, p 581

Brock RC, Whytehead LL (1955) Radical pneumonectomy for bronchial cancer. Br J Surg 43:8–24

Bromley LL, Szur L (1955) Combined radiotherapy and resection for carcinoma of the bronchus. Lancet II:937–941

Le Roux BT (1972) Management of bronchial carcinoma by segmental resection. Thorax 27:70–74

Levison VB (1980a) What is the best treatment for early operable small cell carcinoma of the bronchus? Thorax 35:721–724

Levison V (1980b) Pre-operative radiotherapy and surgery in the treatment of oat cell carcinoma of the bronchus. Clin Radiol 31:345–348

Miller AB, Fox W, Tall R (1969) Five year follow-up of the Medical Research Council comparative trial of surgery and radiotherapy, for the primary treatment of small or oat celled carcinoma of the bronchus. Lancet II:501–505

Monk I, Woods W (1975) Pre-operative irradiation for carcinoma of the bronchus. Aust J Surg 45:37–41

Overholt RH, Neptune WB, Ashraf MM (1975) Primary cancer of the lung: a 42 years' experience. Ann Thorac Surg 20:511–519

Sensenig DM, Rossi NP, Ehrenhaft JL (1966) Pulmonary resection for bronchogenic carcinoma in geriatric patients. Ann Thorac Surg 2:508–513

Shields TW, Higgins GA Jr (1974) Minimal pulmonary resection in treatment of carcinoma of the lung. Arch Surg 108:420–422

Shields TW, Higgins GA, Lawton R, Hellbrunn A, Keehn RJ (1970) Pre-operative X-ray therapy as an adjuvant in the treatment of bronchogenic carcinoma. J Thorac Cardiovasc Surg 59: 49–61

Shields TW, Yee J, Conn JH, Robinette CD (1975) Relationship of cell type and lymph node metastasis to survival after resection of bronchial carcinoma. Ann Thorac Surg 20:501–510

Shore DB, Paneth M (1980) Survival after resection of small cell carcinoma of the bronchus. Thorax 35:819–822

Thompson Evans EW (1973) Resection for bronchial carcinoma in the elderly. Thorax 28:86–88

Chapter 12

Surgical Resection as an Adjunct to Chemotherapy for Small Cell Carcinoma of the Lung

John A. Meyer

Introduction

The second edition of the World Health Organisation's classification of lung tumours (World Health Organisation 1982) divides small cell carcinoma into three subtypes: oat cell carcinoma, intermediate cell type and combined oat cell carcinoma (see p. 135). Both oat cell and intermediate cell tumours grow rapidly and disseminate widely. Labelling indices are the highest among lung tumours (Muggia and DeVita 1972). It is generally accepted that volume-doubling times are short, with median values in the range of about 23–40 days (Chahinian 1972; Meyer 1973; Bhaskar et al. 1977); one study did report a median doubling time for small cell carcinomas of 77 days (Brigham et al. 1978) but the authors did not give measurements or define their calculations. The discrepancy between these findings is not easily explainable. Considering that median doubling times of all lung cancers have been reported to be in the range of about 80–90 days (Schwartz 1961; Garland et al. 1963; Spratt et al. 1963), one would expect doubling times of this most malignant tumour to be considerably shorter (see pp. 226, 233).

Ultrastructural demonstration of intracytoplasmic neurosecretory granules is a reliable diagnostic sign, but is shared with other APUD tumour cells, including bronchial carcinoids (Bensch et al. 1968). All small cell carcinomas seem to share a deletion involving sites 14–21 of the p (short) arm of chromosome #3, known as the 3p deletion (Whang-Peng et al. 1981). However, diagnostic confirmation of every case by electron microscopy or chromosome analysis is hardly feasible, and the WHO diagnostic criteria are intended to be applicable by light microscopy.

Historical Notes

A mountain range known as the Erzgebirge, or the Ore Mountains, separates the German province of Saxony from the Czech province of Bohemia. Pitchblende for the Curies' laboratory was mined here, and uranium and cobalt are the foremost products of these mines today. A lethal lung disease of the miners, the *Bergkrankheit*, or mountain sickness, has been recognised since the nineteenth century as clearly being of occupational origin. Studies of the Bergkrankheit showed that there were two histological types of malignancy: squamous cell carcinoma and a highly cellular sarcoma which was felt to be akin to 'lymphosarcoma'. Barnard noted that the latter tumour differed in several ways from sarcomas, and proposed that it be classified as a highly anaplastic carcinoma instead (Barnard 1926).

Studies of the miners' cancer were centered especially on the towns of Schneeberg in Saxony and Joachimsthal in Bohemia (now renamed Jáchymov). The review by Lorenz (1944) may have been the last definitive study in English. The area of the mines at first spanned the border between Germany and Austria–Hungary, and after the Treaty of Versailles, the border between Germany and Czechoslovakia. Following the Munich agreement of 1938 the area came entirely under the control of Hitler, and after World War II it passed under the control of the German Democratic Republic and the Peoples' Republic of Czechoslovakia. It is still a major source of uranium in the atomic age, and the Bergkrankheit of the nineteenth century remains an occupational health problem; thus a postwar review of the subject in German listed 55 cases (Horacek 1969). Lung cancer among uranium miners is an occupational hazard in the western United States as well (Saccomanno et al. 1971, 1974). Smoking and inhalation of radioactive dust appear to be strongly synergistic as causative factors, and provided that they do not smoke, even uranium miners may not be at much added risk (Saccomanno et al. 1974).

In the United States generally, cigarette smoking is the prime and almost sole causative mechanism. Thus of 112 consecutive patients treated for small cell carcinoma of the lung at the National Cancer Institute, Bethesda, Maryland, only one had never smoked (Johnston-Early et al. 1980). The epidemic of lung cancer is gaining speed and momentum among women, and small cell carcinoma is no exception. Currently, it appears that approximately a third of the patients are women.

In the 1950s and 1960s, the extreme biological malignancy of this tumour was defined, and it became quite apparent that surgical resection by itself did nothing to alter its rapidly lethal course. Over a 12-year period, 1960 through 1971, 161 patients were treated for small cell carcinoma at the Roswell Park Memorial Institute, Buffalo, New York, by all modalities then available (Takita et al. 1973). Median patient survival was 4.6 months, and the authors noted that no patient could be said to have been cured. One patient treated by radiation therapy and the drug hexamethylmelamine remained in complete remission after 38 months, however, and may have had eradication of his disease.

The Medical Research Council of Great Britain conducted a prospective clinical trial of surgical resection versus radiation therapy (Miller et al. 1969; Fox and Scadding 1973). Criteria for acceptance of patients into the study were (a) that a biopsy diagnosis of small cell carcinoma was available, and (b) that the patient's tumour must have been declared operable by the surgical consultants. We must note that at that time the available diagnostic and staging techniques were limited in comparison to those of today. All told, 71 patients were randomised to undergo surgical resection as definitive treatment, and 73 to be treated by radiation therapy. Four patients treated by radiotherapy survived for more than 5 years, and three for 10 years. Of the patients assigned to surgical treatment, only one, who had refused resection and been treated by radiotherapy instead, survived for more than 5 years.

Rightly or wrongly, this study convinced oncologists everywhere that surgical resection was of no value for this disease, while the other 'local' modality, radiation therapy, possessed at least some curative potential. The study criteria may, however, have placed surgical treatment at a disadvantage, for only relatively advanced and

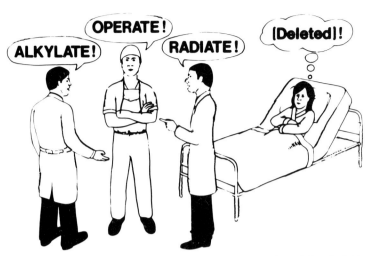

Fig. 1. Treatment strategy for cancer, in the past, has often depended on individual points of view. We have aimed instead to combine our treatment efforts, in accordance with an agreed plan. (Meyer et al. 1983, reproduced with permission from the Annals of Thoracic Surgery).

central primary tumours would have been accessible for direct biopsy through rigid bronchoscopes, which were then the sole type. Moreover, clinical methods for identification of disseminated disease were relatively primitive at the time of the study. We believe that this study has had a lasting adverse effect on the formulation of new treatment strategies against small cell carcinoma (Fig. 1).

Several reports have called attention to the importance of early disease stage for the patient's chance of long-term survival after surgical resection. (We discuss staging under a separate heading below.) While Mountain (1978) found no long-term survivors after resection among 15 patients classifiable retrospectively as having had stage I disease, or among five more with stage II disease, other reports have disagreed somewhat. An appreciable impact of surgical resection on patient survival, however, has been noted only among those presenting with stage I disease (Lennox et al. 1968; Higgins et al. 1975; Shore and Paneth 1980; Shields et al. 1982; Mayer et al. 1982); in fact, very few patients present with disease in stage I (Weiss et al. 1980). Shields et al. (1982) reported that of those patients undergoing resection of the earliest identifiable lesions, $T_1 N_0 M_0$, less than half are still alive after 5 years. So we must all agree that surgical resection by itself is without exception inadequate treatment for small cell carcinoma of the lung, of any histological subtype and in any TNM stage grouping. Microscopic tumour dissemination plainly is responsible for the failure of surgical resection.

During the 1960s, the US Veterans' Administration Lung Group treated large numbers of patients with inoperable lung cancer, of all histological types, by randomisation to single-drug chemotherapy regimens. Green et al. (1969) reported that treatment with cyclophosphamide did not prolong survival in the patient group as a whole; however, when treated patients were separated by cell type a significant prolongation of median survival from 1.7 to 4.0 months was noted among those with small cell carcinoma. This and other studies established the principle that this tumour is generally responsive to chemotherapy.

Staging of Disease

For the patient with a given type of cancer, many things depend on the extent of disease at presentation: the possibility of curative treatment, the possibility of effective palliation if the disease is incurable, and the probable length of survival if it is incurable. Results of treatment at different centres or using different methods cannot be compared unless the patients are matched by stage of disease. In the United States, oncologists for the most part have classified patients with inoperable lung cancer into the simple categories of 'limited' or 'extensive' disease (Hyde et al. 1965). Limited disease is defined as being restricted to one hemithorax plus the ipsilateral supraclavicular nodes, while extensive disease includes all those cases with more distant involvement. Almost all reviews of treatment for small cell carcinoma have divided the patients into these two categories.

The American Joint Committee for Cancer Staging developed a more precise staging system based on the extent of the primary tumour, the lymph nodes and metastases (Mountain et al. 1974). The TNM system, as it is known, gained immediate acceptance as a means of briefly defining those factors of disease extent which affect the patient's prognosis. Currently, the two American journals of thoracic surgery will reject manuscripts dealing with lung cancer unless disease stage is defined according to the TNM system. Originally, the scheme classified all small cell carcinomas as stage III, noting that 'the survival curves for patients with undifferentiated small cell carcinoma indicate a disastrous clinical course regardless of the demonstrable anatomic extent of disease' (Mountain et al. 1974). Our group in Syracuse, however, found it necessary to use the TNM system from the beginning, in order to specify the lesions for which surgical treatment seemed to be appropriate (Meyer et al. 1979). The scheme as recently revised (American Joint Committee for Cancer Staging and End-Results Reporting 1979) takes note of the accumulating evidence that survival is closely linked to stage, even in small cell carcinoma, and recommends that the TNM system be used for all tumour types. Since disease staging is important to our hypothesis, we must briefly outline the system here.

The Primary Tumour (T Factor)

T_1 signifies a solitary tumour, 3.0 cm or less in greatest diameter, surrounded by lung or uninvolved visceral pleura. There must be no extension proximal to a lobar bronchial orifice, and no atelectasis or obstructive pneumonitis.

T_2 tumours are over 3.0 cm in greatest diameter, or they may be of any size if: (a) involving visceral pleura, or (b) producing atelectasis or obstructive pneumonitis extending to the hilum. The proximal margin of tumour must be at least 2.0 cm distal to the carina. Atelectasis or pneumonitis must involve less than the entire lung, and there must be no pleural effusion.

T_3 designates a tumour of any size that (a) approaches to less than 2.0 cm from the carina; or (b) shows direct extension into the chest wall, mediastinum or diaphragm; or (c) causes atelectasis or pneumonitis of an entire lung; or (d) is associated with identifiable pleural effusion.

The Lymph Nodes (N Factor)

This factor may not always be defined precisely until after examination of the surgical specimen.

N_0 specifies that no nodes are involved by tumour.
N_1 signifies that peribronchial and/or ipsilateral hilar nodes are involved.
N_2 indicates that mediastinal nodes are involved.

Metastatic Disease (M Factor)

M_0 indicates that no metastatic disease can be identified.
M_1 indicates involvement of cervical or supraclavicular nodes, or the presence of distant blood-borne metastases.

The Stage Groupings

Stage I disease includes those tumours classified as $T_1 N_0 M_0$, $T_2 N_0 M_0$ and $T_1 N_1 M_0$.

Stage II lesions are relatively few in number, made up only of those classified as $T_2 N_1 M_0$. Translated, this signifies a primary tumour confined to lung, not closely approaching the carina, more than 3.0 cm in diameter if peripheral, and associated with involvement only of peribronchial or, at most, hilar nodes.

Stage III includes all T_3 primary tumours, with any N or M factors; all N_2 disease (mediastinal nodes involved), with any T or M factors; and all M_1 disease (metastatic disease), with any T or N factors.

We should note here that stage III factors do not *necessarily* indicate incurability in lung cancer, except for the M_1 factor. With this point in mind, the National Cancer Center of Japan adopted a TNM system which includes a stage IV, defined by the M_1 factor. Such a distinction is rational and may be adopted eventually in the United States.

Some Points of Oncological Theory

It seems clear that small cell carcinoma responds better to combinations of effective drugs than to a single drug given to maximum tolerance. There is, however, at least one reported instance of a patient whose disease apparently was eradicated by treatment with a single drug, without radiotherapy (Vosika 1979a, b). Many chemotherapeutic drugs work by different mechanisms, and on theoretical grounds it seems rational to attack a highly malignant tumour by several mechanisms simultaneously. The drugs clearly active against small cell carcinoma number no more than eight or so, and may be classified as follows.

A. *Alkylating agents:*
Cyclophosphamide, marketed as Cytoxan in the United States
Chloroethyl-cyclohexyl-nitrosourea (CCNU) marketed as Lomustine in the United States
Hexamethylmelamine

B. *Plant alkaloids:*
Vincristine (Oncovin)

C. *Antibiotics:*
Doxorubicin (Adriamycin)

D. *Antimetabolites:*
Amethopterin or methotrexate

E. *Agents which (like alkylating agents) act by scission and cross-linkage of deoxyribonucleic acid):*
cis-Diamine-dichloro-platinum (*cis*-platin)
The epipodophyllotoxin VP-16-213, now marketed in the United States as Etoposide.

A curious feature of the bewildering number of reports and treatment programmes is that, provided combinations of the effective agents and modalities are used, response rates appear to be almost independent of the specific regimen. The 'optimal' treatment regimen has not yet been defined; possibly this means that the most essential mechanisms for control of the disease are still beyond our understanding.

Treatment to the absolute limit of patient tolerance is not necessarily the answer. A regimen of incredible ferocity, under which 24% of the patients died of treatment-related causes, concluded with an 'actuarial' estimate of 30% long-term survivors in limited disease. This figure of course exceeds the true percentage of long-term survivors. No patient with extensive disease achieved long-term survival (Johnson et al. 1978). Conversely, regimens designed for reasonable patient tolerance on an out-patient basis have achieved essentially the same rates of response and survival — and even one long-term survivor in the group with extensive disease — without treatment-related mortality (Ginsberg et al. 1979).

Those of us who are not oncologists may have difficulty understanding the primary characteristic of chemotherapy: that no matter how effective a given drug regimen may be against a given tumour, it kills tumour cells by a pattern of first-order kinetics. This means that a dose or a cycle of chemotherapy will kill, at best, a given percentage or proportion of the patient's tumour cells, never a given bulk or mass of the tumour. As a tumour responds, its mass diminishes; hence the number of tumour cells killed by subsequent cycles will also diminish. The scheme outlined in Table 1 may help to define this point. We must note that the chemotherapeutic effect required to reduce a microscopic burden of 1000 surviving tumour cells to one cell is equal to that required to reduce a gross tumour 10 cm in diameter to a residual tumour 1 cm in diameter. Each response constitutes a 'three-log' or thousand-fold reduction of tumour burden. Unfortunately, in the end it is likely that pre-existing or mutant clones of tumour cells, resistant to the chemotherapy, will grow out again and result in relapse.

Zeno of Elea (ca. 490–410 B.C.) knew nothing of cancer chemotherapy, but formulated a paradox which may be instructive to us. An archer stands up to the line, draws his bow and looses an arrow at the target. The arrow first travels half the

Table 1. Theoretical scheme of the logarithmic reduction of tumour burden by perfectly effective chemotherapy[a]

Tumour cells	Tumour bulk	Tumour weight
10^{12} cells	10 cm tumour diameter	1 kg
10^9 cells	1 cm diameter	1 g
(Complete remission)[b]		
10^6	1 mm diameter	1 mg
10^3 cells	1000 cells	
10^0	1 cell	
10^{-1}	Tumour eradication in 90% of cases	
10^{-2}	Tumour eradication in 99% of cases	

[a] A patient with a far advanced incurable malignancy carries a tumour burden roughly in the order of 10^{12} cells. In the aggregate, this is equivalent to a tumour mass approximately 10 cm in diameter, weighing approximately 1 kg.
[b] A three-log or greater reduction of initial tumour bulk is generally sufficient to induce clinically complete remission, since visceral tumours ordinarily are not detectable clinically at a diameter of less than 1 cm. (A 'three-log reduction' means that 99.9% of the tumour cells have been killed.)

distance to the target, then half the remaining distance, and so on. It follows that the arrow can never reach the target. For the medical oncologist, Zeno's paradox is not just an intriguing fallacy of logic, but a hard and inescapable fact of life. The few exceptions only go to prove the rule.

While surgeons love to speak of 'cure', oncologists speak more realistically of disease control. Whether or not a patient's malignant disease is actually eradicated, the distinction is immaterial if the patient can be given a normal life expectancy. 'Complete remission' after chemotherapy is defined as disappearance of all clinical evidence of residual disease. 'Partial remission' or partial response is used variably; most commonly it is defined as a 50% reduction in the *product* of two perpendicular diameters of a measurable lesion. Partial remission can also be applied to marked clearing of non-measurable disease, such as lymphangitic spread within the lung. 'Relapse' is defined as reappearance of gross disease after complete remission, or a 50% increase in the product of two diameters after partial response.

Among all patients with tumours responsive to chemotherapy, it is clear that responders live longer than do non-responders or untreated patients. It is clear also that clinically complete remission is an absolute prerequisite for long-term disease-free survival.

Treatment Strategy: Continuing Problems

Only a decade ago, the first systematic trial of combined-modality therapy for small cell carcinoma was reported (Eagan et al. 1973). Treatment strategy visualised reduction of the large mass of tumour at the primary site and in the mediastinal nodes by irradiation, while intensive combination chemotherapy was used with the intent of controlling disseminated disease. In many variations, this general plan of a 'local' plus a 'systemic' modality has governed treatment since that time. Radiation therapy has always been chosen as the local modality, of course, as the result of the Medical Research Council study which we have already noted. The study fostered a conviction among oncologists that radiation therapy by itself possesses at least some curative potential, while surgical resection possesses none (Miller et al. 1969; Fox and Scadding 1973).

It seems clear that radiation therapy does not prolong survival if gross disease is present outside the treatment field. As a result, its use is restricted mainly to patients with 'limited' disease; patients with 'extensive' disease seem to benefit primarily from intensive chemotherapy. Radiotherapy may give effective palliation for severe local symptoms such as bone pain or cerebral metastases. It follows that prior to treatment patients must be carefully staged for extent of disease. Most institutions in the United States require a histological biopsy specimen, and isotope scans of the liver and skeletal system are obtained in all cases, as are computerised tomographic scans of the central nervous system. In the absence of known skeletal metastases, bone-marrow aspiration and biopsies are obtained from both iliac crests.

Even among patients whose disease appears localised at diagnosis, the incidence of brain metastases increases progressively with longer survival. In one review, the combined (clinical and autopsy) intracranial failure rate reached 80% among patients who survived for more than 24 months (Nugent et al. 1979). Prophylactic cranial irradiation seems to control this increasing risk. In a study by Komaki et al. (1981), of 131 patients initially without evidence of metastases to the central nervous system, 74 did not receive prophylactic cranial irradiation at the time of initial treatment. Of these, 28% had developed brain metastases by 1 year and 58% by 2 years after the initiation of treatment. On the other hand, of 57 patients who received prophylactic cranial irradiation, 11% had developed brain metastases by 1 year, and still only 11% by 2 years (Komaki et al. 1981). Prophylactic cranial irradiation is a necessity if we are to aim for total disease control.

Combined treatment by chemotherapy and irradiation of patients with 'limited' disease achieves significant response in almost all, and clinically complete remission in perhaps 70%. These response rates are not so high if radiotherapy is omitted from the treatment regimen. Approximately 10%–15% of limited disease patients achieve long-term disease-free survival, off treatment, and may have had their disease eradicated. Accumulated experience from many centres suggests that patients who remain in *complete remission* at 2 years after the start of treatment are most unlikely to suffer relapse thereafter.

Patients presenting with 'extensive' disease do much less well, and perhaps 25%–30% may achieve complete remission. As we have noted, radiation therapy does not prolong survival in this group, since its effects are limited to the treatment field. It can, however, be of considerable palliative value in the relief of severe local symptoms. Median patient survival after treatment averages perhaps 7–8 months, and long disease-free survival is almost non-existent in this group. Until fundamentally different modes of treatment evolve, our efforts towards disease control must necessarily be directed at those patients with clinically localised disease.

We have noted that only a small minority of responding patients remain clinically disease-free at 2 years. But among limited-disease patients who achieve complete remission, the most common site of relapse is *within the chest* (60%–77% of relapses in a number of series) (Figs. 2–5). This remains true whether treatment was by alternating regimens of intensive chemotherapy (Cohen et al. 1979), or by combination chemotherapy plus irradiation of the primary and the mediastinum (Johnson et al. 1978; McMahon et al. 1979). The role of surgical eradication of the primary site and mediastinal nodes must be re-examined within the context of combined modality therapy. We should consider separately its application to early localised disease (stages I and II) and to more advanced but still clinically localised disease, stage III-M_0.

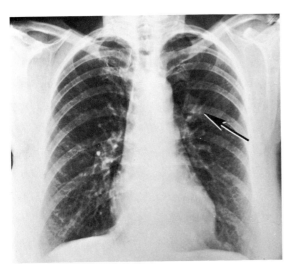

Fig. 2. Frontal chest film of a 56-year-old woman, a long-time smoker. A poorly defined 3-cm mass density is present in the left upper lobe. At thoracotomy, a 1.5-cm hilar node was found to be involved by small cell carcinoma. At that time (1975) surgical resection was thought unwarranted, and the procedure was abandoned. (Reproduced with permission from Ann Thorac Surg 30:608)

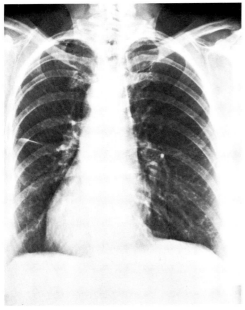

Fig. 3. Same patient as in Fig. 2. Following thoracotomy, the patient was treated by chemotherapy and irradiation of the primary site, with clinically complete remission. Chest film during remission, 7 months after diagnosis. (Reproduced with permission of Ann Thorac Surg 30:608)

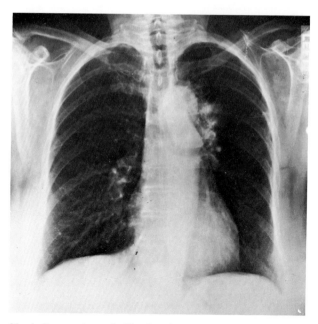

Fig. 4. Same patient as in Figs. 2 and 3. A recurrent density appeared at the site of the primary tumour 19 months after the start of treatment. Bronchoscopic biopsy confirmed that this lesion represented recurrent small cell carcinoma. (Reproduced with permission from Ann Thorac Surg 30:608)

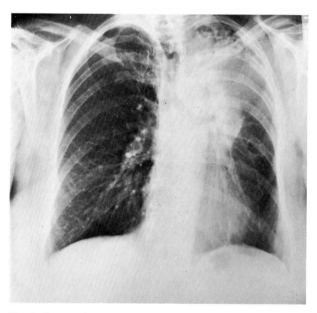

Fig. 5. Same patient as in Figs. 2–4. Progressing disease in spite of alternative chemotherapy, at 23 months after the start of treatment. The patient died at 27 months; at autopsy, no distant metastatic disease could be identified. (Reproduced with permission from Ann Thorac Surg 30:608)

Surgical Resection plus Chemotherapy for Stage I and II Lesions

Reviewing briefly, stage I and II tumours are for the most part peripheral, confined to the lung, and associated with involvement only of bronchopulmonary or hilar nodes, or of no nodes at all. My associates and I have adopted two minor amendments to the TNM scheme, for use only in our small cell carcinoma study. First, to be classified as stage I or II, a tumour must be peripheral, be surrounded by clear lung and be undetectable by mediastinoscopy. Most such lesions will not have been diagnosed pre-operatively unless routine percutaneous needle biopsies are made of all peripheral pulmonary densities. Secondly, small cell tumours causing lobar atelectasis (ordinarily classifiable as T_2) cannot be distinguished from the mediastinum by radiography or computed tomography. For our study only, they are considered as presumptive T_3, hence stage III, and are treated as outlined in the next section (Meyer et al. 1982).

Theoretical considerations favouring initial surgical resection of the stage I and II lesions might be listed as follows.

1. Grossly complete excision of intrathoracic disease would have the effect of establishing complete remission immediately. The patient's bone marrow and haematological reserve would so far have remained untouched. Chemotherapy then could deal more effectively with an expected small burden of microscopic disseminated disease.
2. Therapeutic irradiation of disease in the chest and mediastinum has often required reduction of the chemotherapy dosage, because of diminished patient tolerance for a time thereafter (Meyer et al. 1982).
3. Clean surgical eradication of the commonest site of relapse should offer a better chance of ultimate disease control.

Following resection of gross disease, and completion of staging studies if necessary, prolonged intensive chemotherapy appears to be indispensable. The residual tumour burden at this time is lowest, and chances for disease control are best. We do not know how long a patient should be treated, but our practice is to treat for 1 year if the patient will tolerate it. We do not know, either, whether prophylactic cranial irradiation must be given to all patients after resection of stage I or II tumours, but we do know that relapse in the brain signifies incurability. As a result, we now treat all patients.

Ten patients have undergone resection of stage I or II lesions more than 2 years ago, followed by intensive chemotherapy for the full course thereafter (Meyer et al. 1983). One patient died of a pulmonary embolus on the 7th postoperative day. One patient presented at 35 months after resection with disseminated prostatic carcinoma, and died at 50 months. At autopsy, no residual small cell carcinoma could be identified. One patient has had relapse in the lumbar spinal cord at 14 months after resection, the only instance of recurrence. The other seven patients remain well at more than 2 years since resection, and five have passed 5 years. We have concluded that almost all patients with stage I or II small cell carcinoma of the lung may be rendered disease-free by surgical resection followed by the full course of chemotherapy.

Chemotherapy plus Surgical Resection for More Advanced Local Disease (Stage III-M$_0$)

The question naturally arose whether surgical resection could be combined with chemotherapy in treatment of more advanced local disease. We believed that if T$_3$ or N$_2$ factors could be identified at staging, clean surgical eradication of intrathoracic disease probably could not be accomplished. Grossly incomplete surgical excision is unlikely to benefit the patient. However, patients who achieve a quick initial response to chemotherapy might be suited for clean surgical resection of the primary tumour and the mediastinal nodes. Chemotherapy would, of course, have to be continued thereafter, and prophylactic cranial irradiation would be a necessity. We have administered this to all patients in a dose of 3000 rads over a 2-week period, coinciding with resumption of chemotherapy after a successful surgical resection.

The appropriate timing of the surgical procedure was not clear. A review of our limited-disease patients who achieved complete remission after chemotherapy plus irradiation showed a pattern of relapse beginning only 4 months after the start of treatment (Meyer et al. 1982). This pattern seemed to indicate that if surgical resection were to be included rationally as the 'local' modality, it should be undertaken early. We have aimed to evaluate the patients for resection as soon as possible after 6 weeks from the start of treatment.

The statement that grossly incomplete excision is unlikely to benefit the patient may raise objections; in the United States, at any rate, there are surgeons who still believe in the value of 'palliative resection' or in 'de-bulking'. Let us remember that continuing treatment will have to be by chemotherapy. A surgeon who manages to excise 90% of the gross bulk of a tumour may leave the operating room feeling that he has accomplished a very great thing, that he has done 90% of the job and the remainder can easily be taken care of by the chemotherapist. On the contrary, the logarithmic reduction principle (Table 1) indicates that he has accomplished, at best, a one-log reduction of tumour burden out of a necessary 13 or more. He may have in fact facilitated gross dissemination, at considerable risk to the patient and it is unlikely that he has aided the chemotherapist at all. But a grossly clean resection may easily accomplish a five- or six-log reduction, or more; and if so, it might significantly improve the chances of disease control by chemotherapy.

Since this treatment plan aims for improved local tumour control, the problem of treatment failure resulting from ineffective chemotherapy must be considered as well. Not all patients will respond to a generally effective chemotherapy regimen. As a result of bad experiences early in our trial (Meyer et al. 1982), we have concluded that patients who do not show significant response by 6 weeks should not undergo surgical resection. One could have predicted reasonably that if chemotherapy alone did not induce significant initial response, it could not be expected to control disseminated disease following resection (Figs. 6–9).

We have planned the pulmonary resections to remove the same amount of lung tissue as was involved before treatment; a dramatic response to chemotherapy would not alter this principle. Also, we have aimed to dissect the hilar, subcarinal and (on the right side) paratracheal nodes in all patients.

Given all the above considerations, certain groups of patients should not be considered candidates for surgical resection. Our tentative criteria for exclusion amount to: carinal involvement, severe superior vena caval syndrome, contralateral

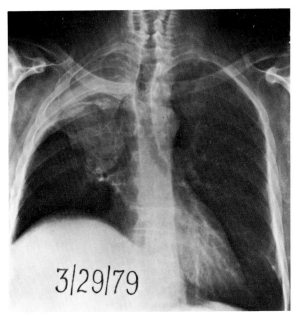

Fig. 6. Initial chest film of a 63-year-old man. Bronchoscopic and mediastinal node biopsies were diagnostic of small cell carcinoma. Studies for distant metastatic disease were unrevealing. Stage T_3N_2: primary tumour invading the mediastinum; the mediastinal nodes are also involved. (Reproduced with permission from J Thorac Cardiovasc Surg 83:14)

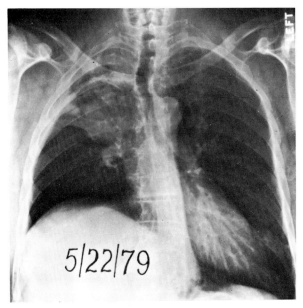

Fig. 7. Same patient as in Fig. 6. No appreciable response after 6 weeks of chemotherapy. At this early stage in our clinical trial, we felt it necessary to accomplish resection at all costs. The patient was accordingly treated by radiation therapy, to a dose of 2400 rads. (Reproduced with permission from J Thorac Cardiovasc Surg 83:14)

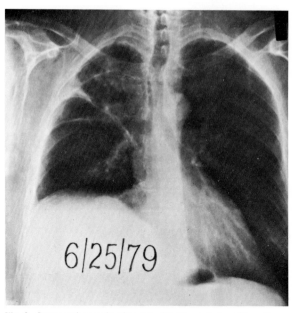

Fig. 8. Same patient as in Figs. 6 and 7. Frontal chest film after completion of radiotherapy. Significant response induced by irradiation, after lack of response to chemotherapy. The patient then underwent right pneumonectomy and dissection of the mediastinal nodes.

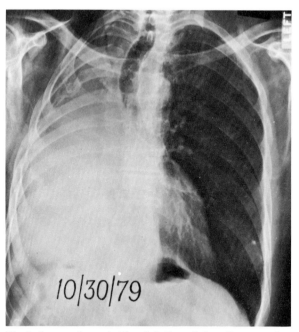

Fig. 9. Same patient as in Figs. 6–8. Frontal chest film approximately 4 months after pneumonectomy. Four months after this, the patient presented with massive recurrent disease in the liver. We now believe that if the chemotherapy regimen does not induce a significant initial response, it cannot be expected to control disseminated disease after resection.

mediastinal node involvement, malignant pleurisy, inadequate physiological status, insufficient response to allow clean resection and refusal of the operation by the patient. Alternative modes of treatment are explained to all patients, and informed consent is sought. Patients excluded from resection for any of these reasons continue to receive standard non-operative treatment: radiation therapy and continued chemotherapy.

Abstinence from smoking is urged on all patients, since it appears to make a difference even if only from the time of diagnosis (Johnston-Early et al. 1980). Our chemotherapy regimens have been reviewed in detail (Meyer et al. 1982). At present the regimen includes four drugs, cyclophosphamide, vincristine, doxorubicin and etoposide, on a 3-week cycle. A set of rules for dose reduction is a necessary part of this regimen. Potential sites of infection, such as decayed or broken teeth, require correction prior to the start of treatment.

It is difficult at present to give a coherent summary of the results of treatment. In the jargon of American cancer research, our study is a phase II trial; that is, the study accepts for treatment all patients meeting the criteria of eligibility. There is no simultaneous control group. The role of surgical resection for this patient group will not be defined until a phase III study has been done, with randomisation of patients to alternative modes of treatment. Such a study could accumulate a sufficient number of cases only if several institutions joined co-operatively; at present our colleagues in Oncology are seeking to organise such a clinical trial.

A brief account of some of our patients may be instructive. Early in the study, two patients ($T_3 N_2$, $T_2 N_2$) had not responded at the 6-week evaluation. Both then responded to radiation therapy at a dose of 2400 rads and underwent resection, by

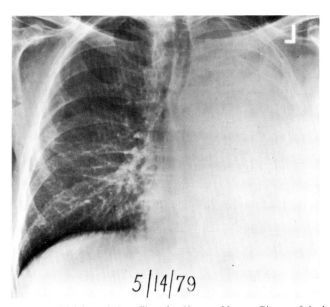

Fig. 10. Initial frontal chest film of a 65-year-old man. Biopsy of the lesion in the left main bronchus revealed small cell carcinoma. Mediastinoscopy showed no abnormalities, and studies for distant metastatic disease were unrevealing. Stage $T_1 N_1$. (Reproduced with permission from J Thorac Cardiovasc Surg 83:16)

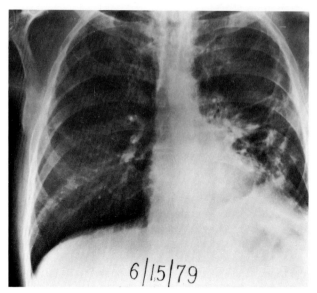

Fig. 11. Same patient as in Fig. 10. Dramatic response after only a month of chemotherapy, with partial re-aeration of left lung. The patient underwent left pneumonectomy after the 6-week evaluation. (Reproduced with permission from J Thorac Cardiovasc Surg 83:16)

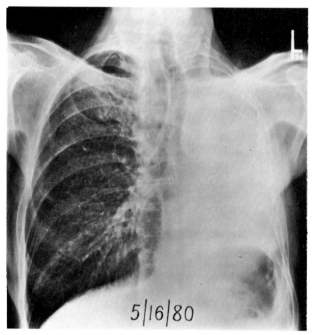

Fig. 12. Same patient as in Figs. 10 and 11. Frontal chest film, 1 year after the start of treatment. Chemotherapy was discontinued at this time. The patient died of a myocardial infarction at 35 months. At autopsy, no residual tumour could be identified.

pneumonectomy and lobectomy respectively. Both died of recurrent tumour at 8 and 10 months. Since that time, as we have noted above, patients not showing a response at 6 weeks are no longer considered eligible for surgical treatment.

Two patients achieving minimal and moderate response underwent thoracotomy but no resection. In the former, the main pulmonary artery could not be isolated or controlled at the hilum, and resection was abandoned; the patient remains in partial remission at 9 months. The other patient had severely limited pulmonary reserve and lower lobectomy was planned; but an involved node was found densely adherent to the pulmonary artery and bronchus at a level which would have required pneumonectomy for removal. It was plain that the patient could not tolerate pneumonectomy and the procedure was abandoned; the patient died of meningeal recurrence at 16 months after the start of treatment.

All told, 11 more patients have responded and undergone successful resection, some of them recently so that significant follow-up is not available. Resection has required pneumonectomy in almost all the patients in this group. Dissection of involved mediastinal nodes has been found to be feasible after response. We should say, however, that in general the resections are laborious and involve extreme technical difficulty.

One patient ($T_3 N_1$) died of a massive myocardial infarction at 34 months after the start of treatment; at autopsy, no residual tumour could be found (Figs. 10–12). Two other patients ($T_3 N_1$ and $T_2 N_2$) remain disease-free at 35 and 25 months respectively, off all treatment since 12 months. Other patients remain in remission after shorter periods. Five patients have died of recurrent disease. So far at any rate, no patient undergoing resection plus continued chemotherapy has shown relapse within the chest.

In summary, small cell carcinoma of the lung remains a highly lethal disease. Surgical treatment is obviously inappropriate in the presence of known dissemination. Chemotherapy remains the key to disease control. Whether surgical resection may aid control in selected patients remains unproved, but a careful clinical trial appears to be warranted.

References

American Joint Committee for Cancer Staging and End-Results Reporting (1979) Staging of lung cancer, 1979. Chicago, Illinois

Barnard WG (1926) The nature of the 'oat-celled sarcoma' of the mediastinum. J Pathol Bacteriol 29:241–244

Bensch KJ, Corrin B, Pariente R, Spencer H (1968) Oat cell carcinoma of the lung: Its origin and relationship to bronchial carcinoid. Cancer 22:1163–1172

Bhaskar D, Maldonado A, Ng A, Selawry O (1977) Volume doubling time of small cell carcinoma of the lung. Proc Am Soc Clin Oncol 18:335 (Abstr)

Brigham BA, Bunn PA, Minna JD, Cohen MH, Ihde DC, Shackney SE (1978) Growth rates of small cell bronchogenic carcinoma. Cancer 42:2880–2886

Chahinian P (1972) Relationship between tumour doubling time and anatomo-clinical features in 50 measurable pulmonary cancers. Chest 61:340–345

Cohen MH, Ihde DC, Bunn PA et al. (1979) Cyclic alternating chemotherapy for small cell bronchogenic carcinoma. Cancer Treat Rep 63:163–170

Eagan RT, Maurer LH, Forcier RJ, Tulloh M (1973) Combination chemotherapy and radiation therapy in small cell carcinoma. Cancer 32:371–379

Fox W, Scadding JG (1973) Medical Research Council comparative trial of surgery and radiotherapy for primary treatment of small-celled or oat-celled carcinoma of the bronchus: Ten year follow-up. Lancet II:63–65

Garland LH, Coulson W, Wollin E (1963) The rate of growth and apparent duration of untreated primary bronchogenic carcinoma. Cancer 16:694–707

Ginsberg SJ, Comis RL, Gottlieb AJ et al. (1979) Long-term survivorship in small cell anaplastic carcinoma. Cancer Treat Rep 63:1347–1349

Green RA, Humphrey E, Close HM, Patno ME (1969) Alkylating agents in bronchogenic carcinoma. Am J Med 46:516–525

Higgins GA, Shields TW, Keehn RJ (1975) The solitary pulmonary nodule: Ten year follow-up of the Veterans' Administration–Armed Forces co-operative study. Arch Surg 110:570–575

Horacek J (1969) Der Joachimstaler Lungenkrebs nach dem zweiten Weltkrieg (The lung cancer of Joachimsthal since the Second World War). Zeitschr Krebsforsch 72:52–56

Hyde L, Yee J, Wilson R, Patno ME (1965) Cell type and the natural history of lung cancer. JAMA 193:52–54

Johnson RE, Brereton HD, Kent CH (1978) 'Total' therapy for small cell carcinoma of the lung. Ann Thorac Surg 25:510–515

Johnston-Early A, Cohen MH, Minna JD et al. (1980) Smoking abstinence and small cell lung cancer survival: an association. JAMA 244:2175–2179

Komaki R, Cox JD, Whitson W (1981) Risk of brain metastasis from small cell carcinoma of the lung related to length of survival and prophylactic irradiation. Cancer Treat Rep 65:811–814

Lennox SC, Flavell G, Pollock DJ, Thompson VC, Wilkins JL (1968) Results of resection for oat-cell carcinoma of the lung. Lancet II:925–927

Lorenz E (1944) Radioactivity and lung cancer: Critical review of lung cancer in miners of Schneeberg and Joachimsthal. J Natl Cancer Inst 5:1–15

Mayer JE, Ewing SL, Ophoven J, Sumner HW, Humphrey EW (1982) Influence of histology on survival after curative resection for undifferentiated lung cancer. J Thorac Cardiovasc Surg 84:641–648

McMahon LJ, Herman TS, Manning MR, Dean JC (1979) Patterns of relapse in patients with small cell carcinoma of the lung treated with adriamycin–cyclophosphamide chemotherapy and radiation therapy. Cancer Treat Rep 63:359–362

Meyer JA (1973) Growth rate versus prognosis in resected primary bronchogenic carcinomas. Cancer 31:1468–1472

Meyer JA, Parker FB (1980) Small cell carcinoma of the lung (Collective Review). Ann Thorac Surg 30:602–610

Meyer JA, Comis RL, Ginsberg SJ, Ikins PM, Burke WA, Parker FB (1979) Selective surgical resection in small cell carcinoma of the lung. J Thorac Cardiovasc Surg 77:243–248

Meyer JA, Comis RL, Ginsberg SJ et al. (1982) Phase II trial of extended indications for resection in small cell carcinoma of the lung. J Thorac Cardiovasc Surg 83:12–19

Meyer JA, Comis RL, Ginsberg SJ et al. (1983) The prospect of disease control by surgery combined with chemotherapy in stage I and II small cell carcinoma of the lung. Ann Thorac Surg36:37–41

Miller AB, Fox W, Tall R (1969) Five year follow-up of the Medical Research Council comparative trial of surgery and radiotherapy for the primary treatment of small-celled or oat-celled carcinoma of the bronchus. Lancet II:501–505

Mountain CF (1978) Clinical biology of small cell carcinoma: Relationship to surgical therapy. Semin Oncol 5:272–279

Mountain CF, Carr DT, Anderson WAD (1974) A system for the clinical staging of lung cancer. Am J Roentgenol 120:130–138

Muggia FM, DeVita VT (1972) In vivo tumor cell kinetic studies: Use of local thymidine injection followed by fine-needle aspiration. J Lab Clin Med 80:297–301

Nugent JL, Bunn PA, Matthews MJ (1979) CNS metastases in small cell bronchogenic carcinoma: Increasing frequency and changing pattern with lengthening survival. Cancer 44:1885–1893

Saccomanno G, Archer VE, Auerbach O, Kuschner M. Saunders RP, Klein MG (1971) Histologic types of lung cancer among uranium miners. Cancer 27:515–523

Saccomanno G, Archer VE, Auerbach O, Saunders RP, Brennan LM (1974) Development of carcinoma of the lung as reflected in exfoliated cells. Cancer 33:256–270

Schwartz M (1961) A biomathematical approach to clinical tumour growth. Cancer 14:1272–1294

Shields TW, Higgins GA, Matthews MJ, Keehn RJ (1982) Surgical resection in the management of small cell carcinoma of the lung. J Thorac Cardiovasc Surg 84:481–488

Shore DF, Paneth M (1980) Survival after resection of small cell carcinoma of the bronchus. Thorax 35:819–822

Spratt JS, Spjut HJ, Roper CL (1963) The frequency distribution of the rates of growth and the estimated duration of primary pulmonary carcinomas. Cancer 16;687–693

Takita H, Brugarolas A, Marabella P, Vincent RG (1973) Small cell carcinoma of the lung: Clinicopathologic studies. J Thorac Cardiovasc Surg 66:472–477

Vosika G (1979a) Large cell bronchogenic carcinoma: Prolonged disease-free survival following chemotherapy. JAMA 241:594–595

Vosika G (1979b) Large cell-small cell bronchogenic carcinoma (Letter to the Editor). JAMA 241:1813

Weiss RB, Minna JD, Glatstein E, Martini N, Ihde DC, Muggia FM (1980) Treatment of small cell undifferentiated carcinoma of the lung: Update of recent results. Cancer Treat Rep 64:539–547

Whang-Peng J, Bunn PA, Kao-Shan E, Lee E, Minna J, Gazdar A (1981) Non-random chromosomal abnormalities (3p) in continuous cultures of small cell lung cancer. Proc Am Assoc Cancer Res 22:45 (Abstr)

World Health Organization (1982) The World Health Organisation histological typing of lung tumours. Am J Clin Pathol 77:123–136

Chapter 13

Postoperative Pain and Its Relief

Barry Ross

Surgical operations are painful, and doctors experiencing the suffering that they inflict will undoubtedly be more concerned with the postoperative welfare of their patients. Graphic accounts of the pain of thoracic surgery have been described and in particular the dread of the arrival of the physiotherapist (Donald 1976; Gallon 1982). It therefore behoves all medical practitioners to alleviate pain whenever possible, and the control of postoperative pain is a major problem to the thoracic surgeon and his staff.

Brock (1936), in pre-antibiotic days, demonstrated the problem of postoperative chest complications, particularly after upper abdominal surgery. He identified that pain was the most important cause of impaired ventilation and subsequent atelectasis in this type of operation. Surgery has made considerable advances since 1936, and thoracic surgery particularly has been born and bred in the years following. Surgeons, anaesthetists and all concerned with the postoperative patient are forced to steer between the Scylla of intense respiratory depression produced by complete analgesia and the Charybdis of pulmonary complications described by Brock. This chapter reviews the various methods of pain relief available, anticipating that there is a reasonable margin of safety allowing neither of these extremes to consume the patient.

The time-honoured analgesic is morphine given on a patient-demand, nurse-response basis. The classical prescription of morphine 15 mg i.m. 4 hourly × 6 has probably killed more patients who have undergone thoracic surgery than any other form of analgesia. The intramuscular administration of such a dose of this drug provides an unpredictable rate of absorption, particularly in the patient who is peripherally vasoconstricted after recovering from a 3-h operation. The timely improvement of tissue perfusion may result in a hitherto poorly absorbed agent suddenly being released into the circulation. This bolus of morphine may just be sufficient to induce respiratory depression.

The combination of an opiate premedication, opiates during the operation and morphine postoperatively may produce superb analgesia. It may at the same time be followed by significant respiratory depression and even the persistence of an unconscious state so that either intubation and ventilation or morphine antagonist or both will be required.

Analgesia following thoracic surgery is particularly critical for many patho-physiological reasons. Patients after pulmonary resection need to expectorate their secretions in order to maintain ventilation of residual lung tissue. Their ventilatory reserve may have been significantly compromised by the resection of the offending lobe or the whole lung.

The greatest cause of postoperative mortality following oesophagectomy is respiratory, the patients surviving operation being additonally faced with morbidity from the same cause (Jackson et al. 1979). In an attempt to reduce respiratory complications our service maintains intermittent positive pressure ventilation (IPPV) for 16–24 h after oesophagectomy. The mortality of the operation has fallen from 25% (Ross 1981) to 5% over the last 4 years. Similarly, following cardiac surgery many patients are ventilated until the circulation is stable, allowing the administration of intravenous opiates without risk of respiratory depression.

The greatest difficulty related to any discussion on analgesia is an objective assessment of the efficacy of the various agents available and the routes of administration. The disturbance of single breath analysis of lung function is hardly applicable following lobectomy or pneumonectomy although these estimations are often used for assessment of pain relief after other surgical procedures. Assessment of an analgesic regime relies to a great extent on subjective information by either the patient or an observer aided by a linear analogue pain score.

Routes of Administration

Table 1 shows the various routes of drug administration available. Table 2 presents some of the drugs available for administration by these routes.

Table 1. Routes available for the administration of analgesia

1. **Oral**
   a) Swallowed
   b) Sublingual

2. **Parenteral**
   a) Intramuscular
   b) Intravenous

3. **Intravertebral**
   a) Epidural
   b) Spinal

4. **Local Anaesthetic**
   a) Local infiltration — intercostal nerves

5. **Operative**
   a) Intercostal nerve section
   b) Rhizotomy
   c) Cryoneurolysis

6. **Miscellaneous**
   a) Acupuncture
   b) Transcutaneous nerve stimulation
   c) Rectal drugs
   d) Inhalation

Table 2. Some of the drugs available for each of the routes of administration. (The list is not intended to be comprehensive)

Route of administration	Drugs available
Oral	Aspirin, paracetamol, dihydrocodeine, dextropropoxyphene (Distalgesic), pentazocine, pethidine, diamorphine etc.
Sublingual	Buprenorphine
Intramuscular	Morphine, papaveretum, pethidine etc.
Intravenous	Morphine, papaveretum, fentanyl etc.
Rectal	Oxymorphone, aspirin, dextromoramide etc.
Epidural	Morphine, methadone, fentanyl, local anaesthetics etc.
Spinal	As for epidural
Inhalation	Entonox, trichlorethylene, enflurane etc.
Local anaesthetics	Lignocaine, bupivacaine etc.
Neurolytics	Aqueous phenol, alcohol etc.

Oral

Administration of drugs by mouth is hardly applicable to patients recovering from lung resection. However, all patients having reached the stage in the postoperative period when more potent analgesics are no longer required or desirable can be maintained in a pain-free state by oral agents. Aspirin, paracetamol, dextropropoxyphene (Distalgesic) and a host of other compounds are available and effective. The choice of drug is governed by patient tolerance, many finding pentazocine and dihydrocodeine hallucinogenic.

Sublingual

Buprenorphine (Temgesic) is a potent analgesic given sublingually and has proved effective in the relief of post-thoracotomy pain usually from 72 h after the operation.

Intramuscular

For thoracic surgical operations this time-honoured route of administration of narcotic drugs should be abandoned during the first 24–48 h after operation. The dose absorbed is critical and may not bear any relation to the dose administered. The main advantage of this method is nursing economy and possibly financial savings compared with other methods to be discussed below. Although controlled drugs must be administered in the presence of a State Registered nurse, the formalities involved in the 'extended role of the nurse' do not apply. Hard-pressed junior medical staff do not have to be available for routine analgesia, making the intramuscular route very convenient.

Intravenous

To obtain rapid and guaranteed analgesia the intravenous route had been practised on my service for many years. The dose is titrated against the patient's pain or discomfort, small doses (2.5–5 mg papaveretum) being given initially in the recovery room by a member of the surgical or anaesthetic team. The patient having been made comfortable, a similar dose can be administered at hourly intervals or more frequently if required. The injection is given into the existing infusion tubing and can be given by an SRN in the general ward. The allowance of this procedure is covered by the implementation of the extended role of the nurse and demands a signed recognition that the nurse has been trained in this particular procedure.

Nayman (1979) advocated continuous infusion of intravenous analgesics, measuring pain on a linear analogue. The infusion rate was varied by the nursing staff, maintaining a conscious, pain-free patient. The rate of infusion could be varied for painful interventions such as physiotherapy. Nayman showed a reduction in postoperative respiratory complications using this technique compared with the intramuscular route. In addition, serum levels of morphine were determined, postulating that a blood level of morphine could be sought which would render the patient pain-free yet fully conscious and co-operative. Thus the guesswork is removed from analgesic dosage. This route is also favoured by Dodson (1982). Fentanyl is conveniently used in an infusion pump to achieve analgesia; however, this apparatus is expensive and its use is usually confined to intensive therapy units or an area in which there is a higher nurse to patient ratio than on the general ward.

Rectal

This route is not commonly used in the United Kingdom although it finds favour in other European countries. Suppositories of potent analgesics such as pentazocine or oxycodone pectinate have been used but the rate of absorption cannot be guaranteed. The use of rectal analgesia is mainly in the management of chronic pain in patients whose upper gastro-intestinal tract is sensitive to standard oral analgesics.

Epidural

The administration of analgesic drugs through the epidural space has presented the most exciting development in postoperative care in the last decade. This route for administration of local anaesthetic drugs has of course been used for over half a century.

Single injections of an agent can be given into the epidural space, but following thoracotomy all patients require pain relief for days rather than hours. For continued relief of pain it is therefore necessary to insert a catheter into the epidural space. This can be achieved in the thoracic epidural space at the level of the incision but the insertion of the catheter can be difficult due to the obliquity of the thoracic spinous processes. James et al. (1981) described the use of this technique in patients undergoing thoracotomy but admitted a failure rate to introduce the catheter of 11%.

A catheter is more easily passed into the lumbar epidural space and advanced 2–4 cm into the space. This route has now been used on our service with such success that further description is warranted. The technique has been detailed by Welch and Hrynaszkiewicz (1981) and is used on most adult thoracotomies and the majority of patients admitted to our service with chest injuries. Gross skin contamination by infection is the commonest contra-indication to its use. All patients are on subcutaneous heparin at the time of insertion of the catheter.

The catheter is inserted in the operating room, preferably prior to operation. Methadone, the analgesic of choice, in a dose of 4 mg is diluted in 20 ml saline for a 70-kg patient, the dose and volume being adjusted according to the size and weight of the patient. Methadone is used in preference to morphine as it is pure and free from preservatives which are potentially harmful in the extradural or subarachnoid spaces. The injection is given through a filter, protected subsequently in a plastic bag suspended from the patient's shoulder. Registered nurses 'top-up' the dose in the ward on a patient-demand, nurse-response basis, the effect of each dose lasting from 4 to 12 h. Side-effects, including problems of catheter insertion, have been encountered but are rare. The level reached by the opiate is determined by the level of injection and particularly by the volume of fluid injected. The mid-thoracic nerve roots are reached without difficulty after injecton of approximately 20 ml of the diluted methadone through a lumbar catheter. Respiratory depression and narcosis may follow opiate epidural injection, this effect being readily reversed by intravenous naloxone. Using methadone in preference to bupivacaine or lignocaine, severe hypotension is not seen. The catheter is retained for up to 4 days and is easily removed in the ward.

The production of a pain-free patient after thoracotomy or with multiple rib fractures has greatly improved the ability of the physiotherapist to clear bronchial secretions and has certainly lessened the need for IPPV in the second group. Aspiration bronchoscopy following lung resection has not been performed for 5 years. We believe, in company with Kent Trinkle et al. (1975), that IPPV is often unnecessary and even harmful. Patients with rib fractures are ideally managed by strict control of fluid intake and by rigorous analgesia allowing vigorous physiotherapy, resulting in a pain-free patient who is able to ventilate his lung satisfactorily. Scant attention need be paid to the 'flail segment' of chest wall, so long the sacred cow of closed chest injuries.

Spinal

Spinal analgesia is particularly suited to lower abdominal and lower limb surgery. The level to which the anaesthetic agent reaches can be controlled; however, it is more difficult to control in a patient who is being nursed in the lateral position, when the spinal agent may reach such a height in the sub-arachnoid space that profound hypotension will result. The use of spinal analgesia in the relief of post-thoracotomy pain is therefore limited.

Inhalation

The advantage of inhalation analgesia is that it can provide very acceptable pain relief for short periods of time, making it ideal for short procedures such as dressing of empyema fenestrations, removal of chest drains and physiotherapy. Entonox, a mixture of nitrous oxide and oxygen in equal volumes, can be inhaled from a cylinder through a suitable reducing valve. This gas can be used to drive respiratory-assist devices such as the Bird ventilators.

Other agents include trichlorethylene and enflurane, which have been used with benefit in the aforementioned short procedures. The method does not provide long-term analgesia and therefore its use in the postoperative period is limited.

Local Infiltration

Long-acting local anaesthetics may be used at operation or postoperatively to produce pain relief. Intraoperative injections are very simple, bupivacaine 0.25% being introduced into the subpleural space to block the intercostal nerves above and below the incision to include the drain sites. Satisfactory analgesia may be achieved for up to 12 h, after which the procedure needs to be repeated in the ward. It is therefore time consuming and often distressing for the patient. A single large volume of local anaesthetic, introduced into the sub-pleural space and allowed to spread in the paravertebral gutter, has been used with success. However, disruption of the parietal pleura at operation makes this an unreliable technique. Olivet et al. (1980) described a technique in which multiple catheters left in the intercostal spaces at operation are brought out through the skin, thus enabling repeated injections of bupivacaine to be given as required.

Moore (1975) has advocated local anaesthetic nerve blocks in preference to thoracic epidural analgesia for patients undergoing thoracotomy.

Operative

Transection of intercostal nerves at operation is a method of producing analgesia. However, the effects are permanent and if more than one nerve is divided the area of anaesthesia or hyperaesthesia together with the weakness of the upper abdominal muscles makes this an unacceptable procedure. Some surgeons prefer to divide the intercostal nerve of the incision before it is stretched by the rib spreader, hoping to achieve a reduction in postoperative pain (Belsey, personal communication). There is no doubt that a low thoracotomy incision through the eighth or ninth interspace is more painful than an incision through the fifth or sixth space. Resections for carcinoma of the bronchus, usually performed through the higher incisions, result in a lower incidence of late neuralgia than that found in patients undergoing repair of hiatus hernia. Such incisions are often performed through a seventh rib thoraco-tomy, any lower incision being destined for severe post-thoracotomy neuralgia in the long term.

Recently a technique of neurolysis has been introduced that reduces the medium-term postoperative pain. The details of this technique have been described by Maiwand and Makey (1981). Using a cryoprobe and nitrous oxide as the freezing agent, four or five intercostal nerves above and below the incision are exposed. These nerves should include the intercostal spaces carrying the pleural drains. The nerves are subjected, for 60 s, to an ice ball produced at the tip of the cryoprobe (Spembly Ltd., Andover, England). A temperature of approximately $-60°C$ is reached and the applications are in divided periods of 30 s each.

Cryoneurolysis does not achieve an adequate degree of acute postoperative pain relief for the first 24 h. To cover this period patients have a lumbar epidural catheter inserted as described above. Analgesia achieved during the first few days after operation appears to be ideal, the effect of cryoneurolysis taking over after the removal of the epidural catheter and lasting for up to 12 weeks. The technique leaves the nerve in continuity, allowing regeneration to occur, whereas complete transection is permanent. The whole procedure adds only 15 min to the operation. A further use of neurolysis is for relief of chronic post-thoracotomy pain.

Neurolysis can also be achieved using multiple, percutaneous injections of 6% phenol in water or 50% ethyl alcohol in water or even 95% absolute alcohol. These techniques are used by colleagues in the Pain Relief Service and are not applicable to acute post-operative pain relief. It is possible, however, to use any of these agents at operation and inject each intercostal nerve under direct vision, producing analgesia for about 6 weeks.

Miscellaneous

The relief of chronic post-thoracotomy pain taxes the ingenuity of both surgeons and their colleagues in the Pain Relief Service. Methods of analgesia other than drugs or the various forms of neurolysis can be tried in an attempt to rid the patient of discomfort that on occasions is of such severity that it precludes a return to useful work.

The theories of pain causation are beyond the scope of this chapter and the reader should consult authoritative texts on the subject. However the 'gate control theory' is important when analysing the effectiveness of transcutaneous nerve stimulation. Stimulation of the affected area at a frequency of 2 Hz for short periods — 15 min — can result in pain relief for many hours. The release of endorphins by this stimulation is another reason put forward for the efficacy of this mode of therapy.

Conclusion

Of the various methods and agents available for the relief of pain following pulmonary resection for carcinoma, one or two stand out as being superior to the others. To enable a patient to breathe to the maximum of his ability, expectorate secretions and yet not be mentally obtunded demands a careful appraisal of the needs of each patient, his response to pain and the intervention prescribed for relief. An opiate premedication, supplemented by analgesia throughout the operation, is the ideal starting point for postoperative pain relief. The insertion of a lumbar epidural catheter at the start of thoracotomy enables the first dose of methadone to be administered while the incision is being closed. Also during the operation intercostal nerves above and below the incision are treated with the cryoprobe, producing a neurapraxia imparting analgesia for about 6 weeks. The patient recovering from his operation will be fully conscious, hopefully pain free and thus able to co-operate fully with the nursing and physiotherapy staff. Adequate cryo-neurolysis should render the patient free of pain but not necessarily of discomfort, allowing mobilisaton. Oral analgesic agents can be substituted, the choice being governed by the degree of discomfort and often the emotive decisions of the medical staff.

References

Brock RC (1936) Post-operative chest complications. Guy's Hosp Rep 86:191–247

Dodson ME (1982) A review of methods of relief of post-operative pain. Ann R Coll Surg Engl 64:324–327

Donald I (1976) At the receiving end: a doctor's personal recollection of second time cardiac valve replacement. Scott Med J 21:49–57

Gallon AM (1982) Epidural analgesia for thoracotomy patients. Physiotherapy 68:193

Jackson JW, Cooper DKC, Guvendic C, Reece-Smith H (1979) The surgical mangement of malignant tumours of the oesophagus and cardia. Br J Surg 66:98–104

James EC, Kolberg HL, Iwen GW, Gellatly TA (1981) Epidural analgesia for post-thoracotomy patients. J Thorac Cardiovasc Surg 82:898–903

Kent Trinkle J, Richardson JD, Franz JL, Grover FL, Arom KV, Holmstrom FMG (1975) Management of flail chart without mechanical ventilation. Ann Thorac Surg 19:355–363

Maiwand O, Makey AR (1981) Cryoanalgesia for relief of pain after thoracotomy. Br Med J 282:1749–1750

Moore DC (1975) Intercostal nerve block for post-operative somatic pain following surgery of thorax and upper adbomen. Br J Anaesth 47:284–286

Nayman J (1979) Measurement and control of post-operative pain. Ann R Coll Surg Engl 61:419–426

Olivet RT, Nauss LA, Payne WS (1980) A technique for continuous intercostal nerve block analgesia following thoracotomy. J Thorac Cardiovasc Surg 80:308–311

Ross BA (1981) The present state of thoracic surgery — 5th Coventry Conference. Pitman Medical, London, pp 113–122

Welch DB, Hrynaszkiewicz A (1981) Postoperative analgesia using epidural methadone. Anaesthesia 36:1051–1054

Chapter 14

The Immunology of Bronchial Carcinoma

Bryan H. R. Stack

In the nineteeth century, the first successful attempts to immunise patients against infectious diseases were made. It was probably this concept of active immunisation that led investigators to consider whether it would be possible to immunise patients against tumours that were already established (Currie 1972). The early investigations involved two types of immunological stimulant. The first consisted of cells or extracts taken from the patient's own tumour (autologous) or from one or more tumours extracted from other patients (allogeneic) (Von Leyden and Blumenthal 1902). The second consisted of non-specific bacterial antigens; for example, Loeffler (1901) described injection of staphylococci and later tubercle bacilli in patients with advanced cancer.

The results of these early experiments in humans were variable and in general no attempt was made to monitor their effect by immunological tests, such as delayed hypersensitivity skin tests. Hence the science of tumour immunology did not flourish until the last 30 years, when more satisfactory laboratory work suggested that there is a host defence mechanism against tumours and that this can be enhanced by the administration of tumour extracts or cells and/or non-specific immunological stimulants, particularly bacterial antigens.

The following biological observations suggest that there may be a host defence mechanism against the development and growth of tumours:

1. The varying rate of progress of histologically similar tumours in different individuals. This can be relatively easily assessed in lung cancer by measuring the tumour doubling time on the chest radiograph (Geddes 1979). Tumours can regress completely; Everson and Cole (1956) described 47 patients collected from literature in whom this had occurred, including one patient with lung cancer (Blades and McCorkle 1954).

2. 'Cure' following incomplete removal of tumour. Surgeons are sometimes surprised to find that patients in whom only palliative resection of tumour has been achieved live indefinitely without further progress of the tumour. This has been described in lung cancer by Abbey Smith (1970). In another study, a surprisingly large proportion of patients in whom tumour cells were found along the cut margin of the bronchus in the operation specimen survived (Soorae and Stevenson 1979).

3. Invasion of tumours by cells normally immunologically active. Lymphocytes, plasma cells and macrophages are more abundant in well differentiated lung cancer than in small cell carcinomas and have been seen in relation to destroyed tumour cells (Ioachim et al. 1976).

4. Increased incidence of tumours in immunosuppressed patients. The increased incidence of not only lymphomas but also skin and other tumours in patients taking immunosuppressive drugs following kidney transplantation is now well known (Penn 1978).

Evidence that Lung Cancer Evokes an Immunological Response

1. *Lung Cancer Associated Antigens*. The antigens have been demonstrated by injecting extracts of tumour tissue into laboratory animals. Next the serum from these animals has been absorbed with normal lung and other body tissue components so as to remove antibodies to these components. The presence of the tumour antigen has then been tested using double immunodiffusion in agarose (Frost et al. 1975) or indirect immunofluorescence in tissue sections (Bell and Seetharam 1976).

Using methods based on these techniques, antigens of molecular weight between 40 and 200×10^3 daltons have been isolated. These have a fairly high degree of specificity although antisera against some antigens also react with extracts of tumours of other histological types and with extracts of normal foetal lung. With the use of affinity chromatography and polyacrylamide gel electrophoresis, a highly specific human lung tumour associated antigen has been isolated (Herberman et al. 1978). Tumour antigens can be isolated not only from extracts of the tumour but also from cultures of tumour cells and from malignant pleural effusions.

2. *Inhibitory Substances in Body Fluids from Lung Cancer Patients*. It is now known that serum from lung cancer patients has an inhibitory action in a number of immunological tests. Lymphocytes in culture can be induced to undergo transformation to lymphoblasts under the action of certain 'mitogens', including phytohaemagglutinin (PHA), concanavalin A (Con A), pokeweed mitogen (PWM) and PPD. Serum from lung cancer patients inhibits not only the mitogen-induced transformation of lymphocytes from these patients but also the transformation of normal donor lymphocytes (Guiliano et al. 1979). The serum also inhibits migration of leucocytes under special laboratory conditions and their adherence to glass (Sanner et al. 1980). Inhibitory activity is found in thoracic duct lymph from lung cancer patients (Han and Takita 1976) and in pleural fluid from malignant pleural effusions (Wolf et al. 1981).

3. *Antibodies and Immune Complexes*. Circulating antibodies to lung tumour antigen have been detected infrequently and this is probably because they are produced only in small amounts, because they are combined in immune complexes, because the antibody producing cells are inhibited by circulating tumour factors or because tumour antigen evokes only a cellular response (Kennel 1979).

The presence of immune complexes in animals bearing experimentally induced sarcomas was first described by Sjögren et al. (1971). Evidence of circulating immune complexes has been found in between 90% (Rossen et al. 1977) and 34% (Lowe et al. 1981) of patients with bronchial carcinoma. Their presence in lung cancer may be partly related to associated infection as a high prevalence has also been found in bronchitic patients (Guy et al. 1981).

Immunological Tests in Lung Cancer

Delayed Hypersensitivity Skin Tests

Delayed hypersensitivity skin tests consist of applying to the skin an antigen or a substance which, alone or in combination with body protein, evokes a reaction. The tests are usually read between 48 and 72 h after application. The antigens are listed in Table 1 and can be divided into recall and new antigens. Recall antigens are derived from organisms to which the subject has previously been exposed. With new antigens such as dinitrochlorobenzene (DNCB) a sensitising dose is given first. After 2 weeks serial weak challenge doses are applied and the degrees of erythema and oedema are measured after a further 48 h.

Table 1. Substances used to test delayed hypersensitivity skin reactivity

Recall antigens
  Bacterial:
  Tuberculin, streptokinase/streptodornase
  Viral:
  Mumps
  Fungal:
  Trichophyton, Candida albicans
New antigens
  DNCB
  PHA
  Keyhole limpet haemocyanin

In most reports, the prevalence of positive tests to recall antigen and the mean strength of reaction to these antigens have not been depressed in patients with stage I and II tumours and in series of operable cases (Stack 1982). However, even in operable cases, the prevalence of a positive reaction to DNCB is much lower than that found in a matched control population. Skin reactions to recall and new antigens become depressed with progression of the disease.

The probable mechanism of delayed hypersensitivity skin reactions is detailed in Fig. 1. The discrepancy between the reactivity to recall and new antigens is presumably due to an inability to recognise the latter or to become sensitised to them.

Some authors have injected tumour antigens into the skin of patients with lung cancer. This has produced a positive reaction in between 30% and 50% of cases (Stewart 1969; Marabella and Takita 1975). The incidence and strength of positive reactions to tumour antigen has been greatly enhanced by administration of allogeneic tumour antigen with Freund's complete adjuvant (Hollinshead and Stewart 1981).

Circulating Immunologically Competent Cells

Another potential measure of immunological reactivity is the concentration of lymphocytes, T cells and B cells in the peripheral blood. Thymus-derived lymphocytes (T cells) make up about 70% of peripheral blood lymphocytes. They are recognised by their ability to form rosettes with uncoated sheep red blood cells. T cells play a major role in cell-mediated immunity, including that activated by the

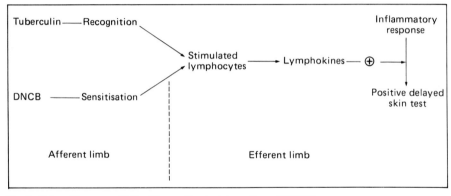

Fig. 1. Delayed hypersensitivity skin reaction to tuberculin and DNCB.

presence of tumour cells. By a number of different techniques it has been possible to divide the T cell population into two main groups:

1. *Helper cells.* These comprise about 70% of the peripheral blood T cells and bear surface markers for IgM. They help proliferation of B cells into plasma cells (Moretta et al. 1980) and the transformation of lymphocytes into lymphoblasts by mitogens such as PHA and Con A.
2. *Suppressor cells.* These comprise about 20% of peripheral blood T cells. They suppress helper T cells, B cells and macrophages and form part of a negative feed-back system which regulates the immunological defence mechanism. Markers for IgG are found on their cell surface.

Bursa-derived lymphocytes (B cells) comprise about 20% of circulating lymphocytes. These cells are coated with immunoglobulin and are recognised by their ability to form rosettes with sheep erythrocytes coated in IgG or the third complement factor (C3). Their concentration is measured by a technique using fluorescent anti-immunoglobulin. B cells are the progenitors of plasma cells and so are mainly concerned with the production of antibodies (humoral immunity).

There has been a wide variation in the results of measurements of peripheral blood immunocompetent cells in bronchial carcinoma. An important reason for this is the frequent failure to use controls matched for age, sex and smoking habits. In general, depression of total and T-lymphocytes occurs in patients with more advanced disease, and depression of T-lymphocytes has even been reported in some series of patients with localised disease. Elevation of the peripheral blood B cell concentration has been reported in squamous cell carcinoma with regional extension (Ritts et al. 1977) and in advanced lung cancer (Anthony et al. 1975). Another recently documented change is elevation of circulating basophils (Anthony 1982).

Lymphocyte Transformation Studies

Transformation of cultured lymphocytes into lymphoblasts stimulated by certain proteins (mitogens) is the basis of a series of non-specific tests of cell-mediated immunity. These mitogens can be classified as follows:

Non-specific	Phytohaemagglutinin (PHA)
	Concanavalin A (Con A)
	Pokeweed mitogen (PWM)
	Helix pomatia haemocyanin (HPH)
Bacterial	PPD
Mixed lymphocyte culture (MLC)	

PHA and Con A are believed to act mainly on T cells whereas PWM is a stimulator of B cells (Ritts et al. 1977). These mitogens stimulate the transformation of lymphocytes whether or not these have been exposed to the mitogens before. In contrast, lymphocytes respond to bacterial antigens and to HPH only when they have previously been sensitised to these. Lymphocyte transformation is usually measured by the uptake of purines labelled with radioisotopes, for example, ^{3}H-thymidine.

In general, lymphocyte transformation in the presence of PHA, PWM and Con A is normal in patients with operable tumours and reduced in patients with more advanced tumours (Saumon et al. 1968). By contrast, significant reduction in lymphocyte transformation by PPD (Stack et al. 1979) and, in sensitised patients, by HPH (Jansen et al. 1979) has been demonstrated in operable cases.

As with other immunological tests, it is essential to use controls matched for age, sex and smoking habits as lymphocyte reactivity may be depressed in older patients (Barnes et al. 1975) and in smokers.

More sophisticated measurement of lymphocyte properties has been carried out in some laboratories. These methods have included the use of flow cytometry (Brzyski et al. 1979) and the measurement of protein synthesis in lymphocytes stimulated by mitogens (Whitcomb and Parker 1977). Such tests have shown defects in the lymphocytes of patients with bronchial carcinoma even when standard transformation tests have been normal.

Tests of the Ability of Lymphocytes to Damage Tumour Cells

As the tests so far described are entirely non-specific, it would seem desirable to obtain more direct evidence of the ability of lymphocytes and macrophages to kill tumour cells. Two groups of lymphocytes have been studied:

1. Antibody-dependent cytotoxic cells (K cells)
2. Natural killer cells (NK cells)

K cells are lymphocytes which possess surface receptors for IgG. They can bind to and damage tumour cells coated with this immunoglobulin. Their presence can thus be detected by using target cells such as K562 cells from a myeloid cell line coated with IgG (Jonsdottir et al. 1979).

NK cells are found among the large granulated lymphocytes and have immunological properties which are similar to those of T-lymphocytes. Their activity is measured by their ability to damage tumour cells in culture in the absence of IgG.

NK cells comprise 1%–2% of all lymphoid cells in the spleen or peripheral blood (Herberman et al. 1980; Mitchison and Kinlen 1980). NK activity is depressed in lymphocytes taken from lung tumour tissue and those found in malignant pleural effusions. It is enhanced by local injection of BCG (Niitsuma et al. 1981), *C.parvum*, interferon and streptococcal antigens.

Measurement of NK and K cell activity is carried out only in research laboratories. The value of these measurements in peripheral blood is uncertain.

Circulating Antigenic Markers and Immunoreactive Hormones

One of the most interesting advances in the study of tumour immunology has been the discovery of immunoreactive peptides in tumour tissue and in the peripheral blood of some patients. These substances are listed in Table 2.

Table 2. Antigenic markers in lung cancer

1. *Oncofoetal*
   Carcinoembryonic antigen
   α-foetoprotein
2. *Placental*
   Human chorionic gonadotrophin and β-subunit
   Human placental lactogen
3. *Ectopic hormones*
   Pro-ACTH
   Calcitonin
   Antidiuretic hormone
   Parathormone
   β-lipotrophin
4. *Others*
   Ferritin
   Lactoferrin
   Casein
   β_2-microglobulin
   Caeruloplasmin
   Pregnancy-associated α_2-glycoprotein

One group, also found in high concentrations in foetal tissue, are known as oncofoetal antigens, e.g. carcinoembryonic antigen (CEA). Several workers have derived the upper limit of the normal range of CEA by studying controls and have then measured the prevalence of CEA levels above this value in lung cancer patients. Unfortunately lack of standardisation of the laboratory methods and the use of poorly matched controls have produced variable and misleading results. For example, raised CEA levels have been found in 13.6% of otherwise healthy cigarette smokers (Stevens et al. 1973). Thus it is essential to have a control population matched for smoking habits.

The prevalence of raised CEA levels in large series of lung cancer patients has ranged from 6% (Ford et al. 1977) to 55% (Broder 1980) where normal values were derived from controls with benign respiratory disease and/or from smokers. Even where several markers were studied, the prevalence of raised levels of one or more of these was only 46% (Stack 1982) and 76% (Reddy et al. 1979).

HLA Status

In the wake of interest in HLA typing in so many immunological disorders, several workers have studied HLA status in bronchial carcinoma patients. Apart from the isolated finding that the prevalence of HLA-B8 was increased in prolonged survivors after operation, no positive findings have been reported (Sengar et al. 1977).

The Value of Immunological Tests in Clinical Management of Lung Cancer

Many of the tests so far described have evolved during research into possible methods of immunotherapy. However, if it had been discovered that one or more of the antigens or other tumour markers produced by lung cancer were present in all cases but not in properly matched controls, their measurement might have been used in the diagnosis of doubtful cases or even in the screening of at risk populations. Unfortunately we have seen that although there are some changes of in vivo and in vitro immunological measurements in series of bronchial carcinoma cases, the prevalence is never enough to make any single test of diagnostic value. Moreover the abnormalities are relatively infrequent and of minor extent in patients with treatable localised tumours; they become more marked only at a stage where the tumour is easily detected and where no effective treatment is available.

Measurement of some tumour markers may have a limited value in assessing prognosis and the response to treatment. For example, a significantly raised CEA level in a patient with operable lung cancer is a bad prognostic sign (Vincent et al. 1979). Where plasma ACTH levels were raised in patients with small cell carcinoma, they fell to normal within 10 days of the start of chemotherapy (Hansen et al. 1980). After an elevated plasma ACTH level has fallen following treatment, a subsequent rise may indicate tumour recurrence and progression (Gropp et al. 1980).

Possible Mechanisms of Immunological Defence Against Tumours

Figure 2 shows a cancer cell coated with different antigens. This is in some way recognised as foreign by the immunological system, leading to the activation of lymphocytes and macrophages which damage the tumour cells. One type of lymphocyte involved is the cytotoxic T-lymphocyte derived from the stem T cell under the influence of tumour antigens. Activated lymphocytes produce substances which act on other cells known as lymphokines. This is probably the mechanism whereby helper T cells promote the maturation of B cells into plasma cells. These produce antibody which may bind with surface antigen and thus coat some of the tumour cells. Helper T cells also produce lymphokines which impart directional mobility to

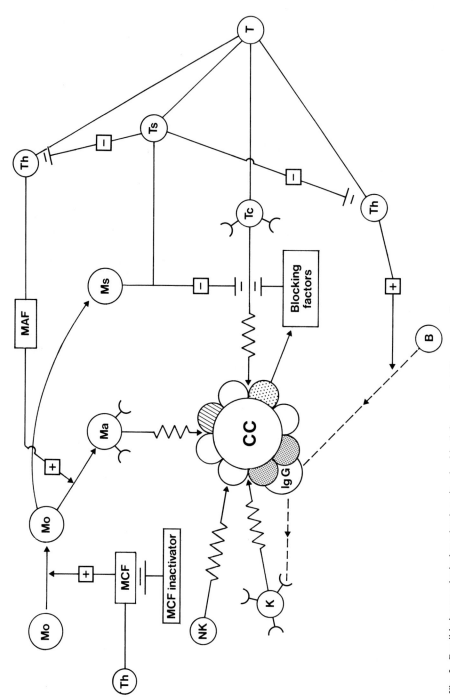

Fig. 2. Possible immunological mechanisms involved in defence against the cancer cell.

monocytes and which activate macrophages. These are known as monocyte chemotactic factor and macrophage activating factor, and are essential in the preparation of macrophages which damage tumour cells. The other cells which kill tumour cells are NK and K cells, to which reference has already been made.

With such an armamentarium of antitumour mechanisms, it is surprising that tumour cells survive and multiply at all. Possible reasons why they do so are as follows:

1. *Failure of recognition*. The discrepancy between delayed hypersensitivity (DHS) reactivity to recall antigens and DHS reactivity to new antigens (e.g. DNCB) suggests some impairment of the surveillance mechanism. Thus the immunological system may not react to 'new' tumour antigen (Holmes and Golub 1976).

2. *Blocking factors*. As has already been shown, serum from bronchial carcinoma patients inhibits various non-specific immunological tests. It is believed that tumour cells produce 'blocking factors' which depress the reactivity of lymphocytes and macrophages and, in particular, their ability to damage tumour cells.

3. *Suppressor cells*. Suppressor T-lymphocytes predominate among lymphocytes infiltrating tumour tissue (Vose and Moore 1979). They also depress the reactivity of peripheral blood lymphocytes to PHA and autologous cells. There are also suppressor cells of the monocyte series. These two groups of suppressor cells are believed to inhibit the killing of tumor cells by lymphocytes and macrophages.

4. *Defects in the monocyte/macrophage system*. Monocyte chemotaxis has been found to be defective in 45% of patients with bronchial and prostatic carcinoma, and in 90% of these cases a monocyte chemotactic factor inactivator was described (Kjeldsberg and Pay 1978). In another study, deficiency of monocyte chemotactic factor was found in patients with advanced bronchial carcinoma but not in those with localised disease (Kay and McVie 1977). Moreover, Dent and Cole (1981) found that in vitro monocyte maturation was reduced in patients with localised squamous cell carcinoma compared with controls and even greater reduction was shown in advanced squamous cell carcinoma. In experimental animals it has been shown that tumours and their metastases develop more readily when macrophages are inactivated by macrophage poisons (Mantovani et al. 1980).

It thus seems that although there is an immunological defence mechanism against tumour cells, this is overcome by other factors, some of which may be produced by the tumour itself.

Immunotherapy

Treatment aimed at increasing the immunological defence against tumours has been known as immunotherapy, although the term 'biological response modification' has recently been introduced (Livingston 1981). While early investigations of immunotherapy in bronchial carcinoma were carried out in patients with advanced tumours, latterly immunotherapy has been used mainly in patients with minimal tumour

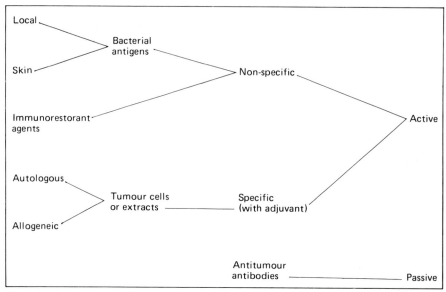

Fig. 3. Methods of immunotherapy used in lung cancer.

burden following surgery or radiotherapy. Unfortunately, while some early results seemed promising, clinicians are now beginning to suspect that these positive findings were due to faults in the design and analysis of clinical trials rather than to the useful effect of treatment. Methods of immunotherapy which have been used in bronchial carcinoma are classifed in Fig. 3.

Non-specific Systemic Immunotherapy

Non-specific systemic immunotherapy consists of introducing agents which cause a generalised stimulation of all cells concerned in the immunological response in the hope that some of the activated immunocompetent cells will then attack 'foreign' tumour cells. Most non-specific stimulants have been bacterial or fungal antigens.

BCG has been the most popular non-specific immunological stimulant, being widely used ever since Halpern et al. (1959) showed that it stimulated the reticulo-endothelial system of rats. BCG has been administered systemically through multiple scarification on the trunk or by percutaneous injection using multiple puncture needles. Variation in the number of organisms, viable or non-viable, the strain of BCG used and the frequency and duration of treatment accounts for the wide variability in the results of this treatment (Wilmott et al. 1979). Although percutaneous BCG produces a 48-h febrile reaction and moderate inflammatory changes at the site of injection in tuberculin-positive patients, serious side-effects, including disseminated infection with BCG, have seldom been reported in bronchial carcinoma patients so treated.

Some of the earlier trials of systemic BCG in unselected series of patients with advanced bronchial carcinoma were encouraging. For example, Hadziev and Kavaklieva-Dimitrova (1969) claimed a clinical response of 50%–71% in patients with stage III and stage IV tumours. However, in the study by Pines (1976) there was no difference in 5-year survival between BCG-treated and control patients with locally advanced carcinomas previously treated with radiotherapy.

The pioneer work on *Corynebacterium parvum* was also performed by Halpern and his colleagues (1964), and early reports of its use in bronchial carcinoma also came from France (Israel 1974). *C. parvum* was said to have more than twice the effect of BCG on phagocytic activity. Patients treated with *C. parvum* combined with cyclophosphamide had a longer median survival time than patients treated with cyclophosphamide alone. Systemic administration of *C. parvum* is usually intra-venous. It produces malaise, nausea and vomiting, an acute febrile illness and occasionally severe hypotension (Fox et al. 1980).

Other immunological stimulants have included schizophyllan, a polysaccharide prepared from a mushroom-like fungus (Oshima et al. 1980), bestatin, derived from *Streptomyces olivoreticuli* (Svanberg et al. 1980), and OK 432, a bacterial extract obtained by innoculating haemolytic streptococci with potassium penicillin (Watanabe et al. 1980). More recently, vitamin A derivatives have been shown to restore DHS reactivity in immunodepressed cancer patients (Serrou et al. 1982). Finally, the possible role of interferon in bronchial carcinoma is under investigation. Early clinical trials in other tumours have shown that human fibroblast interferon has improved DHS reactivity and NK activity of peripheral blood lymphocytes.

Immunorestorant Drugs

Levamisole is an orally administered antihelminthic drug which restores depressed DNCB reactivity in bronchial carcinoma patients (Holmes and Golub 1976). Unfortunately it produces intolerable side-effects, especially gastrointestinal upset, in about a fifth of treated patients (Parkinson et al. 1977). In patients treated with levamisole after resection of bronchial carcinoma, there was an excess of death from cardiorespiratory failure (Anthony et al. 1979). A soluble extract of calf thymus (thymosin fraction 5) has a similar action. Patients with low pre-treatment CEA values who were treated with this fraction survived longer than controls (Lipson et al. 1979).

Non-specific Immunotherapy in Operable Bronchial Carcinoma

Early experience of immunotherapy in bronchial carcinoma suggested that this relatively weak form of treatment was likely to have a place only in patients in whom the tumour cell population was small, as after resection of bronchial carcinoma

(Ritts et al. 1977). The high relapse rate after apparently curative surgery suggests that tumour cells remain at the site of resection and in distant organs. If immunologically active cells could be stimulated to seek out and destroy the latent tumour cells, a substantial improvement in postoperative survival could be expected. Moreover cell-mediated immunity is generally depressed after surgery (Ota et al. 1979), a factor which might favour growth of micrometastases during the postoperative period.

Table 3. Actual or projected (indicated by a) survival after operation of patients treated with non-specific immunotherapy

Authors	Immunotherapy	Time after operation	Percentage patients surviving		
			Treated	Controls	Significance
Djurovic and Decroix (1977)	Heat-killed myco-bacterial suspension	2 years	80	40	$P < 0.001$
Edwards and Whitwell (1978)	Single subdermal BCG Glaxo injection	5 years	30	20	N.S.
Pouillart et al. (1979)[a]	Percutaneous BCG Pasteur	2 years	77	52	$P < 0.02$
Miyazawa et al. (1979)	Percutaneous BCG Japan	2 years	100	69	$P < 0.02$
Millar et al. (1982)	Intradermal and percutaneous BCG Glaxo	5 years	36	37	N.S.
Amery (1980)	Levamisole	2 years	65	57	N.S.
Hadziev et al. (1980)	BCG or soluble fraction F 70	2 years	41	18	$P = 0.01$

The results of systemic non-specific therapy in patients afte resection of bronchial carcinoma are summarised in Table 3. The studies of Djurovic and Decroix (1977) and of Hadziev et al. (1980) were prejudiced by the use of historical controls. Edwards and Whitwell (1978) gave only a single, low-dose subdermal injection of BCG Glaxo. Although their initial results were promising, these were not confirmed by 5-year survival figures. In the study by Millar et al. (1982), BCG Glaxo was administered percutaneously or intradermally on seven occasions during the immediate postoperative period. There was a substantial increase in tuberculin reactivity but none in survival. Two trials with matched controls did produce significant results at 2 years, but the long-term results are still awaited. The early results of the use of levamisole in patients with resected lung cancer were promising, but these were not confirmed subsequently except for patients who had a dose of more than 2.1 mg/kg (Amery 1980).

Local Non-specific Immunotherapy

If tumour cells shed surface antigen, this must pass to the draining regional lymph nodes. One might expect these lymph nodes to show signs of intense immunological activity, particularly in those areas believed to be the source of cytotoxic lymphocytes. This was not in fact the case in one study of lymph nodes draining bronchial carcinoma (Syrjanen 1979), although lymphocytes from regional lymph nodes have been shown to mount a significant cytotoxic attack on autologous tumour cells (Kimura et al. 1982). It could be that tumour antigen alone is not enough to activate lymphoid centres in the local lymph nodes but that an 'adjuvant' stimulus such as bacterial antigen is necessary. This would explain the anecdotal observation that patients who develop empyema after resection of bronchial carcinoma survive longer.

In 1976, McKneally and his colleagues reported the effect of intrapleural BCG given 7 days after operation. Those patients in the BCG group who had stage I tumours survived and remained free from tumour recurrence significantly longer than controls. This difference still holds 4 years after completion of the trial, although now the P value for the difference is only 0.048 (Maver et al. 1982). It is now recognised by the authors that the early striking difference was partly due to the worse than average results of surgery in the controls. As routine biopsy of mediastinal lymph nodes was not performed, there may have been an excess of undiagnosed stage III patients in the controls. These results have not been confirmed by a number of other groups (Table 4), including Low et al. (1980) and the U.S. Lung Cancer Study Group (a large multicentre study: Holmes 1982). Intrapleural *C. parvum* has been used in a study of 475 patients carried out by the Ludwig Cancer Study Group in Europe, also without improvement in survival (Karrer 1982). However, there is some evidence of the benefit of intrapleural *C. parvum* (Millar et al. 1980a; Felletti and Ravazzoni 1983) and OK 432 (Uchida and Micksche 1982) in patients with malignant pleural effusions. In this latter study, the clinical improvement was accompanied by enhanced NK activity of intrapleural lymphocytes.

A different form of local immunotherapy has been the injection of BCG into tumours either percutaneously 2–3 weeks before operation or through a fibreoptic bronchoscope (Holmes 1981). In the percutaneous group and their controls, the

Table 4. Results of local non-specific immunotherapy in patients who have undergone resection of lung cancer

Authors	Immunotherapy	Results
Maver et al. (1982)	Intrapleural BCG Tice	6-year survival of stage I BCG cases = 60%, controls = 25%, $P < 0.048$
Lowe et al. (1980)	Intrapleural BCG Glaxo	2-year survival of stage I BCG cases = 59% controls = 66%, N.S.
Karrer (1982)	Intrapleural *C. parvum*	No difference between *C. parvum* group and controls, follow-up > 2 years
Holmes (1981)	Intralesional BCG	Disease-free survival over median follow-up of 14 months: BCG group = 55%, controls = 37%

tumours were excised and NK activity of the tumour-infiltrating lymphocytes was measured. This was found to be vigorous in the tumours which had been injected with BCG (Niitsuma et al. 1981). This treatment also produced some clinical benefit at an early stage of follow-up. Per-bronchoscopic injection of BCG in patients previously treated with percutaneous BCG and intravenous mustine produced radiographic improvement in 6 of 17 and clinical improvement in 9 of 19 patients in another series (Millar et al. 1980b). In general these methods have not appealed to other workers and the significant risk of disseminated BCG infection has discouraged further projects of this nature.

Specific Immunotherapy

Specific immunotherapy can be defined as injection of tumour cells or extracts taken from the same patient (autologous) or other patients (allogeneic). An adjuvant, usually BCG, is given during the same period in order to produce generalised stimulation of immunologically active cells in the draining lymph nodes. This activity is then focused on to residual tumour cells by the addition of further tumour antigen.

When tumour cells are used, they are usually irradiated first in order to prevent growth at the site of implantation. In addition, their immunogenicity may be enhanced by treatment with neuraminidase (Takita et al. 1976). Autologous tumour cells are less likely to be removed by transplant rejection mechanisms and so may be retained within the body for longer periods. There is thus more time for them to evoke an immunological response. On the other hand allogeneic cells, being immunologically different from residual cells, may evoke a response more readily during

Table 5. Some examples of specific immunotherapy in patients who have undergone resection of lung cancer

Authors	Immunotherapy	Clinical measurements	Treated group	Controls	Significance
Perlin et al. (1980)	Irradiated allogeneic tumour cells	Percentage survival at 2 years	72	61	$P = 0.06$
Stewart et al. (1982)	Soluble allogeneic lung cancer antigen homogenised with Freund's adjuvant ± intravenous methotrexate	Percentage survival at 4 years of stage I patients	80	50	$P < 0.01$
Takita et al. (1981)	Pooled allogeneic squamous cell carcinoma with Freund's adjuvant	Projected 3-year survival	89	44	$P < 0.05$
Stack et al. (1982)	Irradiated autologous tumor cells and percutaneous BCG	Percentage stage I patients alive and free from tumour recurrence at 2 years	71	43	N.S.

their shorter period of survival. Whereas the dose of autologous cells is limited by the amount of solid non-necrotic tissue in the patient's own tumour, allogeneic cells can be obtained in virtually unlimited supplies from pools of tumours excised from other patients.

Some reports of specific immunotherapy in bronchial carcinoma are summarised in Table 5. In general this treatment has produced some promising early results in relatively small numbers of patients. In particular, subgroups such as DNCB-positive patients (Stack et al. 1982), those showing a moderate postoperative skin reaction to intradermal tumour antigen (Stewart et al. 1982) and those with depressed lymphocyte transformation in mixed lymphocyte culture (Reid et al. 1982) did appear to benefit from specific immunotherapy.

Passive Immunotherapy

Passive immunotherapy consists of the administration of antibodies to tumour cells. Newman et al. (1971) injected goat antitumour serum into patients who had undergone resection of bronchial carcinoma and who were also receiving anticancer drugs. Although there were more deaths and tumour recurrences in the control group, the difference was not significant. Current interest is centred around the therapeutic use of monoclonal antibodies. These have been raised by immunising mice with a continuous cell line of adenocarcinoma of the lung and fusing the spleen cells of the mice with cells from a mouse non-secretory myeloma. The antibodies to adenocarcinoma produced by the hybrids of this union were found to react with adeno-, squamous cell and large cell carcinomas of the lung (Abrams et al. 1982). At present research workers are investigating the diagnostic and therapeutic possibilities of attaching radioisotope or anticancer drugs to monoclonal antibodies in the hope of demonstrating clinically latent populations of tumour cells and of destroying them.

Conclusions

During the past 25 years, there has been a vast amount of research into the immunology of bronchial carcinoma. This has demonstrated that there is some form of immunological defence against bronchial carcinoma which is largely cell-mediated. Patients with evidence of active cell-mediated immunity have a better prognosis, and conversely cell-mediated immunity becomes depressed in patients with advanced tumours and also in patients following operation and radiotherapy. Unfortunately efforts to restore or stimulate the cell-mediated immunity with immunotherapeutic agents have shown only marginal benefits. In the few instances where a clinical benefit has been achieved, serial immunological tests have failed to show an associated improvement in cell-mediated immunity. The promising early results of several forms of immunotherapy have not been confirmed by other workers. One reason may be that clinical results were assessed from actuarial survival curves which can give a false impression of the progress of a group of patients, especially if the numbers are small. The second reason has been the failure to stage groups of patients accurately. As a result, control groups may have contained larger numbers of patients with more advanced stages of bronchial carcinoma, thus giving the false impression that the treatment used was beneficial.

It seems unlikely that a further search for more potent bacterial antigens or better ways of administering these will produce any worthwhile advance in the treatment of bronchial carcinoma. The future in this field clearly lies with monoclonal antibodies and their application in both diagnosis and treatment.

References

Abbey Smith R (1970) Long term clinical follow-up after operation for carcinoma. Thorax 25:62–76

Abrams PG, Cuttita FC, Kimball E, Minna JD (1982) A monoclonal antibody specific for non-small cell bronchogenic carcinoma. In: Abstracts of the 3rd World Conference on Lung Cancer, IASLC, Tokyo, p 49

Amery WKPC (1980) Adjuvant levamisole in the treatment of patients with resectable lung cancer. Ann Clin Res 12 [Suppl 27]:1–83

Anthony HM (1982) Blood basophils in lung cancer. Br J Cancer 45:209–216

Anthony HM, Kirk JA, Madsen KE, Mason MK, Templeman GH (1975) E and EAC rosetting lymphocytes in patients with carcinoma of bronchus. Clin Exp Immunol 20:41–54

Anthony HM, Mearns AJ, Mason MK et al. (1979). Levamisole and surgery in bronchial carcinoma patients: increase in deaths from cardiorespiratory failure. Thorax 34:4–12

Barnes EW, Farmer A, Penhale WJ, Irvine WJ, Roscoe P, Horne NW (1975) Phytohemagglutinin-induced lymphocyte transformation in newly presenting patients with primary carcinoma of the lung. Cancer 36: 187–193

Bell CE, Seetharam S (1976) A plasma membrane antigen highly associated with oat-cell carcinoma of the lung and undetectable in normal adult tissue. Int J Cancer 18:605–611

Blades B, McCorkle R (1954) A case of spontaneous regression of an untreated bronchogenic carcinoma. J Thorac Surg 27:415–419

Broder LE (1980) Marker substances in bronchogenic carcinoma — emphasis on carcinoembryonic antigen (CEA) and human chorionic gonadotropin (HCG). In: Hansen HH, Dombernowsky P (eds) Abstracts of Second World Conference on Lung Cancer

Brzyski H, Konchanin L, Baustin A, Ruckdeschel JC (1979) Abnormal mitogen-induced lymphocyte proliferation in patients with lung cancer: possible role of the surface modulating assembly. Proc Am Assoc Cancer Res 20:148

Currie GA (1972) Eighty years of immunotherapy: a review of immunological methods used for the treatment of human cancer. Br J Cancer 26:141–153

Dent RG, Cole P (1981) In vitro monocyte maturation as a prediction of survival in squamous cell carcinoma of the lung. Thorax 36:446–451

Djurovic V, Decroix G (1977) Postoperative non-specific immunotherapy in primary bronchogenic carcinoma. Rec Res Cancer Res 62:156–163

Edwards FR, Whitwell F (1978) Use of BCG as an immunostimulant in the surgical treatment of carcinoma of lung: a five year follow-up report. Thorax 33:250–252

Everson TC, Cole WH (1956) Spontaneous regression of cancer: preliminary report. Ann Surg 144:366–383

Felletti R, Ravazzoni C (1983) Intrapleural C. parvum for malignant pleural effusions. Thorax 38:22–24

Ford CHJ, Newman CE, Lakin J (1977) Role of carcinoembryonic antigen in bronchial carcinoma. Thorax 32:582–588

Fox RM, Woods RL, Tattersall MHN, Basten A (1980) A randomised study of adjuvant immunotherapy with levamisole and Corynebacterium parvum in operable non-small cell lung cancer. Int J Radiat Oncol Biol Phys 6:1043–1045

Frost MT, Rogers GT, Bagshawe KD (1975) Extraction and preliminary characterisation of a human bronchogenic carcinoma antigen. Br J Cancer 31:379–386

Geddes DM (1979) The natural history of lung cancer: a review based on rates of tumour growth. Br J Dis Chest 73:1–17

Gropp C, Havemann K, Scheuer A (1980) The use of carcinoembryonic antigen and peptide hormones to stage and monitor patients with lung cancer. Int J Radiat Oncol Biol Phys 6: 1047–1053

Guiliano AE, Rangel D, Golub SH, Holmes EC, Morton DL (1979) Serum-mediated immunosuppression in lung cancer. Cancer 43:917–924

Guy K, Di Mario U, Irvine WJ, Hunter AM, Hadley A, Horne NW (1981) Circulating immune complexes and auto-antibodies in lung cancer. Br J Cancer 43:276–285

Hadziev S, Kavaklieva-Dimitrova J (1969) Application of BCG in cancer in man. Folia Med (Plovdiv) 11:8–13

Hadziev S, Kavaklieva-Dimitrova J, Mandulova P, Madzarova S, Spassova M (1980) Survival of lung cancer patients treated with BCG and/or a soluble BCG fraction (F 70) after surgery, radiotherapy and chemotherapy. Neoplasma 27:83–94

Halpern BN, Biozzi G, Stiffel C, Mouton D (1959) Effect of stimulation of the reticuloendothelial system by injection of BCG on the development of atypical epithelioma 7–8 of Guèrin in the rat. C R Soc Biol (Paris) 153:919–923

Halpern BN, Prévot A-R, Biozzi G et al. (1964) Stimulation of the phagocyte activity of the reticuloendothelial system provoked by *Corynebacterium parvum*. J Reticuloendothel Soc 1:77–96

Han T, Takita H (1976) Inhibition of mixed lymphocyte reaction by thoracic duct lymph: removal of inhibitory effect by thoracic duct drainage in lung cancer. J Surg Oncol 8:237–243

Hansen M, Hammer M, Hummer L (1980) ACTH, ADH and calcitonin concentrations as markers of response and relapse in small-cell carcinoma of the lung. Cancer 46:2062–2067

Herberman RB, McIntire KR, Braatz J et al. (1978) Antigenic markers associated with lung cancer. In: Krebs BP, Lalanne CM, Schneider M (eds) Clinical application of carcinoembryonic antigen assay. Excerpta Medica International Congress Series, vol 439:165–174

Herberman RB, Timonen T, Ortaldo JR, Bonnard GD, Gorelik E (1980) Natural cell-mediated toxicity. In: Fougereau M, Dausset J (eds) Progress in Immunology, vol 4. Academic Press, London New York, pp 691–709

Hollinshead AC, Stewart THM (1981) Specific and non-specific immunotherapy as an adjunct to curative surgery for cancer of the lung. Yale J Biol Med 54:367–379

Holmes EC (1981) The immunotherapy of lung cancer. In: Livingston RB (ed) Lung cancer, vol 1. Mattinus Nijhoff, The Hague, pp 51–62

Holmes EC (1982) Surgical adjuvant intrapleural BCG. In: Abstracts of the 3rd World Conference on Lung Cancer, IASLC, Tokyo, p 10

Holmes EC, Golub SH (1976) Immunologic defects in lung cancer patients. J. Thorac Cardiovasc Surg 71:161–168

Ioachim HL, Dorsett BH, Paluch E (1976) The immune response at the tumor site in lung carcinoma. Cancer 38:2296–2309

Israel L (1974) Non-specific immunostimulation in bronchogenic cancer. Scand J Resp Dis [Suppl] 89:95–105

Jansen HM, Esselink MT, Orie NGM, The TH (1979) Cell-mediated immune response in patients with bronchial carcinoma. Neth J Med 22: 1–9

Jonsdottir I, Dillner-Centerlind M-L, Perlmann H, Perlmann P (1979) Antibody dependent cellular cytotoxicity and mitogen responsiveness of human peripheral blood lymphocytes differing in avidity for sheep erythrocytes. Scand J Immunol 10:525–533

Karrer K (1982) Adjuvant immunotherapy for non-small cell bronchial carcinoma. In: Abstracts of the 3rd World Conference on Lung Cancer, IASLC, Tokyo, p 8

Kay AB McVie JG (1977) Monocyte chemotaxis in bronchial carcinoma and cigarette smokers. Br J Cancer 36:461–466

Kennel SJ (1979) Characterisation of a tumour cell surface protein with heterologous antisera to a spontaneous BALC/c lung carcinoma. Cancer Res 39:2934–2939

Kimura H, Yamaguchi Y, Kadoyama C et al. (1982) Induction and clinical application of specific immune lymphocytes against autologous lung cancer cells. In: Abstracts of 3rd World Conference on Lung Cancer, IASLC, Tokyo, p 142

Kjeldsberg CR, Pay GD (1978) A qualitative and quantitative study of monocytes in patients with malignant solid tumours. Cancer 41:2236–2241.

Lipson SD, Chretien PB, Makuch R, Kenady DE, Cohen M (1979) Thymosin immunotherapy in patients with small cell carcinoma of the lung. Cancer 43:863–870

Livingston RB (1981) Preface. In: Livingston RB (ed) Lung cancer, vol 1. Martinus Nijhoff, The Hague, p 11

Loeffler F (1901) A new method of treating carcinomas. Dtsch Med Wochenschr 27:725–726

Lowe J, Iles PB, Shore DF, Langman MJS, Baldwin RW (1980) Intrapleural BCG in operable lung cancer. Lancet I:11–14

Lowe J, Segal-Eiras A, Iles PB, Baldwin RW (1981) Circulating immune complexes in patients with lung cancer. Thorax 36:56–59

Mantovani A, Giavazzi R, Polentarutti N, Spreafico F, Garattini S (1980) Divergent effects of macrophage toxins on growth of primary tumours and lung metastases in mice. Int J Cancer 25:617–620

Marabella PC, Takita H (1975) Skin test with tumour extract in bronchogenic carcinoma: a preliminary study. J Surg Oncol 7: 299–301

Maver C, Kausel H, Lininger L, McKneally M (1982) Intrapleural BCG immunotherapy of lung cancer patients. In: Mathé G, Bonnadonna G, Salmon S (eds) Adjuvant therapies of cancer. Springer, Berlin Heidelberg New York, pp 227–231

McKneally MF, Maver C, Kausel HW (1976) Regional immunotherapy of lung cancer with intrapleural BCG. Lancet I:377–381

Millar JW, Hunter AM, Horne NW (1980a) Intrapleural immunotherapy with *Corynebacterium parvum* in recurrent malignant pleural effusions. Thorax 35:856–858

Millar JW, Hunter AM, Wightman AJA, Horne NW (1980b) Intralesional injection of BCG using the fibreoptic bronchoscope in the treatment of bronchogenic carcinoma. Eur J Respir Dis 61:162–166

Millar JW, Roscoe P, Pearce S, Ludgate S, Horne NW (1982) The five year results of a controlled study of BCG immunotherapy after surgical resection for bronchogenic carcinoma. Thorax 37:57–60

Mitchison NA, Kinlen LJ (1980) Present concepts in immune surveillance. In: Fougereau M, Dausset J (eds) Progress in Immunology, vol 4. Academic Press, London New York, pp 641–650

Miyazawa N, Suemasu K, Ogata T, Yoneyama T, Naruke T, Tsuchiya A (1979) BCG immunotherapy as an adjuvant to surgery in lung cancer: a randomised prospective clinical trial. Jpn J Clin Oncol 9:19–26

Moretta L, Mingari MC, Moretta A, Haynes BG, Fauci AS (1980) T cell Fc receptor as markers of functional human lymphocyte subsets. In: Fougereau M, Dausset J (eds) Progress in Immunology, vol 4. Academic Press London New York pp 223–238

Newman CE, Ford CHJ, Davies DAL, O'Neill GJ (1977) Antibody-drug synergism: an assessment of specific passive immunotherapy in bronchial carcinoma. Lancet II: 163–166

Niitsuma M, Golub SH, Edelstein R, Holmes EC (1981) Lymphoid cells infiltrating human pulmonary tumours: effect of intralesional BCG injection. J Natl Cancer Inst 67:997–1003

Oshima S, Izumi T, Kado M, Sato A, Honda K (1980) Immunotherapy with schizophyllan of lung cancer. In: Hansen HH, Dombernowsky P (eds) Abstracts of Second World Conference on Lung Cancer, p 193

Ota DM, Copeland EM, Corriere JN, Dudrick SJ (1979) The effects of nutrition and treatment of cancer on host immunocompetence. Surg Gynecol Obstet 148:104–111

Parkinson DR, Cano PO, Jerry LM et al. (1977) Complications of cancer immunotherapy with levamisole. Lancet I:1129–1132

Penn I (1978) Tumours arising in organ transplant recipients. Adv Cancer Res 28:31–36

Perlin E, Oldham RK, Weese JL et al. (1980) Carcinoma of the lung: immunotherapy with intradermal BCG and allogeneic tumour cells. Int J Radiat Oncol Biol Phys 6:1003–1039

Pines A (1976) A 5 year controlled study of BCG and radiotherapy for inoperable lung cancer. Lancet I: 380–381

Pouillart P, Palangie T, Huguenin P et al. (1979) Attempt at immunotherapy with living BCG in patients with bronchus carcinoma. Rec Res Cancer Res 68:260–267

Reddy MN, Rochman H, Hunter RL, Fang VS, De Meester T (1979) Carcinoembryonic antigen, k-casein and β-human chorionic gonadotropin in the staging of lung cancer. In: Lehmann F-G (ed) Carcino-embryonic proteins, vol II. Elsevier/North Holland Biochemical Press, Amsterdam Oxford New York, pp 173–176

Reid JW, Cannon GB, Perlin E, Blom J, Connor R, Herberman RB (1982) Immunologically defined prognostic subgroups as predictors of response to BCG immunotherapy. In: Mathé G, Bonnadonna G, Salmon S (eds) Adjuvant therapies of cancer. Springer Berlin Heidelberg New York, pp 219–226

Ritts RE, Jacobsen DA, Caron J, Weyl KG et al. (1977). Is the lung cancer patient immunologically competent? In: Perspectives in lung cancer. Frederick E Jones Memorial Symposium in Thoracic Surgery, Columbus, Ohio. Karger, Basel, pp 47–56

Rossen RD, Reisberg MA, Hersh EM, Gutterman JU (1977) The CIq binding test for soluble immune complexes: clinical correlations obtained in patients with cancer. J Natl Cancer Inst 58:1205–1215

Sanner T, Kotlar HK, Eker P (1980) Immune responses in lung cancer patients measured by a modified leukocyte adherence inhibition test using serum. Cancer Lett 8:283–290

Saumon G, Dermenghem F, Saint-Paul M, Sors C, Decroix G (1968) Study of the culture of lymphocytes in the course of broncho-pulmonary cancer. Presse Medic 76:1657–1660

Sengar DPS, McLeish WA, Stewart THM, Harris JE (1977) HLA antigens in bronchogenic carcinoma. Oncology 34:143–145

Serrou B, Cupissol D, Rosenfeld C (1982) Immune imbalance and immune modulation in solid tumour patients: new insights. In Mathé G, Bonadonna G, Salmon S (eds) Adjuvant therapies of cancer. Springer, Berlin Heidelberg New York, pp 9–16

Sjögren HO, Hellström I, Bansal SC, Hellström KE (1971) Suggestive evidence that the 'blocking antibodies' of tumour bearing individuals may be antigen-antibody complexes. Proc Natl Acad Sci USA 68:1372–1375

Soorae AS, Stevenson HM (1979) Survival with residual tumour on bronchial margin after resection for bronchogenic carcinoma. J Thorac Cardiovasc Surg 78:175–180

Stack BHR (1982) Immunological investigations and immunotherapy in lung cancer. MD Thesis, University of Edinburgh, pp 105–111

Stack BHR, McSwan N, Stirling JM et al. (1979) Cell-mediated immunity in operable bronchial carcinoma: the effect of injecting irradiated autologous tumour cells and BCG. Thorax 34:68–73

Stack BHR, McSwan N, Stirling JM et al. (1982) Autologus X-irradiated tumour cells and percutaneous BCG in operable lung cancer. Thorax 37:588–593

Stevens DP, Mackay IR, Busselton Population Studies Group (1973) Increased carcinoembryonic antigen in heavy cigarette smokers. Lancet II: 1238–1239

Stewart THM (1969) The presence of delayed hypersensitivity reactions in patients toward cellular extracts of their malignant tumours. Cancer 23:1368–1387

Stewart THM, Hollinshead AC, Harris JE, Raman S (1982) Specific active immunotherapy in lung cancer: the induction of long-lasting cellular responses to tumour-associated antigens. In: Mathé G, Bonadonna G, Salmon S (eds) Adjuvant therapy of cancer. Springer, Berlin Heidelberg New York, pp 232–239

Svanberg L, Widell A, Cronberg S (1980) Clinical and immunological investigation of the effect of bestatin. In: Hansen HH, Domebernowsky P (eds) Abstracts of Second World Conference on Lung Cancer, p 196

Syrjanen KJ (1979) Bronchial carcinoma and its regional lymph nodes in relation to immunological functions. Z Immunitaets Forsch 155: 212–222

Takita H, Minowada J, Han T, Takada M, Lane WW (1976) Adjuvant immunotherapy in bronchogenic carcinoma. Ann NY Acad Sci 277:345–354

Takita H, Hollinshead AC, Edgerton F et al. (1981) Adjuvant immunotherapy of squamous cell lung carcinoma. Proc Am Assoc Cancer Res 22:199

Uchida A, Micksche M (1982) Intrapleural administration of OK-432 in cancer patients: activation of natural killer (NK) cells and reduction of NK suppressor cells. In: Abstracts of the 3rd World Conference on Lung Cancer, IASLC, Tokyo, p 145

Vincent RG, Chu TM, Lane WW (1979) The value of carcinoembryonic antigen in patients with carcinoma of the lung. Cancer 44:685–691

Von Leyden E, Blumenthal F (1902) Preliminary information about results of cancer research from the first medical clinic. Dtsch Med Wochenschr 28:637–638

Vose BM, Moore M (1979) Suppressor cell activity of lymphocytes infiltrating human lung and breast tumours. Int J Cancer 24:579–585

Watanabe Y, Iwa T, Yamamoto K (1980) Clinical value of immunotherapy by streptococcal preparation OK-432 as an adjuvant for resected lung cancer. In: Hansen HH, Dombernowsky P (eds) Abstracts of Second World Conference on Lung Cancer, p 198

Whitcomb ME, Parker RL (1977) Abnormal lymphocyte protein synthesis in bronchogenic carcinoma. Cancer 40:3014–3018

Wilmott N, Pimm MV, Baldwin RW (1979) Quantitative comparison of BCG strains and preparations in immunotherapy of rat sarcoma. J Natl Cancer Inst 63:787–795

Wolf A, Micksche M, Bauer H (1981) An improved antigenic marker of human lung carcinomas and its use in radioimmunoassays. Br J Cancer 43:267–275

Chapter 15

Radiographically Occult Lung Cancer

Stewart Clarke

Introduction

Radiographically occult lung cancer may be defined as that situation in which a patient has sputum positive for cancer cells but a negative chest radiograph (Williams and Cortese 1982). A screening programme for lung cancer was set up in the early 1970s by the U.S. National Cancer Institute involving a collaborative study between Johns Hopkins Hospital, New York Memorial Hospital and the Mayo Clinic. Each centre aimed at enrolling about 10 000 male smokers at risk, 5000 each in the screen and control groups. The majority of the information on radiographically occult lung cancer has been generated therefrom in individual reports (Marsh et al. 1978; Melamed et al. 1981; Williams and Cortese 1982).

The chest radiograph is usually assumed to be a standard posterior–anterior (PA) film with a lateral projection also — the mass miniature radiograph is now rarely used. To improve radiographic screening, attention to the following criteria are suggested by Stitik and Tockman (1978): careful technique, high kVP (about 140 kVP) both PA and lateral views, independent double reading (with a third opinion if the first two disagree) and comparison with previous films. The expected degree of resolution with these methods will pick up lesions down to about 0.5 cm in diameter. More refined methods such as conventional or computerised axial tomography will show smaller lesions but are inapplicable for screening at present. It has been suggested that 'curative' surgical resection is possible in most patients with radiographically detectable but 'pre-symptomatic' lung cancer, with a 5-year survival probability of 40%. By contrast, 'curative' resections are possible in less than 5% of patients with symptomatic visible lesions and their 5-year survival rate is less than 10% (Williams and Cortese 1982).

The diagnostic accuracy of sputum cytology screening depends upon the care with which sputum is collected and the location and cell type of the tumour. Most patients will be smokers who are likely to have chronic cough and sputum satisfying the British Medical Research Council (1965) criteria for the diagnosis of chronic bronchitis. In these patients spontaneous early morning coughing usually produces adequate samples which should be placed in a suitable container. Sputum can be induced by mist inhalation otherwise (Fontana et al. 1965). Three specimens must be examined either separately or pooled. Large, central lesions yield positive sputum cytology in 80% of patients, while peripheral lesions (beyond the fourth and fifth bronchial divisions) are positive in less than 50% (Oswald et al. 1971). Squamous cell carcinoma cells far outweigh cells from adeno-, small (oat) cell and large cell carcinomas. Recent results from the Mayo Lung Project screening 90 patients with lung cancer showed that 31% had positive sputum cytology, of which the proportions were 58% for squamous cell, 16% for adeno-, 21% for small (oat) cell and 13% for large cell carcinomas (Woolner et al. 1981). What emerges is that almost all occult lung cancers are squamous cell in type.

In a further study by the same group, Muhm et al. (1983) reported on 4618 high-risk male smokers ($\geqslant$45 years of age and $\geqslant$1 pack of cigarettes per day) having a chest radiograph and sputum cytology check at 4-monthly intervals. Out of 109 patients found to have lung cancer, 15 had positive sputum cytology alone, whereas 92 had a radiographically visible lesion (0.8 cm to 7.0 cm in diameter); in seven patients both chest radiograph and sputum cytology were positive and in two both were negative, the diagnosis being made by node biopsy and at autopsy respectively.

The authors were surprised that almost six times more cancers were identified by radiographs alone than by sputum cytology alone. At the outset of the study in 1971 they anticipated the reverse would be the case.

Tumour Duration

Occult lung cancer is by definition a small lesion, radiographically invisible, usually asymptomatic and thus potentially curable. Even so, the lesion may have been established for many months prior to cytological diagnosis. The tumour doubling rate for squamous cell cancer is relatively slow at 88 days, whereas it is 29 days for small (oat) cell tumours. In general squamous cell cancer is diagnosed 8.4 years after origination, with death occurring 1.2 years later (total duration 9.6 years) (Geddes 1979). However, during the greater part of this period the patient will be without specific symptoms other than those associated with smoking and chronic bronchitis. Screening is generally applied, therefore, to the population at risk, namely males over the age of 45 years who smoke 20 or more cigarettes daily; with the increase in lung cancer in females (male–female ratio 6.1:1 in 1961 and 3.4:1 1979), screening could now be extended to include them.

Diagnosis and Location

A good deal of effort has gone into the localisation of occult lung cancer as a prerequisite for optimal treatment. The Mayo Lung project experience reveals that between 13% and 18% of patients who develop lung cancer will present with radiographically occult lung cancer if suitably screened (Woolner et al. 1981). All of these are identified by sputum cytology and almost all are squamous cell in type. Between 70% and 80% are shown to be early, confined within the bronchial wall and histologically in situ, with or without micro-invasion. This early stage cancer is reflected in the survival rates, over 82% surviving lung cancer at 4 years (Cortese and Sanderson 1981).

Localising the site of the occult lung cancer involves a careful examination with the flexible fibre-optic bronchoscope, which gives a better view than the rigid bronchoscope (Marsh et al. 1978). Many authors stress the need to rule out a carcinoma in the upper airways (i.e. above the larynx). The bronchoscopy must be painstaking since over 50% of radiographically occult lung cancers are also visually occult at the time of the first bronchoscopy. Furthermore, the subject may have more than one cancer of which one or all may be occult. Therefore a thorough search is indicated, usually under general anaesthetic with selective brushing, curettage and random mucosal biopsy; specimens are accurately labelled and carefully handled subsequently. The localisation may be considered adequate with a single diagnostic biopsy or two separate bronchoscopic examinations resulting in diagnostic brushings from the same bronchopulmonary segment (Williams and Cortese 1982).

Recently a photo-active chemical, haematoporphyrin derivative (HpD), which acts as a tumour marker, has been used to facilitate localisation of radiographically and visually occult lung cancer. The cancer cells take up HpD and fluorescence can be detected during fibre-optic bronchoscopy using standard white light, by the addition of a photo-electric detector. This has substantially reduced the numbers of bronchoscopies required for adequate localisation from up to five in 18 months to one or two.

With these methods Cortese et al. (1982) performed just one bronchoscopy in each of ten patients with occult lung cancer. Three of these patients had two separate but simultaneous cancers. Six of the 13 cancers were visually occult, were localised by HpD fluorescence and were confirmed by biopsy to be entirely in situ or minimally invasive. Four of the 13 cancers were visible bronchoscopically. All fluoresced and all were squamous cell cancers. In one patient, fluorescence was accompanied by positive bronchial brushings; in two patients both visual and HpD bronchoscopies were negative but both patients developed peripheral lesions outside the bronchoscopic range subsequently.

With this method it is possible to localise cytologically detected cancers within a few months, whereas previously the interval between detection and localisation was much longer. HpD is not specific for cancer, and areas of marked squamous metaplasia also concentrate HpD; nevertheless, the levels appear lower and biopsy proof is, of course, always required (see p. 280).

Results

The final results from the U.S. National Cancer Institute collaborative study await completion of the 6-year screen after the end of patient enrolment. In fact, the Mayo Clinic completed enrolment in 1976, and the Johns Hopkins and Memorial Hospitals in 1978.

In the Mayo study chest radiography has surpassed sputum cytology as a means of detecting early lung cancer, except in early squamous cell carcinoma, where up to 50% may be detected by cytology. This latter category is, of course, the 'occult' group, in which survival is excellent, with over 82% at 4 years (Cortese and Sanderson 1981). However, in general the Mayo screening has not yet been shown to reduce overall mortality from lung cancer.

The Johns Hopkins Lung Project has reported on their initial radiographic screening techniques and results, but not on their cytological findings or occult lung cancer.

The results from Memorial Hospital do not mention occult lung cancers as such (Melamed et al. 1981). However, in the initial examination approximately equal numbers of stage 1 (American Joint Committee — tumour < 3 cm without nodes) lung carcinomas were detected by radiographic and cytological techniques whereas subsequently the ratio was 5:1. Those tumours detected by cytology were of the squamous cell type in major bronchi, while those detected by radiography were peripheral and adenocarcinomas in about two-thirds of the cases. Melamed et al. comment that the effect of screening on lung cancer mortality can be estimated only indirectly so far. However, they note that 40% of all lung cancers can be detected early in stage 1 by screening and that more than 90% of such patients will survive for 5 years with resection.

Conclusions

Radiographically occult lung cancer is uncommon and will only be detected by adequate screening of susceptible patients. These tumours are virtually always squamous cell in type and central in position. They may be diagnosed even earlier by new bronchoscopic techniques. The cost-effectiveness of this screening has yet to be shown, as has any reduction in the overall mortality from lung cancer.

There seems no doubt that once diagnosed and localised, surgical removal, probably by wedge resection, is the treatment of choice for the occult lesion. The results appear to be uniformly excellent though the numbers reported so far are relatively small. In the future other methods may be used, including photo-irradiation by laser, and work is already progressing with this treatment mode (see Chap. 18). It seems likely that both radiotherapy and chemotherapy would be rather like the proverbial sledgehammer used to crack a nut, bearing in mind the small localised nature of this type of lesion, and neither is recommended.

References

Cortese DA, Kinsey JH, Woolner LB, Sanderson DR, Fontana RS (1982) Haemotoporphyrin derivative in the detection and localization of radiographically occult lung cancer. Am Rev Respir Dis 126:1087–1088
Cortese DA, Sanderson DR (1981) Localization of occult lung cancer. Semin Respir Med 3:35–36
Fontana RS, Carr DT, Woolner LB, Miller FK (1965) Value of induced sputum in cytologic diagnosis of lung cancer. JAMA 191:134–136
Geddes DM (1979) The natural history of lung cancer: a review based on rates of tumour growth. Br J Dis Chest 73:1–17
Marsh BR, Frost JK, Erozan YS, Carter D (1978) Diagnosis of early bronchogenic carcinoma. Chest 73:716–717 [Suppl]
Medical Research Council (1965) Definition–classification of chronic bronchitis for clinical and epidemiological purposes. Lancet I:775–779
Melamed MR, Flehinger BJ, Muhammad BZ, Heelan RT, Hallerman ET, Martini N (1981) Detection of true pathologic stage 1 lung cancer in a screening programme and the effect on survival. Cancer 47: 1182–1187

Muhm JR, Miller WE, Fontana RS, Sanderson DR, Uhlenhopp MA (1983) Lung cancer detected during a screening program using four-month chest radiographs. Radiology 148:609–615

Oswald NC, Hinson KFW, Canti G, Miller AB (1971) The diagnosis of primary lung cancer with special reference to sputum cytology. Thorax 26:623–631

Stitik FP, Tockman MS (1978) Radiographic screening in the early detection of lung cancer. Radiol Clin North Am 16:347–366

Williams DE, Cortese DA (1982) The present status of screening and diagnosis of early lung cancer. Semin Respir Med 3:210–217

Woolner LB, Fontana RS, Sanderson DR, Miller WE, Muhm JR, Taylor WF, Uhlenhopp MA (1981) Mayo Lung Project: Evaluation of lung cancer screening through December, 1979. Mayo Clin Proc 56:544–555

Chapter 16

The Role of Radiotherapy in Carcinoma of the Bronchus

Adrian R. Timothy

Lung cancer is not a single disease but a heterogeneous group of diseases with differing histological subtypes and patterns of evolution (Seydel et al. 1976; Cox et al. 1979; Gazdar et al. 1983). While it is likely that the majority of patients will ultimately develop distant metastases, the behaviour of individual lung tumours at presentation may be quite different (Spjut and Mateo 1965; Matthews et al. 1973; Rissanen et al. 1968). At one end of the spectrum, small cell carcinomas tend to pursue a rapid course with a high propensity for early dissemination, and traditionally carry the worst prognosis (Kirsh et al. 1972). At the other extreme, a small number of the well differentiated epidermoid tumours will not metastasise until late in the disease — some of these patients may be cured by local therapy, either surgery or radiation, while others will succumb to uncontrolled primary disease but without evidence of distant spread (Spjut and Mateo 1965; Kirch et al. 1972; Matthews et al. 1973; Abadir and Muggia 1975; (Cox et al. 1979; Schaake-Koning et al. 1983). More recently certain histological subsets, in particular small cell carcinoma, have been shown to be responsive to combination cytotoxic chemotherapy, and a number of long-term survivors are now recorded among individuals presenting with clinically localised tumours (Arnold and Williams 1979; Hansen et al. 1980; Greco and Oldham 1979; Smith et al. 1981). With these few exceptions, the long-term outlook for lung cancer patients is poor. In the face of apparent advances in diagnostic and treatment techniques, the overall prognosis has not altered significantly over the past 30 years — less than 10% of all patients may be expected to survive for 5 years after initial diagnosis (Green 1981; Chilvers 1982).

Natural History

Some insight into the problems of lung cancer treatment can be gained from an understanding of the basic biology of the different tumour types. It is generally accepted that, in the early stages of tumour development at least, the individual cells divide at a constant rate and the time taken for a tumour to double in size is constant (Collins et al. 1956). The available human lung cancer data have been reviewed by Geddes (1979) and support this concept of exponential growth. Tumour doubling times show a variation from around 29 days for small cell tumours to 88 and 160 days for squamous cell carcinoma and adenocarcinoma respectively. Some 30 doublings are required to produce a tumour of 1 cm diameter, which is the smallest size likely to be readily detected on routine chest X-ray. Death is estimated to occur at around 40 doublings, when the tumour mass becomes unsupportable (Table 1).

From a knowledge of initial size, doubling time and the size at which death will occur, a description may be obtained of the natural history of a particular tumour (Table 2). For example, a patient presenting with a 1–2 cm well differentiated squamous cell carcinoma which has a doubling time of 80–100 days may survive without treatment for several years. In contrast, the more biologically aggressive small cell tumour of similar size but with a doubling time of only 30 days will pursue a rapid course, causing death within a few months. Data from several series in the literature have estimated the mean tumour size at diagnosis to be around 3 cm, equivalent to approximately 35 cell doublings. In most patients therefore, the clinician is dealing with a disease at a late stage in its evolution, which may have been present in the body for many years and which has had ample opportunity to spread both locally and to distant sites.

Several prognostic factors have been identified for lung cancer patients, among the most important of which are tumour size, histology, weight loss in the preceding 6 months and Karnofsky rating (Stanley 1980; Cox et al. 1983). From the previous discussion it will be appreciated that these are all reflections of the biological behaviour of the tumour, its particular time course and its effect upon the general health of the host.

Patterns of Treatment Failure

Despite the often unsatisfactory outcome, surgery still appears to offer the best hope for cure in lung cancer. Thompson (1966) has examined the progress of over 1000 patients presenting to a large general hospital (Fig. 1). Approximately one-half were inoperable at presentation because of either local tumour extension or the presence of distant metastases, and a further 20% were considered ineligible for surgery on the findings at bronchoscopy. In over two-thirds of the patients therefore, by the time of diagnosis the tumour was too far advanced for any hope of a surgical cure. Of the remaining 300 patients who progressed to thoracotomy, 100 were technically unresectable and in the final analysis, only one in five of the original number were actually candidates for an attempt at "curative" resection. Twelve months after the operation only 90 patients (9% of the total) were alive.

Table 1. Exponential growth patterns in lung cancer (Geddes 1979)

No. of tumour doublings	No. of cells	Tumour size	
0	1	10 μm	Undetectable clinically
20	10^6	1 mm	Undetectable clinically
30	10^9	1 cm	Detectable on chest X-ray
35	10^{10}	3 cm	Average size at initial presentation
40	10^{12}	10 cm	Death

Table 2. Natural history of lung cancer (Geddes 1979)

Histological type	Doubling time (days)	Time in years to		
		Earliest diagnosis (1 cm)	Average diagnosis (3 cm)	Death (10 cm)
Squamous cell	88	7.2	8.4	9.6
Adenocarcinoma	161	13.2	15.2	17.6
Undifferentiated	86	7.1	8.2	9.4
Small cell	29	2.4	2.8	3.2

While other studies from specialist centres may offer variations on these particular figures (Kirsh et al. 1976; Martini and Beattie 1977), the general pattern and outcome are little changed — less than 25% of all lung cancer patients are suitable for radical surgery and of these, less than one-third will survive beyond 5 years (Mountain 1973).

Radical radiotherapy, like surgery, is a local or at best a regional form of treatment. Examination of sites of failure in patients with inoperable tumours treated by irradiation confirms the impression of a high incidence of generalised disease. In over half of all patients metastases will reveal themselves within 6 months of completion of treatment (Rissanen 1968; Eisert et al. 1976). Analysis of patterns of failure after radiotherapy in relation to individual tumour type reinforces the importance of this division when discussing treatment strategy and prognosis. Squamous cell carcinomas consistently appear to have the lowest incidence of distant metastases at post mortem, approximately 30% of patients dying with clinically disseminated disease compared with more than 70% of patients who have small cell carcinomas. Adenocarcinomas run an intermediate course with some 50% of patients dying with metastases. These figures are in close agreement with those obtained following attempted "radical" surgical resection (Table 3) and highlight the limitations of local therapy in lung cancer (Rissanen et al. 1968; Matthews et al. 1973; Abadir and Muggia 1975).

It is clear that for lung cancer patients in general, any significant improvement in survival will only follow the introduction of effective systemic therapy. However, closer examination reveals a small but constant proportion of patients dying with uncontrolled local disease, the majority of these with squamous cell tumours (Matthews et al. 1973; Abadir and Muggia 1975; Cox et al. 1979) (Table 4). This

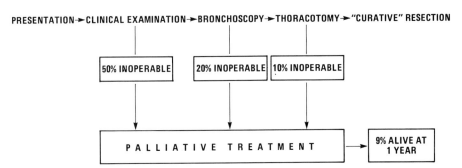

Fig. 1. Progress of patients with carcinoma of the bronchus. (Adapted from Thompson 1966)

Table 3. Patterns of failure following "curative" surgical resection (adapted from Matthews et al. 1973)

Histology	Number treated	Persistent disease	Local/regional failure only	Distant metastases
Squamous	131	44	22/131	22/131 (17%)
Adenocarcinoma	30	13	1/30	12/30 (40%)
Large cell	22	3	0/22	3/22 (14%)
Small cell	19	13	1/19	12/19 (63%)
Total	202	73 (36%)	24 (12%)	49 (24%)

group in particular are likely to benefit from more aggressive local treatment and results are already available showing that improved local control may be mirrored by corresponding improvements in survival (Choi and Doucette 1981; Perez et al. 1982; Cox et al. 1983; Schaake-Koning et al. 1983). In the longer term, with advances in cytotoxic chemotherapy, the ability of radiotherapy to eradicate bulk disease in the thorax or in "sanctuary" sites, for example in the central nervous system, will become a major factor in management.

Though there are now a large number of publications on all aspects of radiotherapy in the treatment of lung cancer, a lack of carefully controlled randomised clinical trials remains. In many reports no clear distinction is made on the basis of histology or other prognostic factors when assessing the results of different treatment regimes. Furthermore many of the early radiotherapy studies were conducted using relatively low radiation doses and old-fashioned equipment, which considerably limits their value in designing modern treatment policies.

The precise role of radiotherapy in the treatment of lung cancer has yet to be clearly defined. Before examining its current place in overall management it is of value to review the developments in radiotherapy equipment and technique that have taken place during the last three decades.

Radiotherapy — Orthovoltage vs Megavoltage

Until the late 1950s the majority of radiotherapy departments were equipped with modified diagnostic X-ray units capable of providing beams with energies in the range of 200–300 kV — so-called orthovoltage or "deep X-ray" therapy. Treatment

Table 4. Local failure alone after radiation therapy (data from Abadir and Muggia 1975, and Cox et al. 1979)

Histology	No of local failures/total number of patients	Local failure only
Squamous cell	17/74	23%
Adenocarcinoma	3/27	11%
Large cell anaplastic	5/17	29%
Small cell	4/24	17%
Total	29/142	20%

with this type of equipment is severely limited on two counts. Firstly, the low energy X-rays are able to penetrate only poorly into tissues; thus deep-seated tumours receive only a fraction of the desired dose. The second major disadvantage with these beams results from the fact that the maximum radiation dose falls on the skin surface; as a consequence severe early and late skin reactions may occur when large doses are directed to a particular area ("radium burns"). The introduction of high energy cobalt units and linear accelerators has transformed the practice of radiotherapy. The megavoltage beams produced from these types of equipment have energies in excess of 1 million eV and not only allow the delivery of tumoricidal doses to sites deep within the body but, because the maximum dose falls below the skin surface, also have a "skin sparing" effect, avoiding the dose-limiting reactions associated with old-fashioned deep X-ray therapy.

In spite of these technical improvements there remains one major factor which may limit the ability of radiation to eradicate many tumours successfully, and that is the tolerance of the adjacent critical normal tissues and mesenchymal stroma. Normal tissue tolerance to ionising radiation depends upon several factors — not only the nature of the tissue itself but also the volume irradiated, the type of radiation, the total radiation dose and the rate at which it is administered. In general, normal tissues are able to repair limited radiation damage better than their malignant counterparts. By splitting the prescribed radiation dose into a number of small daily treatments (fractionation), the non-malignant tissues are allowed to recover between treatments and any major morbidity may be avoided. Even with appropriate fractionation, at the higher dose levels which may be required to sterilise the tumour completely some tissues which cannot be avoided may be irreparably damaged, thus precluding successful treatment. In the case of intrathoracic tumours the critical tissues of interest include the lungs, oesophagus and spinal cord.

With reference to lung tolerance, while small volumes may be subjected to high dose radiation (i.e. 40–60 Gy in daily fractions of 180–200 rads) which inevitably results in irreversible pulmonary fibrosis in the treatment field, the consequences of such treatment will be minimal in terms of symptomatic late effects. Irradiation to more extensive areas of the thorax with large individual or cumulative doses may be followed by severe changes in respiratory function, respiratory failure and even death (Deeley 1966; Salazar et al. 1976a). Every effort is therefore made to minimise the amount of normal tissue included in the radiation field, while at the same time not compromising the chance of local tumour control by missing disease. Careful consideration must also be given to irradiation in the presence of long-standing pulmonary disease, previous surgery or concurrent administration of chemotherapy, all of which may further reduce lung tolerance to radiation (Phillips and Margolis 1972; Libshitz and Southard 1974). The interaction of radiation and chemotherapy and the possible potentiation of normal tissue damage has particular implications for the evolving strategy of combining the two types of treatment as, at present, in small cell carcinoma (Phillips et al. 1975; Greco and Oldham 1979; Cohen et al. 1980; Feld 1981).

The second structure which is intimately involved in the treatment of intrathoracic tumours is the spinal cord. Experience over the years has produced clearly defined dose limits for spinal cord tolerance; failure to respect these may ultimately result in radiation myelitis with progressive neurological deterioration often presenting as a Brown-Séquard syndrome with motor impairment on one side and decrease in pain and temperature sensation on the other. As with the lung, spinal cord tolerance is related to total radiation dose, overall time, volume (length) of cord irradiated and, to some extent, individual fraction size (Wara et al. 1975; Wigg et al. 1981). The latter is of special importance when treatment time is truncated and the dose of each treatment increased (as in the some "split-course" regimens), since there is evidence of an increased risk of late cord damage at higher doses with such schedules (Dische et al. 1981; Petrovich et al. 1981).

The increasing use of CAT scanning in radiotherapy treatment planning in conjunction with high energy treatment beams allows better localisation of the tumour volume, with clearer demarcation of the critical normal tissues to be avoided, thus minimising radiation dose to these structures (Emami et al. 1978; Vandyk et al. 1982; Gunterseydel et al. 1980). With modern techniques and equipment, careful treatment planning and a proper understanding of tumoricidal dose, external beam irradiation may now be regarded as a safe and increasingly effective form of treatment (Choi et al. 1980; Cox et al. 1983).

In practice there are three situations which most commonly confront the radiotherapist and in which radiation may have a part to play:

1. As an adjunct to surgery in those patients with unfavourable features such as hilar or mediastinal node involvement and in whom there is a high risk of residual tumour after resection.

2. As primary treatment where tumour is confined to the thorax but is technically unresectable or the patient is medically unfit for operation.

3. As palliation in patients with distressing symptoms caused either by uncontrolled intrathoracic disease or by distant metastases.

Postoperative Radiotherapy

The continuing failure of radical surgery to eradicate intrathoracic disease in a significant proportion of patients with lung cancer has led to much interest in the possible benefits which may result from the addition of radiotherapy to control residual local or regional tumour. External beam irradiation may be given before or after surgery. With pre-operative therapy the intention is not only to increase local cure rates by improving the chance of successful resection but also to affect the viability of any tumour cells released into the circulation at the time of operation with the hope of reducing the incidence of metastases and ultimately improving survival. It is not proposed to discuss pre-operative irradiation further in this chapter except to note that in some studies, while survival figures have not shown a benefit with radiotherapy compared with surgery alone, in 25%–45% of resected specimens no viable tumour cells have been found after radiation doses of between 37 and 60 cGy given in daily doses of 180–200 cGy over periods of 4–6 weeks (Bromley and Szur 1955; Bloedorn et al. 1961).

This evidence that well tolerated doses of radiotherapy are capable of sterilising small lung tumour deposits has prompted studies on radiation given after apparently "curative" resection, particularly in situations where the risk of local failure is high, for example, where disease has spread to adjacent lymph nodes (Paterson and Russell 1962; Bangma 1971; Green et al. 1975; Kirsh et al. 1976; Choi et al. 1980) (Table 5).

Table 5. Clinical trials of postoperative radiotherapy in lung cancer

	Randomised	Node status	Therapy	No.	Survival		Significance
Paterson and Russell (1962)	Yes	Not given	Surgery	99	36%	3 years	N.S.
			Surgery + XRT	103	33%		
Bangma (1971)	Yes	Not given	Surgery	37	68%	>1 year	N.S.
			Surgery + XRT	36	53%		
Green et al. (1975)	No	Node −	Surgery	64	22%	5 years	N.S.
			Surgery + XRT	59	27%		
		Node +	Surgery	30	3%	5 years	Significant benefit for XRT (<0.01)
			Surgery + XRT	66	35%		
Kirsh et al. (1976)	No	Node +	Surgery	20	0%	5 years	N.S.
			Surgery + XRT	69	23%		
Choi et al. (1980)	No	Node +	*Adenocarcinoma*				
			Surgery	21	8%	5 years	Significant benefit for XRT (<0.01)
			Surgery + XRT	40	43%		
			Squamous				
			Surgery	29	33%	4 years	N.S.
			Surgery + XRT	46	42%		

Only two authors have compared surgery with post-operative irradiation in a random fashion, and in both trials the number of patients was small. Paterson and Russell (1962), in a study involving 202 patients with varying histological tumour types, employed 4 MeV X-rays to doses of 45 Gy after resection in 103 patients and compared the outcome with that in 99 patients treated by surgery alone. At 3 years there was no survival difference between the two groups, although there was a suggestion of a possible benefit for more anaplastic tumours. For the squamous cell carcinomas, however, it appeared that irradiation might actually have an adverse effect on survival. No information on tumour size or mediastinal node status was available in this study. Bangma (1971), in a similar trial using comparable radiation doses but with only 73 patients, also showed no advantages for the irradiated group. On the contrary, there was again a higher mortality in those receiving radiotherapy for squamous cell carcinoma during the first post-operative year.

An uncontrolled study of radiotherapy to doses of 50–60 Gy, given after resection, reported by Green could demonstrate no effect on 5-year survival in patients with negative mediastinal or hilar nodes, whereas in those with lymph node metastases at the time of surgery there was a significant improvement in survival, with figures of 3% for surgery alone against 35% for surgery and radiotherapy. By far the greatest benefit was observed in those node-positive cases with adenocarcinoma, with no survivors after surgery alone compared with 10 of 16 patients (62%) who received postoperative radiotherapy and who were followed for 5 years or more (Green et al. 1975). Choi et al., in the search for new treatment strategies for locally advanced lung cancer, have analysed the results of adjuvant radiotherapy in 93 surgically treated patients with T_3, N_1 or N_2 tumours and 55 similar patients undergoing resection but without further treatment. This was a retrospective study and consequently the more advanced tumours tended to appear in the irradiated group. At 4 years there was no difference in survival for squamous cell tumours; however, the imbalance in staging between the two groups suggests some beneficial effect of radiotherapy in patients with the more extensive local disease. For adeno-carcinomas, the findings were similar to those reported by Green et al. in that a significant improvement in survival was recorded at 5 years, 43% of the irradiated group remaining alive compared with only 8% of those receiving surgery alone.

One interesting feature of patients with adenocarcinoma of the lung is the high incidence of brain metastases compared with other tumour types, with a significant proportion failing in the brain only, without evidence of disease elsewhere (Shin et al. 1980; Choi et al. 1980; Komaki et al. 1983) (Table 6). This raises the question of a place for prophylactic cranial irradiation in a subgroup of non-small cell tumours. Cox et al. have demonstrated the ability of modest dose radiotherapy (20 cGy in ten fractions over 14 days to the whole brain) to reduce the incidence of CNS metastases although without any alteration in median survival rates (Cox et al. 1981).

Table 6. Brain metastases as the only site of failure in adenocarcinoma of the lung

	No.	Total no. of failures	Brain only	Brain only as % of total failures
Shin et al. (1980)	121	47	10	10/47 (21%)
Choi et al. (1980)	61	34	12	12/34 (35%)

In conclusion, the only two trials which have investigated the role of post-operative irradiation in a randomised fashion contain few patients, a high percent-age of anaplastic tumours and insufficient detail with regard to tumour size and regional node involvement. No benefit has been demonstrated in these trials for adjuvant irradiation, but a review of other uncontrolled data indicates that radio-therapy in "radical" doses may influence survival in the subgroup of patients with mediastinal node involvement, particularly those with adenocarcinomas.

The paucity of accurate data together with the high observed incidence of CNS relapse in some non-small cell carcinomas demands a proper assessment of adjuvant radiotherapy to both thorax and brain after resection in carefully controlled trials.

Radical Radiotherapy for Locally Unresectable Lung Cancer

Patients with clinically localised but technically unresectable tumours represent a major problem for the radiotherapist, accounting for an estimated 40% of all lung cancer cases seen in the clinic (Roswit et al. 1968).

In occasional series of small and highly selected patient populations, impressive results have been recorded following radiotherapy, comparing favourably in terms of survival with those obtained by surgery (Smart and Hilton 1956). However, these are very much the exception — in most reports the outlook for patients receiving "radical" radiotherapy is uniformly poor, less than 10% surviving for 5 years or more (Table 7). The median time to relapse after treatment is around 6 months, with the majority of patients who will demonstrate metastases doing so within 18 months (Eisert et al. 1975). This underlines the misleading nature of 12-month survival

Table 7. Survival for inoperable lung cancer following radiotherapy alone

Radiation	No.	Survival		
		1 year	3 years	5 years
Orthovoltage				
Smithers (1955)	171	39%	9%	4%
Schultz (1957)	385	15%	3%	1%
Morrison and Deeley (1960)	176	24%	2%	1%
Megavoltage				
Continuous:				
Guttman (1965)	103	57%	17%	9%
Deeley (1967)	513	36%	8%	6%
Holsti and Mattson (1980)	158	27%	11%	6%
Split course:				
Abramson and Cavanaugh (1973)	271	38%	7%	–
Aristizabal and Caldwell[a](1976)	200	50%	19%	16%
Holsti and Mattson (1980)	205	29%	7%	3%

[a] Well differentiated early tumours

figures in any assessment of a particular treatment policy and explains the discrepancy between 1- and 3-year survival rates.

This lack of improvement in survival despite the apparent technical advantages associated with the introduction of megavoltage radiotherapy emphasises not only the high incidence of metastases but also the continued failure to control local disease.

The success of radiotherapy depends upon several critical factors, including total radiation dose, treatment technique and the schedule of administration.

In a study of tumour response to varying radiation schedules, Salazar (1976b) has shown a positive correlation between increasing tumour dose and early tumour regression. One month after treatment the response rate was only 15% with doses of 1360 rets compared with 50%–60% when the dose was increased to above 1650 rets. Radioresponsiveness should not, however, be confused with radiocurability; in particular, the more rapid initial regression seen with small cell tumours should not be misinterpreted as an indication that these require smaller radiation doses than other tumour types to achieve the maximum chance of local control (Choi et al. 1976).

Several reports have demonstrated the ability of carefully planned high dose megavoltage irradiation to eradicate tumour within the thorax and in some cases this has been associated with improvement in survival. Rissanen et al. (1968) found no viable tumour at autopsy in 18 of 60 patients (30%) who had received radiation dose of more than 48 Gy, and Abadir and Muggia, in a second autopsy series, found local "cures" in 8 of 21 patients (38%) following a minimal tumour dose of 40 Gy (Abadir and Muggia 1975).

In separate reviews Eisert et al. and Choi and Doucette have reported local control rates of 29% in patients receiving less than 1500 rets (approximately 50 Gy in 25 treatments over 5 weeks), compared with 50%–60% with doses above 1500 rets (Eisert et al. 1976; Choi and Doucette 1981) (Table 8). While similar observations have been made by others demonstrating a clear relation between increasing radiation dose and local control, above a radiation dose level of 50 Gy the gains are only modest while the risks of significant treatment-related morbidity begin to rise steeply

Table 8. Local control as a function of radiation dose

	< 1500 ret	> 1500 ret
Eisert et al. (1976)	18/61	71/136
Choi et al. (1980)	4/14	21/33
	22/75 (29%)	92/169 (54%)

(Salazar 1976a; Eisert et al. 1976; Sherman et al. 1981; Choi et al. 1980; Choi and Doucette 1981; Perez 1982; Schaake-Koning et al. 1983; Cox et al. 1983).

The response of a tumour to radiotherapy is not solely a function of radiation dose, however, but is also dependent on tumour size. It has been well documented in other tumour sites such as the breast and the head and neck region that local control rates for a given radiation dose decline with increasing tumour size and consequently larger tumours require larger doses for sterilisation (Fletcher 1979; Bataini et al. 1978). Although data already exist for lung cancer to show that local control is most likely with small tumours (< 3 cm) and with high radiation doses (50–60 Gy), many tumours are at least 3 cm in diameter at presentation (Sherman et al. 1981; Perez et al. 1982). On the basis of experience in other sites it seems unlikely that, even with optimum treatment planning, a large percentage of patients will have their thoracic disease eradicated by doses of 50–60 Gy, yet higher doses are precluded by the certain complications that will follow excessive exposure to adjacent normal tissues. The search for ways of improving the efficacy of irradiation has been taxing radiotherapists and radiobiologists for many years. One of the major obstacles to the success of conventional radiotherapy is thought to be the presence of hypoxic but still viable malignant cells within most solid tumours (Gray et al. 1953). These hypoxic cells require two to three times the dose of radiation needed to sterilise their well oxygenated counterparts and are therefore considerably more resistant to therapeutically acceptable levels of radiation, providing a ready source for "recurrence". Much effort has gone into exploring methods of reoxygenating the hypoxic portion of tumours and thereby increasing their sensitivity. Churchill-Davidson in the 1950s pioneered treatment in high pressure oxygen as a possible means of raising the oxygen tension in hypoxic regions of the tumour (Churchill-Davidson et al. 1966). A subsequent trial using hyperbaric oxygen and radiotherapy by Cade and McEwen established a small (though not significant) improvement in survival for lung cancer patients treated with this technique over those treated in air (Cade and McEwen 1978). Hyperbaric therapy has several disadvantages. It is labour intensive and time consuming and may be stressful to some patients who are necessarily confined in an enclosed space for long periods. In the absence of a clearly defined major benefit, high pressure oxygen therapy is no longer considered a practical proposition for widespread use and attention has transferred to other possible mechanisms of sensitising hypoxic cells.

In the past 10 years interest has centered on certain "electron affinic" compounds such as metronidazole and misonidazole which have been shown to sensitise hypoxic tumour cells to radiation in vitro and in vivo (Adams et al. 1979; Dische et al. 1979). Unfortunately, preliminary clinical results have been disappointing. Misonidazole has produced a significant benefit in local control in only one trial and its clinical use has been severely curtailed by dose-limiting neurotoxicity (Dische et al. 1978; Overgaard J, personal communication, 1984). Nonetheless, the development of an easily administered, non-toxic chemical radiosensitiser offers great possibilities for increasing the effectiveness of radiotherapy and this has prompted the continuing search for other drugs with radiosensitising properties (Phillips 1981; Overgaard et al. 1983).

As with other tumours, treatment technique, in this case adequate coverage of all potential sites of disease in the thorax, is of major importance in determining treatment outcome. Failure to include the regional lymphatics in treatment portals will be followed inevitably by a high incidence of local failure and poor survival prospects (Choi and Doucette 1981; Sherman et al. 1981; Perez et al. 1982).

The final consideration with irradiation is the timing of treatment. "Standard" radiotherapy schedules employ daily tumour doses of 1.8–2.0 Gy, five days per week to total doses of 40–60 Gy given in a continuous fashion over a period of 4–6 weeks. For a patient with a probable survival of only 6–8 months this represents a severe intrusion into their already short life expectancy, especially if there is little evidence of a substantial benefit in terms of quality of life. Efforts to reduce the overall time taken to complete the radiotherapy course and also where possible to increase treatment efficacy have led to the investigation of many alternative radiation schedules (Table 9).

Among the most common are "split–course" regimes in which the prescribed radiation dose is given with daily doses of 2–4 Gy in two abbreviated courses of 1–2 weeks separated by a treatment-free interval of 3–4 weeks. These regimen have several possible advantages. Firstly, acute reactions such as oesophagitis are minimised and the patient has time to recover between courses. Secondly, the total

Table 9. Randomised trials of split-course and continuous radiotherapy in inoperable lung cancer

	Treatment regime	Number	Dose (Gy)/fractions/time (days)	Survival	
Levitt et al. (1967)	XRT (cont)	14	60/ 30 /42	7%	} 1 year, N.S.
	vs				
	XRT (split)	15	18/ 3-28-18/ 3	20%	
Guthrie et al. (1973)	XRT (split)	46	30/10-28-30/10	2%	} 2 years, N.S.
	vs				
	XRT (split)	51	20/ 5-28-20/ 5	0%	
Lee et al. (1976)	XRT (cont)	86	50/ 25/35	<10%	} 5 years, N.S.
	vs				
	XRT (split)	102	25/12-21-25/12	<10%	
Holsti and Mattson (1980)	XRT (cont)	158	50/ 25 /35	6%	} 5 years, N.S.
	vs				
	XRT (split)	205	30/15-16-25/12	3%	
Petrovich et al. (1981)	XRT (cont)	191	50/ 25 /35	38/52	} Median survival, N.S.
	vs				
	XRT (cont)	152	42/ 15 /21	38/52	
Perez et al. (1982)	XRT (cont)	97	40/ 20 /28	11%	
	vs				
	XRT (cont)	92	50/ 25 /35	19%	} 2 years, N.S.
	vs				
	XRT (cont)	85	60/ 30 /42	19%	
	vs				
	XRT (split)	93	20/ 5-14-20/ 5	10%	
Sealy et al. (1982)	XRT (split)	137	20/ 5-21-20/ 5	31/52	} Median survival, N.S.
	vs				
	XRT (split)	132	30/15-14-20/10	32/52	

number of treatments and overall treatment times are considerably reduced. Lastly, between 10% and 25% of patients will not require the second half of the split course, either because of a deterioration in their general condition or the appearance of distant metastases (Guthrie et al. 1973; Lee et al. 1976; Sealy et al. 1982). In comparisons of split-course against continuous schedules, opinions are divided as to the efficacy and the incidence of late complications with each type of treatment. Levitt, using two courses of three high dose fractions (6 Gy) separated by a 4-week break, found no difference in survival or symptom relief when compared with a continuous schedule (60 Gy in 6 weeks). As might have been anticipated with these high dose fractions, lung fibrosis was more marked with the split course (Levitt et al. 1967). Holsti reported on 363 patients treated either with a continuous schedule of 50 Gy in 5 weeks (daily fractions) or 55 Gy divided into two courses separated by a 2- to 3-week treatment-free interval over a total of 8 weeks. One-year survival was slightly better for the split course but by 2 years no difference was seen. Lung fibrosis was milder and appeared later with the interrupted treatment (Holsti and Mattson 1980).

Lee, using the same order of radiation dose, found no difference in either survival or complication rates between two similar schedules with the exception of a small group of patients with large cell tumours where there was a significant survival benefit for the split-course treatment at 5 years (Lee et al. 1976).

In a recent study the Radiation Therapy Oncology Group has compared 40 Gy given in a split course, against 40, 50 and 60 Gy given continuously (Perez et al. 1980, 1982). The split-course patients had a reduced complete response rate and a correspondingly higher incidence of local failure compared with patients receiving the highest dose, continuous treatment. There was no difference in the occurrence of distant metastases between any of the groups, and 2-year survival rates were not significantly different, with 10% alive after the split-course treatment compared with 19% after 50 or 60 Gy in continuous fashion. Pulmonary fibrosis and pneumonitis were slightly more common and severe in the split-course and highest dose, continuous treatment (60 Gy) groups.

The appalling prospects for most patients with inoperable lung cancer following treatment raises doubts over the routine use of radiotherapy with its attendant discomfort and inconvenience. Surprisingly, only two studies have attempted to address the question of a possible advantage in survival of immediate over delayed treatment, and in only one was any effort made to assess the quality of life. Roswit has reported the results of a V.A. lung group trial comparing radiotherapy against "no treatment" (placebo) in a prospective fashion in 542 patients (Roswit et al. 1968). Irradiation was given to tumour doses of 40–50 Gy in 4–6 weeks using mainly orthovoltage therapy (DXR). Supportive treatment including antibiotics and blood transfusion was available for both groups. At 12 months, 18% of the treated patients were alive compared with 14% receiving the placebo, with median survival times of 142 and 112 days respectively giving little apparent support to the continued use of routine radiotherapy. There are, however, many deficiencies in this study (including the use of orthovoltage irradiation), and on close examination an early, though not significant, advantage for some subgroups (particularly the epidermoid tumours) is seen following treatment. These authors have again underlined the importance of the biological behaviour of an individual tumour in prognosis — those patients surviving for more than 1 year had symptoms for 10 months on average before presentation, compared with less than 5 months in those who died within 6 months.

In a second study, the Oxford group randomly allocated patients with carcinoma of the bronchus into four treatment arms. In one, treatment was withheld until symptoms appeared, but in the other three groups immediate treatment was given whether or not symptoms were present. Patients received either radiotherapy alone or chemotherapy with or without radiotherapy (Durrant at al. 1971). Again, orthovoltage irradiation was used with minimum tumour doses of 40 Gy in 14 fractions over 28 days given to the primary tumour, hilar and mediastinal nodes. The median survival times were practically identical in all four groups, ranging between 8.3 and 8.8 months. More surprising, perhaps, were the results of the "quality of life" assessed by a simple palliative index based on alterations in each patient's normal activity. Although no direct comparison was made of the acute side-effects, no differences could be identified in the quality of survival, suggesting that for some patients without troublesome symptoms at presentation, radiotherapy may reasonably be delayed until such time as problems develop.

In summary, despite advances in radiotherapy equipment and treatment techniques, the outlook for patients with clinically localised but inoperable lung cancer remains poor. While developments in hyperthermia and chemical radiosensitisers which may enhance the tumouricidal effects of radiation offer exciting possibilities for the future, at present the best chance for cure with irradiation lies with the few patients who have small tumours amenable to high dose treatment (Field and Bleehen 1979, Phillips 1981). Those tumours situated in the periphery (particularly in the upper lobes) which, coincidentally, appear to have a reduced incidence of metastases, are the most suitable for a "radical" approach since for these it is possible to administer maximum radiation doses with minimal risk of significant late effects (Komaki et al. 1981).

For the majority of patients there appears to be little justification on the basis of current results for the continued use of prolonged radiotherapy schedules. Split-course treatment does not appear inferior in terms of survival when compared with continuous treatment but has the obvious advantage for the patient of a reduction in treatment time without any increase in morbidity. The question of immediate against delayed treatment for asymptomatic patients must be considered on an individual basis, although there appears to be no disadvantage in terms of quality of life or survival in delaying active treatment. Further studies are required, particularly in terms of quality of life for these patients.

Palliative Radiotherapy

The failure of radiotherapy to influence significantly the relentless course of lung cancer should not detract from its major contribution in alleviating distressing symptoms caused either by uncontrolled intrathoracic disease or by distant metastases (Slawson and Scott 1979). The prime objective of any palliative treatment is to provide the maximum chance of symptom relief with the minimum of inconvenience to the patient. In most palliative situations, protracted courses of daily treatment are both unnecessary and unjustified, and attention should be directed toward more rapid, high dose per fraction techniques.

The principal symptoms caused by uncontrolled intrathoracic disease include haemoptysis, cough, dyspnoea, chest pain and superior vena caval obstruction. Slawson has assessed the response of patients with such symptoms to thoracic irradiation and has confirmed the high rate of improvement that may be expected, particularly with split-course treatment (Table 10).

Superior Vena Caval Obstruction

Superior vena caval (SVC) obstruction occurs in approximately 5% of all patients with lung cancer but represents one of the few real radiotherapeutic emergencies. Compression of the SVC is characterised by oedema of the face and arms, with venous congestion and a variety of symptoms including dyspnoea and, less commonly, cough and hoarseness of the voice (Scaratino et al. 1979; Lokich and Goodman 1975). Failure to institute rapid treatment in these patients may result in total occlusion of the SVC by either thrombus or tumour and prompt action is therefore required (Longacre and Schockman 1968). For some years it was felt that radiation might itself cause worsening obstruction in the initial stages of treatment by producing oedema in the irradiated tissues (Geller 1963). Subsequent studies of high initial daily radiation doses have suggested that such oedema does not occur or if it does, is not of clinical importance. Scaratino et al., using 4 Gy on each of the first 3 days of treatment, reducing to daily doses of 2 Gy for the remainder of the course, reported relief of symptoms in 26 of 43 patients (60%) within 2 days and 37 of 43 (86%) within 4 days. With standard fractionation (2 Gy per day) improvement was slower, with only 16% responding within 2 days and 50% within 4 days of treatment (Scaratino et al. 1979). Although no comparative studies of low against high initial dose therapy have been undertaken, the value of high doses has been supported by others and is currently to be recommended as the optimal approach to SVC obstruction (Rubin et al. 1963; Levitt et al. 1969; Davenport et al. 1976; Perez et al. 1978). Response to treatment can to some extent be related to onset of symptoms, those with an acute presentation responding less well than those with a subacute onset (Kanji et al. 1980). The outlook for patients with this syndrome is similar to other cases of inoperable lung cancer, those with limited local disease having the best prognosis (Cox et al. 1983).

Extrathoracic Metastases

The high incidence of metastases in lung cancer makes it inevitable that many patients will present with troublesome symptoms due to tumour deposits at sites distant from the thorax, including the brain, liver and bones.

Table 10. Symptomatic response to thoracic irradiation (Slawson and Scott 1979)

	Haemoptysis	Chest pain	SVC obstruction	Dyspnoea	Total
Response	95/113 (84%)	66/108 (61%)	36/42 (86%)	51/85 (60%)	248/348 (71%)

The frequency of cerebral metastases varies depending upon the histological tumour type from 10%–15% for squamous cell carcinomas up to 50% for adeno-carcinomas, and, as previously discussed, for some patients the brain may be the only apparent site of spread. The median survival time for brain metastases is 3–4 months but these patients may exhibit some of the most distressing symptoms and demand maximum effort at palliation despite the short prognosis (Kurtz et al. 1981).

Chu and Hilaris reported substantial benefit in over 60% of patients treated with conventional radiation fractionation schedules (Chu and Hilaris 1961). Anxiety over the possible induction of radiation oedema initially prompted the use of small daily doses of 25–50 cGy gradually increasing to 2 Gy per fraction up to total doses of 30–40 Gy in 3–5 weeks. Subsequent reports have demonstrated the effectiveness of shorter treatment courses using higher individual dose fractions in producing excellent palliation (Shehata et al. 1974; Harwood and Simpson 1977; Borgelt et al. 1980; Kurtz et al. 1981).

In a prospectively randomised trial, the Radiation Therapy Oncology Group have examined five different fractionation schedules for palliative brain irradiation, varying from 20 Gy in 1 week (1103 ret) to 40 Gy in 4 weeks (1357 ret). Results from all treatment groups were comparable with respect to symptom relief, duration of response and survival, while the shortest radiation schedules tended to produce more rapid benefit (Borgelt et al. 1980).

A separate study by Harwood and Simpson compared the relative merits of a single fraction of 10 Gy with 30 Gy given in ten fractions over 2 weeks and again showed no major difference between the two regimes although the acute side-effects (headache, nausea and vomiting) were more marked with the single treatment (Harwood and Simpson 1977).

The concurrent use of corticosteroids during irradiation improves not only the speed but also the overall rate of symptom relief, particularly in those with more severe neurological impairment at the start of treatment (Borgelt et al. 1980). Despite the short-term benefits, over half of patients receiving palliative cranial irradiation will die of uncontrolled cerebral disease. Efforts to improve local control using higher total doses of radiation (50 Gy in 4 weeks) in patients in whom brain metastases are the only site of failure have been disappointing, with no obvious advantage over short-course treatments (Kurtz et al. 1981).

The optimum palliative management for the majority of patients with symptomatic brain metastases is a high dose per fraction treatment course (20–30 Gy in 1–2 weeks) to the whole brain under steroid cover. Over 75% of patients will respond satisfactorily to such a regime, which offers only minimal inconvenience (including total alopecia) but has the advantage that retreatment, if needed, is both possible and often beneficial (Shehata et al. 1974).

Bone metastases may produce dull unremitting pain often worsened by movement and accompanied by local tenderness. Where the vertebrae or ribs are involved, infiltration of the dorsal roots may result in referred pain along the pathway of the involved nerves. Most commonly the responsible lesion is visible on plain X-ray, although bone pain may be present without demonstrable radiological evidence of bone destruction. In a comprehensive review of radiotherapy in the treatment of bone metastases, Ford and Yarnold concluded that for single fraction treatments there is no clear dose-response relationship, tumour doses of 3–4 Gy producing comparable pain relief to higher dose fractions (Ford and Yarnold 1983). Furthermore, from the retrospective data available, single fractions of 4 Gy appear no less effective than multiple treatment schedules with regard to either the probability or the duration of pain relief. Where fracture of long bones is feared (as judged by destruction of more than half the thickness of the cortex) or already established, internal fixation is the initial treatment of choice followed by radiotherapy to prevent further bone destruction and instability (Galasko 1980). Properly designed trials comparing single against multiple dose schedules are required in these patients, but until more data are available there can be little justification for palliative courses of more than 30 Gy in ten fractions for bone metastases and much support for even shorter treatment regimes (Delclos 1976; Tong et al. 1982). In the last few years large field, hemibody irradiation (HBI) has been investigated as palliation in patients with widespread metastases (Urtasun 1983). Single doses of irradiation between 6 and 8 Gy produce pain relief within 48 h in approximately half of those treated and in up to 80% within a week, with a mean duration of relief of 14 weeks (Salazar et al. 1981). The major toxicity of HBI has been the late onset of radiation pneumonitis, with a steep dose-response curve above doses of 7 Gy, but this complication has been significantly reduced by fractionating treatment (Belch 1982). HBI is currently undergoing further study both for palliation and as "systemic" therapy in small cell carcinoma (Urtasun 1983).

Metastatic involvement of the liver may be accompanied by a variety of signs and symptoms, including abdominal pain, nausea and vomiting, fever and night sweats, ascites, anorexia and jaundice. While patients with solitary metastases or more slowly growing adenocarcinomas may have a modest prognosis, the more extensive infiltration associated with abnormal biochemical parameters or ascites or jaundice has an extremely poor outlook, with median survivals of less than 1 month (Jaffe et al. 1968). Whole liver irradiation is of proven value in relieving symptoms such as pain, nausea and vomiting, approximately 50% of patients responding satisfactorily to rapid fractionation schedules (21 Gy in seven fractions). This type of treatment appears as effective as more prolonged schedules, with no evidence of an increased risk of radiation-induced hepatitis or other acute complications, although the median survival and therefore follow up for these patients is only short (Sherman et al. 1978; Borgelt et al. 1981).

Finally, another "emergency" situation that may arise in patients with metastatic lung cancer results from extradural compression of the spinal cord. In many ways this resembles SVC obstruction in that immediate action is required if optimum palliation, i.e. preservation of limb and bowel and bladder function, is to be obtained. The outcome of treatment for spinal cord compression may often be predicted from the findings at presentation — patients with established paraplegia are unlikely to recover function whereas those who are still able to walk will continue to do so after treatment in 70% of cases (Tomita et al. 1983). In very radiosensitive tumours such as the malignant lymphomas it may be appropriate to treat cord compression with high dose per fraction irradiation and corticosteroids since tumour response will be rapid and obstruction quickly relieved (Rubin et al. 1969). With many lung tumours, however, compression is often secondary to bony involvement and radiotherapy alone is insufficient to relieve the obstruction. Furthermore, whatever the histology, tumour response to irradiation is unlikely to be sufficiently rapid to avoid permanent cord damage.

Unless there is an obvious medical contraindication, where some degree of function is preserved, surgical decompression is advisable in all patients with extradural metastases from lung tumours even if the ultimate prognosis is poor. Radiotherapy to the involved area of the spine should be considered after surgery to relieve pain and prevent further bone erosion.

Radiotherapy and Small Cell Lung Cancer

One area of major interest in lung cancer at the present time concerns the optimum management of small cell carcinoma. The medium survival for patients with untreated disease limited to the thorax is approximately 3 months; with radiotherapy this figure rises to 5-6 months. It is now well established that the addition of either single agent or combination chemotherapy to radiotherapy further improves the short-term survival rates for patients with limited disease (Bergsagel et al. 1972; Host 1973; Petrovich et al. 1977; M.R.C. 1979) (Table 11).

With the increasing remission rates being reported for small cell lung cancer (SCLC) treated with chemotherapy alone, the question arises as to the place of radiotherapy in any treatment programme. In a review of the literature by Salazar, between 20% and 40% of patients with limited disease relapsed in the thorax after radiotherapy, compared with 80% of those treated by chemotherapy alone. With a combination of radiation and chemotherapy the local failure rate was around 28% (Salazar and Creech 1980). A further analysis by Bleehen et al. (1983) concluded that in terms of survival the results of the addition of thoracic irradiation to chemotherapy were conflicting (Table 12). Of the two largest trials, the Copenhagen study involving 154 patients randomised between four-drug chemotherapy alone or chemotherapy with split course thoracic radiation to 40 Gy reported median survival times of 12 months and 10.5 months for chemotherapy and combined treatment respectively (Dombernowsky et al. 1980). The reduction in survival for the radiotherapy group was not statistically significant. By contrast, while the trial by Fox et al. was originally reported as showing no difference in median survival times with the addition of thoracic radiation to chemotherapy, on further follow up there was a significant improvement in 2-year disease-free survival for the combined treatment, with a corresponding reduction in relapse rate at the primary tumour site (Fox et al. 1980; Bleehen et al. 1983).

Similar results from the NCI trial comparing chemotherapy (cyclophosphamide, methotrexate and CCNU) alone against chemotherapy with thoracic and cranial irradiation have again confirmed higher complete response rates and improved median survival times with adjuvant radiotherapy. However, further observation on all these trials is required before any firm conclusion can be drawn on the contribution of local irradiation to survival.

With the high observed incidence of brain metastases in patients with SCLC consideration must also be given to the place of prophylactic cranial irradiation (PCI) with chemotherapy in improving long-term survival. Several randomised

Table 11. Radiotherapy vs radiotherapy and chemotherapy in small cell carcinoma

	No.	Median survival (months)	
		Radiotherapy	Radiotherapy + chemotherapy
Bergsagel et al. (1972)	41	5	9.5
Host (1973)	75	5.5	8.5
Petrovich et al. (1977)	59	5	9.5
M.R.C. (1979)	236	6	10.5

Table 12. Chemotherapy vs chemotherapy plus thoracic radiotherapy in small cell carcinoma

	Therapy	Total no.	Median/survival (months)

Williams et al.
(1977)
	CT CYCLO
	        VCR
	        CCNU
	        PROCARB
		25	11

	CT + RT		9

Stevens et al.
(1979)
	CT CYCLO
	        VCR
	        ADR
		32	12

	CT + RT		11.5

Fox et al.
(1980)
	CT CYCLO
	        VCR
	        ADR
		84	14.5

	CT + RT		14.5

Dombernowsky et al.
(1980)
	CT CYCLO
	        VCR
	        CCNU
	        MTX
		154	12

	CT + RT		10.5

Bunn et al.
(1983)
	CT CYCLO
	        MTX
	        CCNU
		63	12

	CT + RT		17

CYCLO, cyclophosphamide; VCR, vincristine; PROCARB, procarbazine; ADR, adriamycin; MTX, methotrexate

studies have explored the potential benefits of PCI with total radiation doses between 20 and 40 Gy, and while some have shown a significant reduction in CNS relapse rates, others have shown no benefit (Table 13). More importantly, none of these trials have demonstrated any significant improvement in survival with the addition of whole brain irradiation.

For patients with SCLC who do not achieve a complete remission with chemotherapy, the chance of developing CNS metastases is high whether or not they have received PCI (Rosen et al. 1981); for these patients it seems appropriate to withhold treatment until symptoms occur since therapeutic cranial irradiation at the time of relapse will produce relief in over 90% of patients (Nugent et al. 1979). In patients with limited disease at presentation who show a complete response to initial

Table 13. Prophylactic cranial irradiation in small cell carcinoma

		Patients with CNS relapse (%)		
	No.	PCI	No PCI	Survival difference
Jackson et al. (1977	29	0	27	N.S.
Maurer et al. (1980)	163	4	18	N.S.
Beiler et al. (1979)	54	0	16	N.S.
Cot et al. (1978)	45	17	24	N.S.
Seydel et al. (1982)	217	5	22	N.S.

treatment, the reduced incidence of CNS metastases suggests a benefit in the quality of survival and in these prophylactic treatment may be justified although no advantage in long-term survival may accrue from PCI. Further trials randomising complete responders to receive PCI or not at the time of remission are required to assess properly any potential benefit in survival for patients with SCLC.

In all regimes where chemotherapy and radiation are combined, much caution should be exercised in the scheduling of treatment and with escalation of doses to avoid undue toxicity (Feld 1981; Goodman 1983).

As new and more effective chemotherapeutic drugs and combinations become available, other studies will be required to define more clearly the exact role of radiotherapy in "curative" treatment. In addition, novel radiation techniques such as total or hemi-body irradiation are currently being assessed in SCLC, although to date the results are not especially promising (Bleehen et al. 1983; Urtasun 1983).

In any study, precise details of radiation therapy should be recorded and careful documentation made of any toxicity. Furthermore, results should in future be reported on the basis of 2-year survival or disease-free survival rates and not in terms of median survival times if a true assessment of any new treatment strategy is to be made (Bleehen et al. 1983).

Summary

Despite improvements in equipment and treatment techniques, the results of radiotherapy for lung cancer have not altered significantly over the past 30 years. Analysis of patterns of failure in these patients reveals that the majority will ultimately develop distant metastases and for these, survival will only improve with the introduction of effective systemic therapy. On closer examination, however, certain patient subgroups can be identified who appear to relapse in the thorax or brain alone and who may therefore benefit from better local tumour control. The continuing failure of radiotherapy to eradicate intrathoracic disease requires that further investigation be undertaken with other techniques such as hyperthermia or the use of chemical hypoxic cell sensitisers which may increase the efficacy of local irradiation.

The high response rates following chemotherapy in patients with small cell carcinoma has raised the question of the place of thoracic and cranial irradiation in overall management, and carefully controlled randomised studies of chemotherapy and radiation are required to assess properly any potential benefit in terms of survival.

Finally, for the large number of lung cancer patients who present with troublesome symptoms due to uncontrolled intrathoracic disease or to metastases at distant sites, radiotherapy has an established place in providing rapid and effective palliation.

Acknowledgements. I would like to acknowledge the invaluable assistance of Miss Linda Mather in the preparation of this manuscript.

References

Abadir R, Muggia FM (1975) Irradiated lung cancer: an autopsy analysis of spread pattern. Radiology 114:427–430

Abramson N, Cavanaugh PJ (1973) Short course radiation therapy in carcinoma of the lung. Radiology 108:685–687

Adams GE, Clarke ED, Flockhart IR et al. (1979) Structure-activity relationships in the development of hypoxic cell radiosensitisers. Int J Radiat Biol 35:133–138

Aristizabal SA, Caldwell WL (1976) Radical irradiation with the split-course technique in carcinoma of the lung. Cancer 37:2630–2635

Arnold AM, Williams CJ (1979) Small cell lung cancer: a curable disease. Br J Dis Chest 73:327–348

Bangma PJ (1971) Post operative radiotherapy. In: Deeley TJ (ed) Modern radiotherapy. Carcinoma of the bronchus. Appleton-Century Crofts, New York, pp 163–170

Bataini JP, Picco C, Martin M, Calle R (1978) Relation between time-dose and local control of operable breast cancer. Cancer 42:2059–2065

Beiler DD, Kane RC, Bernath AM et al. (1979) Low dose elective brain irradiation in small cell carcinoma of the lung. Int J Radiat Oncol Biol Phys 5:941–945

Belch AR, Urtasun RC, Bodnar D (1982) Fractionated sequential hemi-body irradiation (HBI) in small cell lung cancer. Proc Am Soc Clin Oncol 1:139

Bergsagel DE, Jenkin RDT, Pringle JF et al. (1972) Lung cancer: clinical trial of radiotherapy alone vs radiotherapy plus cyclophosphamide. Cancer 30:621–627

Bleehen NM, Bunn PA, Cox JD et al. (1983) Role of radiation therapy in small cell anaplastic carcinoma of the lung. Cancer Treat Rep 67:11–19

Bloedorn FG, Cowley RA, Cuccia CA, Mercado R (1961) Combined therapy: irradiation and surgery in the treatment of bronchogenic carcinoma. Am J Roentgenol 85:875–885

Borgelt B, Gelber R, Kramer S, Brady LW (1980) The palliation of brain metastases: final results of the first two studies by the RTOG. Int J Radiat Oncol Biol Phys 6:1–9

Borgelt BB, Gelber R, Brady LW, Griffin T et al. (1981) The palliation of hepatic metastases: result of the RTOG pilot study. Int J Radiat Oncol Biol Phys 7: 587–591

Bromley LL, Szur L (1955) Combined radiotherapy and resection for carcinoma of the bronchus. Lancet II:937–941

Bunn P, Cohen M, Litcher A et al. (1983) Randomised trial of chemotherapy versus chemotherapy plus radiotherapy in limited stage small cell lung cancer. Proc Am Soc Clin Oncol 2:200

Cade IS, McEwan JB (1978) Clinical trials of radiotherapy in hyperbaric oxygen at Portsmouth 1964–1976. Clin Radiol 29:333–338

Chilvers C (1982) Cancer mortality in England and Wales: time, area and social class patterns. Cancer Topics 4:5–8

Choi CH, Carey RW (1976) Small cell anaplastic carcinoma of lung. Reappraisal of current management. Cancer 37:2651–2657

Choi NCH, Doucette JE (1981) Improved survival of patients with unresectable non-small cell bronchogenic carcinoma by an innovative high-dose en bloc radiotherapeutic approach. Cancer 48: 101–109

Choi NCH, Grillo HC, Gardiello M, Scannell JG et al. (1980) Basis for new strategies in post-operative radiotherapy of bronchogenic carcinoma. Int J Radiat Oncol Biol Phys 6:31–35

Chu FCH, Hilaris BB (1961) Value of radiation therapy in the management of intracranial metastases. Cancer 14:577–581

Churchill-Davison I, Foster CA, Wiernik G et al. (1966) The place of oxygen in radiotherapy. Br J Radiol 39:321–331

Cohen MH (1983) Is immediate radiation therapy indicated for patients with unresectable non-small cell lung cancer? No. Cancer Treat Rep 67:333–336

Cohen MH, Lichter AS, Bunn PA, Glatstein EJ et al. (1980) Chemotherapy-radiation therapy versus chemotherapy in limited small cell lung cancer. Proc Am Assoc Cancer Res and ASCO 21:448

Collins VP, Loeffler RK, Tivey H (1966) Observations on growth rates of human tumours. Am J Roentgenol 76:988–1000

Cox JD, Petrovich Z, Pagi G, Stanley K (1978) Prophylactic cranial irradiation in patients with inoperable carcinoma of the lung. Cancer 42:1135–1140

Cox JD, Yesner R, Mietlowski W, Petrovich Z (1979) Influence of cell type on failure pattern after irradiation for locally advanced carcinoma of the lung. Cancer 44:94–98

Cox JD, Stanley K, Petrovich Z, Paig C et al. (1981) Cranial irradiation in cancer of the lung of all cell types. JAMA 245:469–472

Cox JD, Byhardt RW, Komaki R (1983) The role of radiotherapy in squamous, large cell and adenocarcinoma of the lung. Semin Oncol 10:81–94

Cox JD, Komaki R, Byhardt RW (1983) Is immediate chest radiotherapy obligatory for any or all patients with limited stage non-small cell carcinoma of the lung? Yes. Cancer Treat Rep 67:327–331

Davenport D, Ferree C, Balke D, Raben M (1976) Response of superior vena cava syndrome to radiation therapy. Cancer 38:1577–1580

Deeley TJ (1966) A clinical trial to compare two different tumour dose levels in the treatment of advanced carcinoma of the bronchus. Clin Radiol 17:299–301

Deeley TJ (1967) The treatment of carcinoma of the bronchus. Br J Radiol 40:801–822

Delclos L (1976) New and old concepts in radiotherapeutic treatments. Int J Radiat Oncol Biol Phys 1: 1217–1220

Dische S, Saunders MI, Anderson P et al. (1978) The neurotoxicity of misonidazole: pooling of data from five centres. Br J Radiol 51:1023–1024

Dische S, Saunders MI, Flockhart IR, Lee ME, Anderson P (1979) Misonidazole — a drug for trial in radiotherapy and oncology. Int J Radiat Oncol Biol Phys 5:851–860

Dische S, Martin WMC, Anderson P (1981) Radiation myelopathy in patients treated for carcinoma of bronchus using a six-fraction regime of radiotherapy. Br J Radiol 54:29–35

Dombernowsky P, Hansen HH, Hansen M et al. (1980) Treatment of small cell anaplastic bronchogenic carcinoma. Results from two randomised trials. II World Conference on Lung Cancer, Amsterdam. Excerpta Medica, Amsterdam, p 149

Durrant KR, Berry RJ, Ellis F, Black JM et al. (1971) Comparison of treatment policies in inoperable bronchial carcinoma. Lancet I:715–719

Eisert DR, Cox JD, Komaki R (1976) Irradiation for bronchial carcinoma: reasons for failure. Cancer 37:2665–2670

Emami B, Melo A, Carter BL, Munzenrider JE (1978) Value of computed tomography in radiotherapy of lung cancer. Am J Roentgenol 131: 63–67

Feld R (1981) Complications in the treatment of small cell carcinoma of the lung. Cancer Treat Rev 8:5–25

Field SB, Bleehen NM (1979) Hyperthermia in the treatment of cancer. Cancer Treat Rev 6:63–94

Fletcher GH (1979) Basic principles of the combination of irradiation and surgery. Int J Radiat Oncol Biol Phys 5:2091–2096

Ford HT, Yarnold JR (1983) Radiation therapy — pain relief and recalcification. In: Stoll BA, Parbhoo S (eds) Bone metastases: monitoring and treatment. Raven Press, New York, pp 343–345

Fox RM, Woods RL, Brodie GN et al. (1980) A randomised study: small cell anaplastic lung cancer treated by combination chemotherapy and adjuvant radiotherapy. Int J Radiat Oncol Biol Phys 6:1087–1092

Galasko CSB (1980) The management of skeletal metastases. J R Coll Surg Edinb 3:148–151

Gazdar AF, Carney DN, Minna JD (1983) The biology of non-small cell lung cancer. Semin Oncol 10:3–19

Geddes DM (1979) The natural history of lung cancer: a review based on rates of tumour growth. Br J Dis Chest 73:1–17

Geller W (1963) The mandate for chemotherapeutic decompression in superior vena cava obstruction. Radiology 81:385–387

Goodman GE, Miller TP, Manning MM et al. (1983) Treatment of small cell lung cancer with VP-16, vincristine, adriamycin, cyclophosphamide and high-dose radiotherapy. Clin Oncol 1:483–488

Gray LH, Conger DA, Ebert M, Hornsey S et al. (1953) The concentration of oxygen dissolved in tissues at the time of irradiation as a factor in radiotherapy. Br J Radiol 26:638–648

Greco FA, Oldham RK (1979) Current concepts in cancer: small cell lung cancer. N Engl J Med 301: 355–358

Green N (1981) Lung cancer — post-resection irradiation. In: Livingston RB (ed) Lung cancer. Matinus Nijhoff, The Hague Boston London, pp 75–111

Green N, Kurohara SS, George FW, Crews QE (1975) Postresection irradiation for primary lung cancer. Radiology 116:405–407

Gunterseydel H, Kutcher GJ, Steiner RM, Mohiuddin M et al. (1980) Computed tomography in planning radiation therapy for bronchogenic carcinoma. Int J Radiat Oncol Biol Phys 6:601–606

Guthrie RT, Ptacek JJ, Hass AC (1973) Comparative Analysis of two regimens of split course radiation in carcinoma of the lung. Am J Roentgenol 117:605–608

Guttman RJ (1965) Results of radiation therapy in patients with inoperable carcinoma of the lung whose status was established at exploratory thoracotomy. Am J Roentgenol 93:99–103

Hansen M, Hansen HH, Dombernowsky P (1980) Long term survival in small cell carcinoma of the lung. JAMA 244:247–250

Harwood AR, Simpson WJ (1977) Radiation therapy of cerebral metastases: a randomised prospective clinical trial. Int J Radiat Oncol Biol Phys 2:1091–1094.

Holsti LR, Mattson K (1980) A randomised study of split-course radiotherapy of lung cancer: long term results. Int J Radiat Oncol Biol Phys 6: 977–981

Host H (1973) Cyclophosphamide as adjuvant to radiotherapy in the treatment of unresectable bronchogenic carcinoma. Cancer Chemother Rep 4: 161–164

Jackson DV, Richards F, Cooper MR et al. (1977) Prophylactic cranial irradiation in Small cell carcinoma of the lung: a randomised study. JAMA 237:2730–2733

Jaffe BM, Donegan WL, Watson P, Spratt JS (1968) Factors influencing survival in patients with untreated hepatic metastases. Surg Gynecol Obstet 127:1–11, 1968

Kanji AM, Chao JH, Liebner EJ, Lobo P et al. (1980) Extrinsic compression of superior vena cava. An analysis of 41 patients. Int J Radiat Oncol Biol Phys 6:213–215

Kirsh MM, Prior M, Gago D, Moores WY et al. (1972) The effect of histological cell type on the prognosis of patients with bronchogenic carcinoma. Ann Thorac Surg 13:303–310

Kirsh MM, Rotman H, Argenta L, Bove E et al. (1976) Carcinoma of the lung: results of treatment over ten years. Ann Thorac Surg 21:371–377

Komaki R, Roh J, Cox JD et al. (1981) Superior sulcus tumours: results of irradiation in 36 patients. Cancer 48: 1563–1568

Komaki R, Cox JD, Stark R (1983) Frequency of brain metastases in adenocarcinoma and large cell carcinoma of the lung: correlation with survival. Int J Radiat Oncol Biol Phys 9:1467–1470

Kurtz JM, Gelber R, Brady LW, Carella RJ et al. (1981) The palliation of brain metastases in a favourable patient population: a randomised clinical trial by the RTOG. Int J Radiat Oncol Biol Phys 7:891–895

Lee RE, Carr DT, Childs DS (1976) Comparison of split-course radiation therapy and continuous radiation therapy for unresectable bronchogenic carcinoma: 5 year results. Am J Roentgenol 126: 116–122

Levitt SH, Bogardus CR, Ladd G (1967) Split course intensive radiation therapy in the treatment of advanced lung cancer. Radiology 88:1159–1161

Levitt SH, Jones TK, Kilpatrick SJ, Bogardus CR (1969) Treatment of malignant superior vena caval obstruction. Cancer 24:447–451

Libshitz HI, Southard ME (1974) Complications of radiation therapy: the thorax. Semin Roentgenol 9:41–49

Lokich JJ, Goodman R (1975) Superior vena cava syndrome. JAMA 231:58–61

Longacre AA, Schockman AT (1968) The superior vena cava syndrome and radiation therapy. Radiology 91:713–718

Martini N, Beattie EJ (1977) Results of surgical treatment in stage I lung cancer. J Thorac Cardiovasc Surg 74:499–505

Matthews MJ, Kanhouwa S, Pickren J, Robinette D (1973) Frequency of residual and metastatic tumour in patients undergoing curative surgical resection for lung cancer. Cancer Chemother Rep 4:63–67

Maurer LH, Tulloh M, Weiss RB et al. (1980) A randomised combined modality trial in small cell carcinoma of the lung. Cancer 45:30–39

Morrison R, Deeley TJ (1960) Inoperable cancer of the bronchus treated by megavoltage X-ray therapy. Lancet II:618–620

Mountain CF (1973) Keynote address on surgery in the therapy for lung cancer: surgical prospects and priorities for clinical research. Cancer Chemother Rep 4:19–24

M.R.C. Lung Cancer Working Party (1979) Radiotherapy alone or with chemotherapy in the treatment of small cell carcinoma of the lung. Br J Cancer 40:1–10

Nugent JL, Bunn PA, Matthews MJ et al. (1979) CNS metastases in small cell bronchogenic carcinoma. Cancer 44:1885–1893

Overgaard J, Overgaard M, Timothy AR (1983) Studies of the pharmacokinetic properties of nimorazole. Br J Cancer 48: 27–34

Paterson R, Russell MH (1962) Clinical trials in malignant disease. Part IV — lung cancer. Value of post-operative radiotherapy. Clin Radiol 13:141–144

Perez CA (1977) The critical need for accurate treatment planning and quality control in radiation therapy. Int J Radiat Oncol Biol Phys 2:815–818

Perez C, Presant CA, Van Amberg III AL (1978) Management of superior vena caval syndrome. Semin Oncol 5:123–134

Perez CA, Stanley K, Rubin P, Kramer S et al. (1980) A prospective randomised study of various irradiation doses and fractionation schedules in the treatment of inoperable non-oat cell carcinoma of the lung. Cancer 45:2744–2753

Perez CA, Stanley K, Grundy G et al. (1982) Impact of irradiation technique and tumour extent in tumour control and survival of patients with irresectable non-oat cell carcinoma of the lung. Cancer 50:1091-1099

Petrovich Z, Mietlowski W, Ohanian M, Cox J (1977) Clinical report on the treatment of locally advanced lung cancer. Cancer 40: 72-77

Petrovich Z, Stanley KM, Cox JD, Paig C (1981) Radiotherapy in the management of locally advanced lung cancer of all cell types. Cancer 48:1335-1340

Phillips TL (1981) Sensitisers and protectors in clinical oncology. Semin Oncol 8:65-82

Phillips TL, Margolis L (1972) Radiation pathology and the clinical response of lung and oesophagus. In: Front Radiat Ther Oncol 6. Karger, Basel and University Park Press, Baltimore, pp 254-273

Phillips TL, Wharam MD, Margolis LW (1975) Modification of radiation injury to normal tissues by chemotherapeutic agents. Cancer 35:1678-1684

Rissanen PM, Tikka U, Holsti LR (1968) Autopsy findings in lung cancer treated with megavoltage radiotherapy. Acta Radiol Ther Phys Biol 7:433-442

Rosen S, Bunn P, Lighter A et al. (1981) Prophylactic cranial irradiation in small cell lung cancer: benefit restricted to patient in complete response. Proc Am Assoc Cancer Res and ASCO 22:499

Roswit B, Patno ME, Rapp R et al. (1968) The survival of patients with inoperable lung cancer: a large-scale randomised study of radiation therapy versus placebo. Radiology 90:688-697

Rubin P, Green J, Holzwasser G, Gerle R (1963) Superior vena cava syndrome: slow dose versus rapid dose schedules. Radiology 81:388-401

Rubin P, Mayer E, Poulter C (1969) High daily dose experience without laminectomy. Radiology 93:1248-1260

Salazar O, Creech RH (1980) "The state of the art" toward defining the role of radiation therapy in the management of small cell bronchogenic carcinoma. Int J Radiat Oncol Biol Phys 6:1103-1117

Salazar OM, Rubin P, Brown JC, Feldstein ML et al. (1976a) The assessment of tumour response to irradiation of lung cancer: continuous versus split-course regimes. Int J Radiat Oncol Biol Phys 1:1107-1118

Salazar OM, Rubin P Brown JC, Feldstein ML et al. (1976b) Predictors of radiation response in lung cancer. Cancer 37:2636-2650.

Salazar OM, Rubin P, Hendrickson FR et al. (1981) Single dose half-body irradiation for the palliation of multiple bone metastases from solid tumours: a preliminary report. Int J Radiat Oncol Biol Phys 7:773-781

Scaratino C, Salazar OM, Rubin P, Wilson G et al. (1979) The optimum radiation schedule in treatment of superior venal caval obstruction: importance of ^{99m}Tc scintigrams. Int J Radiat Oncol Biol Phys 5:1987-1995

Schaake-Koning C, Schuster-Uitterhoeve L, Hart G, Gonzalez DG (1983) Prognostic factors of inoperable localised lung cancer treated by high dose radiotherapy. Int J Radiat Oncol Biol Phys 9:1023-1028.

Schultz MD (1957) The results of radiotherapy in cancer of the lung. Radiology 69:494-498

Sealy R, Lagakos S, Barkley T et al. (1982) Radiotherapy of regional epidermoid carcinoma of the lung. Cancer 49:1338-1345

Seydel G, Chait A, Cmelich JT (1976) The natural history of cancer of the lung. In: Seydel CR (ed) Cancer of the lung. Wiley, New York, pp 51-63

Seydel HG, Creech R, Pagano M et al. (1982) Elective irradiation of the brain in complete responders to combined radiation and chemotherapy for localised oat cell carcinoma. Int J Radiat Oncol Biol Phys 8 (Suppl):70

Shehata WM, Hendrickson FR, Hindo WA (1974) Rapid fractionation technique and re-treatment of cerebral metastases by irradiation. Cancer 34:257-261

Sherman DM, Weichselbaum R, Order SE et al. (1978) Palliation of hepatic metastases. Cancer 41:2013-2017

Sherman DM, Weichselbaum R, Hellman S (1981) The characteristics of long-term survivors of lung cancer treated with radiation. Cancer 47:2575-2580

Shin KH, Birdsell J, Geggie PHS, Scott Brown I (1980) Adenocarcinoma of the lung: ten years experience in Southern Alberta Cancer Centre. Int J Radiat Oncol Biol Phys 6:835-840

Slawson RG, Scott RM (1979) Radiation therapy in bronchogenic carcinoma. Radiology 132:175-176

Smart J, Hilton G (1956) Radiotherapy of cancer of the lung: results in a selected group of cases. Lancet 1:880-881

Smith IE, Sappino AP, Bondy PK, Gilby ED (1981) Long term survival five years or more after combination chemotherapy and radiotherapy for small cell lung carcinoma. Eur J Cancer 17:1249-1253

Smithers DW (1955) Carcinoma of the bronchus — a radiotherapy view point. J Fac Radiol Lond 6:174-181

Spjut HJ, Mateo LE (1965) Recurrent and metastatic carcinoma in surgically treated carcinoma of lung. Cancer 18:1462–1466

Stanley KE (1980) Prognostic factors for survival in patients with inoperable lung cancer. J Natl Cancer Inst 65:25–32

Stevens E, Einhorn L, Rohn R (1979) Treatment of limited small cell lung cancer. PRoc Am Assoc Cancer Res and ASCO 20:435

Thompson DT (1966) Conservative resection in surgery for bronchogenic carcinoma. J Thorac Cardio-Vasc Surg 53:159–162

Tomita T, Galicich JH, Sundaresan N (1983) Radiation therapy for spinal epidural metastases with complete block. Acta Radiol Oncol Radiat Phys Biol, 22:135–143

Tong D, Gillick L, Hendrickson FR (1982) The palliation of symptomatic osseous metastases. Final results of the study by the RTOG. Cancer 50:893–899

Urtasun RC (1983) Hemibody irradiation technique: a wider use in oncology. Int J Radiat Oncol Biol Phys 9:1585–1586

Vandyk J, Keane TJ, Rider WD (1982) Lung density as measured by computerised tomography: implications for radiotherapy. Int J Radiat Oncol Biol Phys 8:1363–1372

Wara WM, Phillips TL, Sheline GE, Schwade JG (1975) Radiation tolerance of the spinal cord. Cancer 35:1558–1562

Wigg DR, Koschel K, Hodgson GS (1981) Tolerance of the mature human central nervous system to photon irradiation. Br J radiol 54:787–798

Williams C, Alexander M, Glatstein ES et al. (1977) Role of radiation therapy in combination with chemotherapy in extensive oat cell cancer of the lung: a randomised study. Cancer Treat Rep 61:1427–1431

Chapter 17

Chemotherapy for Bronchial Carcinoma

Edna Matthews and Nicholas Plowman

Introduction

The high incidence and fatality of bronchial carcinoma make it a subject of extreme importance. Regrettably, despite the advances in thoracic surgery and the widespread availability of megavoltage radiotherapy in the last two decades, neither of these modalities has made a significant impression on the survival of the majority of patients. Meanwhile, knowledge and experience in the use of chemotherapy have accumulated and, with the improved clinical results in leukaemia, lymphoma and some other malignancies, there has been an impetus to search for effective drug regimes for bronchogenic cancer. So far, this chemotherapeutic attack has had only limited success, but that success is sufficiently important to justify this full review of the subject.

Bronchogenic carcinoma consists of a number of differing histological types, each with its own natural history. They may be broadly divided into non-small cell and small cell carcinoma, and in the discussion which follows these will be considered separately.

Non-Small Cell Carcinoma of Bronchus

This heterogeneous histological group of bronchial carcinomas is more chemoresistant and radio-resistant than small cell carcinoma and, if localised, they are best managed by surgical resection. This is the only modality of therapy currently with a consistent chance, albeit a slim one, of cure. Unfortunately, only approximately one in five adequately evaluated patients will be candidates for operation, as evidence of local extension into the chest wall or mediastinal structures (including nodes), evidence of metastases, poor respiratory function or advanced age or frailty are all contra-indications for surgery. There are almost 25 000 patients per year in the United Kingdom with non-small cell carcinoma of bronchus in whom surgery is not possible or who have relapsed after surgery, and this figure is 90 000 per year in the United States; the median survival for this group of patients from diagnosis varies from 3 to 10 months depending on the prognostic variables discussed later. If an effective systemic therapy could be found for non-small cell carcinoma of bronchus, it could potentially benefit 115 000 people in the United Kingdom and the United States every year.

The quest for effective chemotherapy regimes is now being carried out methodically in many centres of radiotherapy and oncology. At first, single agent activity is sought amongst the ever-increasing number of cytotoxic drugs available. The criteria for activity of a drug are strict and the drug dose is escalated in early phase trials to tolerance. A 50% volume reduction in all sites of measurable disease and an absence of progression to other sites, sustained for two or more cycles, quantifies as a partial response. Complete disappearance of all disease maintained for at least 3 months constitutes a complete response.

Unlike small cell carcinoma, there are no currently available drugs which, when given singly, cause a response in over 30% of patients with non-small cell carcinoma of bronchus. This statement applies to all the three main histological types of non-small cell cancer, viz. squamous (epidermoid), large cell anaplastic and adenocarcinoma of bronchus. However, there are an increasing number of drugs which, when given singly, will consistently cause a response rate of $18\% \pm 5\%$ (almost always a partial response). These include nitrogen mustard, cyclophosphamide, adriamycin, CCNU, methotrexate, procarbazine, vindesine and hexamethylmelamine. Other drugs with slightly lower response rates are *cis*-platinum, bleomycin and vincristine.

Extrapolating from animal studies and clinical successes in the management of leukaemias, lymphomas and paediatric tumours, it is next customary to combine agents from the top of the single agent activity tables and (ideally) with non-overlapping toxicities, to create a combination chemotherapy regime — initially with two or three agents. Many such studies have been performed. Early studies show that adriamycin and nitrogen mustard or cyclophosphamide (used as once 3 weekly bolus injections in doses sufficient to cause a moderately severe leucopenic and thrombocytopenic nadir at 7–12 days) was as good as any other two drug combination but that the additional response rate over cyclophosphamide alone was not great. This combination showed most promise in squamous carcinoma of bronchus.

The subsequent studies in squamous carcinoma are of interest. Livingston et al. (1976) reported a 42% response rate when using a five drug combination (nitrogen mustard, adriamycin, CCNU, bleomycin and vincristine), but when these workers repeated this study the response rate fell to 21% with an insignificant advantage in response rate over a second group of randomised patients who received only three of the drugs (nitrogen mustard, adriamycin and CCNU) (Livingston et al. 1977). This pattern of early enthusiasm with a high response rate for a particular chemotherapy regime followed by a much lower response rate in subsequent usage of the same regime, even by the same workers, is not uncommon and Aisner and Hansen (1981) have called attention to the misleading implications of the premature publication of results in this work. In a Cambridge study, using a four drug combination (cyclophosphamide 750 mg/m^2, adriamycin 50 mg/m^2, vincristine 1.5 mg/m^2 and bleomycin 30 mg, all i.v. 3 weekly), an initial response was obtained in 14 of the first 49 patients (29%) with squamous carcinoma (Wiltshire et al. 1981, unpublished data). However, after 65 patients with squamous carcinoma of bronchus had been treated, the response rate had dropped to 24%, which was felt to be nearer the true rate (Jones et al. 1983).

Recently, *cis*-platinum has been shown to have activity against squamous carcinoma of bronchus, and as it has some non-overlapping toxicities with the front-line drugs discussed above, it has been introduced into combination chemotherapy regimes by several groups of investigators. Again on a basis of adriamycin and cyclophosphamide by intermittent bolus injection, the addition of *cis*-platinum

(40–50 mg/m²) has led to response rates near 40% in the hands of some workers (Eagan et al 1977; Knost et al. 1981). Gralla et al. (1982) found the two drug combination of vindesine and *cis*-platinum to be active in 30% of patients and it was disappointing when this group recently reported that the four drug combination of adriamycin, cyclophosphamide, vindesine and *cis*-platinum did not improve the response rate (Kelsen et al. 1982); it is interesting that they found no loss of activity when bleomycin was substituted for adriamycin in this regimen (Itri et al. 1983). In the Cambridge study, the addition of *cis*-platinum to the four drug combination regime for squamous cancer did not increase the response rate but did increase toxicity (Jones et al. 1983). Three or four drug combination chemotherapy regimes incorporating methotrexate, hexamethylmelamine and/or procarbazine usually together with adriamycin or adriamycin and cyclophosphamide have not produced response rates superior to the studies just cited.

The conclusions of this brief synopsis of current chemotherapy trials in squamous carcinoma of bronchus are that combination chemotherapy can cause significant tumour regression (Fig. 1) and does modestly increase the response rate over single agents. However, these responses are usually partial and not very durable, so that these drug regimes have not yet led to increases in the overall survival, although some analytical methods may purport to demonstrate this (see below). The toxicity of most effective regimes is often (but not always) marked with nausea, vomiting and languor, which may be prolonged. Unlike tumours which respond well to chemotherapy, severe chemotherapy side-effects add to the general ill-health of malignant disease and the quality of life of many patients on chemotherapy regimes suffers. The combined chemoradiotherapy studies in squamous carcinoma of bronchus have not been reviewed but do not appear promising; not surprisingly, the local chest response rate is higher in these studies (e.g. Trovo et al. 1982).

Many of the foregoing remarks also apply to primary bronchial adenocarcinoma and indeed some of the above studies studied adenocarcinoma together with squamous carcinoma. Knost et al. (1981) and Evans et al. (1981) found response

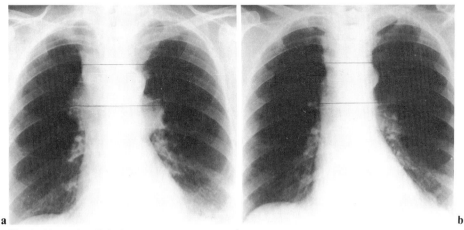

a   b

Fig. 1. Unusual radiological appearance of biopsy-proven squamous cell carcinoma of bronchus **a** before and **b** after combination chemotherapy (cyclophosphamide, adriamycin, bleomycin and vincristine).

rates in the range 24%–28% for cyclophosphamide, adriamycin and *cis*-platinum, while Broder et al. (1982) recently reported a 40% response rate in a small trial using rotating regimes (of mitomycin, vinblastine, procarbazine and methotrexate, vincristine, cyclophosphamide) and involving only patients with adenocarcinoma of bronchus. Overall the current conclusions for primary adenocarcinoma of bronchus are similar to those for squamous cell carcinoma, i.e. current combination chemotherapy regimes can cause tumour regression (Fig. 2) and have a response rate (usually partial only) of 20%–30%; however, the same caveats regarding drug toxicity and no demonstrable survival advantage also apply.

Although large cell anaplastic carcinoma shows no evidence of cellular maturation, this tumour type does share certain similarities with adenocarcinoma in its more peripheral origin, its statistically slightly later dissemination and its pattern of metastases (Matthews et al. 1983). Regrettably, its chemotherapy responsiveness and prognosis are no better than those of adenocarcinoma.

There are a number of prognostic factors in non-small cell carcinoma which may skew survival and possibly response data obtained during chemotherapy studies. The most important factors at diagnosis that will prognosticate for the survival time of a patient with non-small cell carcinoma are: (1) performance status (usually assessed by the scale of Karnofsky et al. 1948), (2) the extent of weight loss and (3) the extent of the disease (and perhaps the sites of any metastases, e.g. brain) (Stanley 1980). With regard to assessing a chemotherapeutic response, a history of prior cytotoxic chemotherapy is important as second remissions are more difficult to achieve. Any analysis of chemotherapeutic effect on survival must take note of the mixture of initial prognostic factors in the patients studied, as the median survival time for patient groups with different initial prognostic loadings varies enormously, as stated above.

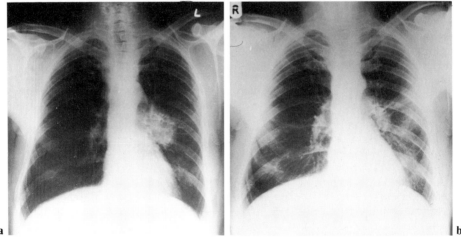

Fig. 2. Radiological appearance of adenocarcinoma of bronchus **a** before and **b** after combination chemotherapy (cyclophosphamide, methotrexate, CCNU and procarbazine).

This brings us lastly to discuss the widespread habit in the oncological literature of plotting survival curves for responders to chemotherapy versus non-responders to chemotherapy, for a single-arm study. Almost invariably, the responders to chemotherapy live longer than non-responders and a positive effect of chemotherapy is deduced. However, more careful analysis will often show that non-responders had a heavier loading of adverse prognostic factors at diagnosis and tolerated chemotherapy worse (perhaps with lower total drug doses administered). Viewed another way, response rate has correlated with performance status. For these reasons, we believe that the interpretation of these curves is very difficult indeed and that to demonstrate a positive effect of chemotherapy on survival a two-arm trial is needed. As stated above, chemotherapy has yet to be proven to prolong life significantly in non-small cell bronchogenic carcinoma, but one early two-arm trial has suggested that it may (Cormier et al. 1982).

The current authors believe that carefully conducted chemotherapy studies are essential for progress in non-squamous carcinoma of bronchus but that routine chemotherapy or 'occasional patient chemotherapy' outside a major study centre has no place in present therapeutics.

Small Cell Bronchial Carcinoma (Oat Cell Carcinoma)

Small cell bronchial carcinoma (SCBC) accounts for 20%–25% of all cases of lung cancer and differs substantially from the other histological types, notably in the more rapid tumour cell proliferation, the early tendency to metastasise and the greater responsiveness to both chemotherapy and radiotherapy. SCBC originates from the amine precursor uptake and decarboxylase (APUD) series of cells (as do bronchial carcinoid tumours), and this lineage is quite distinct from that of other primary lung tumours. The important impact of chemotherapy upon the survival of patients with SCBC justifies the separate consideration of this group of patients.

The historical surgical data demonstrated that although surgical resection of the primary tumour was possible in perhaps one-third of patients who appeared to have localised disease with a 25% 5-year survival rate (Shore and Paneth 1980), nevertheless the 5-year survival figures in another series (Mountain 1978) were very low — less than 5%; the recent reawakened interest in surgical resection of the primary tumour in no way contradicts these early data but rather suggests a debulking role for surgery in occasional patients with early stage disease (Meyer et al. 1979). Similarly, radiotherapy to the primary tumour was effective in local control — in one series one-third of primary tumours irradiated were found at autopsy to be eradicated (Rissanen et al. 1968) — but the patients generally died of distant metastases (Bersagel et al. 1972; Fox and Scadding 1973; Laing et al. 1975). The commonest sites for distant metastases from SCBC are: liver (62%), abdominal lymph nodes (57%), adrenals (39%), bone (38%), brain (37%), pancreas (31%) and kidneys (22%) (Hansen 1974).

Although TNM staging classification exists for SCBC, it has not proved more useful than the Veterans' Administration Lung Cancer Study Group's simple classification into patients with 'limited disease' (confined to one hemithorax including ipsilateral scalene nodes) and those with 'extensive disease' (all the others). Approximately one-third of patients will be staged as limited disease at presentation and two-thirds as extensive disease. The staging investigations are: clinical examination, chest X-ray, liver function tests and technetium bone scan (liver ultrasound and bone marrow sampling are optional).

In untreated SCBC, the natural history is shorter for extensive disease (median survival 5–7 weeks, very few patients surviving longer than 5 months) than for limited disease (median survival 12–18 weeks, most patients being dead by 9 months) (Green et al. 1969). This staging system has been retained, although it is now possible to pick out prognostic subgroups within each category, e.g. extensive disease patients who are 'extensive' only because of a single hot spot on bone scanning or a contralateral supraclavicular node or microscopic evidence of bone marrow infiltration. These patients will do better than average with modern therapy, whereas those with liver or brain metastases tend to fare worse. Thus stage and location of metastases are both important pretreatment prognostic factors, and presentation performance status and age are also determinants of survival (Maurer and Pajak 1981). A history of previous cytotoxic drug therapy for the tumour is an adverse feature for a chemotherapy response, whatever the regime. The WHO histological subtypes of SCBC are not useful prognostic indicators for chemotherapeutic response or survival (Matthews et al. 1980).

Modern chemotherapeutic regimes have led to a four- to fivefold increase in median survival for SCBC patients and a significant proportion (perhaps 10%–15%) of long-term disease-free survivors — almost all from the limited disease group of patients. At first, single agent activity was assessed and there are a considerable number of drugs with a 30% response rate or higher (e.g VP16, vincristine and other vincas, cyclophosphamide and other mustards, adriamycin, methotrexate, CCNU). *Cis*-platinum and procarbazine are only slightly less active. There is no doubt that single agents can be highly effective in causing tumour regression (Fig. 3), and in one controlled clinical study cyclophosphamide was found to be statistically superior to placebo in prolonging survival (Roswit et al. 1968). Combining several (usually up to three or four) drugs from this list into an intermittent adminstration scheme has led to greater success.

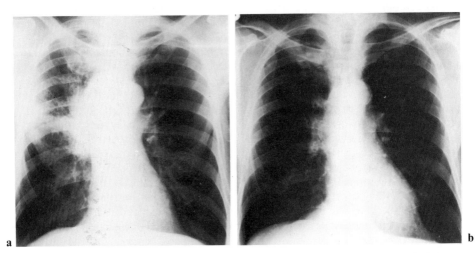

Fig. 3. Radiological appearance of small cell bronchial carcinoma **a** before and **b** after single agent chemotherapy (cyclophosphamide 1.5 g/m² q 3/52).

   Chemotherapy has tended to fall into two types of triple drug regime. In the cyclophosphamide, methotrexate, CCNU (CMC) type of regime explored by the National Cancer Institute workers and Medical Research Council, cyclophosphamide in once 3 weekly intravenous bolus doses of 500–1000 mg/m^2 has been combined with methotrexate (either twice weekly e.g. 15 mg/m^2 or once 3 weekly, e.g. 50 mg/m^2 without folinate rescue) and CCNU (e.g. 50 mg/m^2 once 6 weekly). In the other popular regime (CAV), cyclophosphamide in the previous dose range has been combined with adriamycin (e.g. 40–50 mg/m^2 once 3 weekly) and vincristine (e.g. 2 mg once 3 weekly). In the last few years, with the realisation of the high single agent activity of VP16 (more than 40% responses), this drug has been incorporated into variant schedules of CMC and CAV. There are now multiple publications on this type of therapy that demonstrate a 75%–85% response rate with a complete response rate of 50%–67% for limited disease patients and a 20%–25% complete response rate for extensive disease patients (Figs. 4–6). The

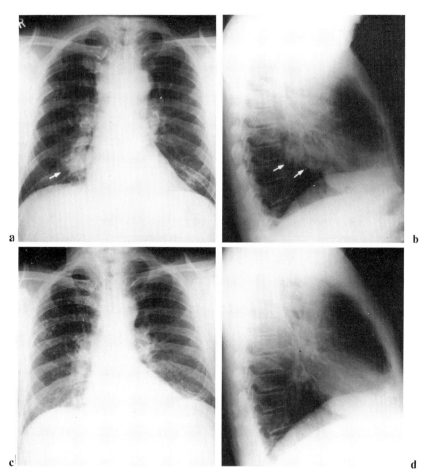

Fig. 4. Radiological appearance of small cell bronchial carcinoma **a, b** before and **c, d** after combination chemotherapy (cyclophosphamide, methotrexate and CCNU)

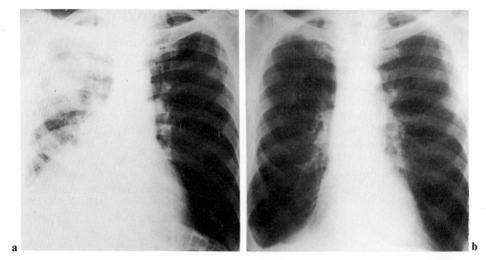

a   b

Fig. 5. Radiological appearance of extensive consolidation and atelectasis throughout the right lung caused by a proximal endobronchial small cell bronchial carcinoma, **a** before and **b** after combination chemotherapy (cyclophosphamide, methotrexate and CCNU).

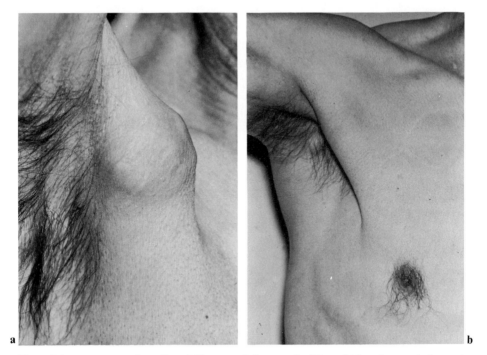

a   b

Fig. 6. Subcutaneous, anterior axillary fold metastasis from small cell bronchial carcinoma **a** before and **b** after combination chemotherapy (cyclophosphamide, methotrexate and CCNU). Note also the greater resilience of axillary and chest hair to the depilatory effects of CMC chemotherapy.

median survival of limited disease patients with these therapies is 12–15 months, with a significant minority of long-term disease-free survivors; the median survival of extensive disease patients is 8–10 months (Greco and Oldham 1979; Hansen 1980, 1982). The toxicity of these therapies includes variable degrees of nausea to vomiting over the 24–48 h following each chemotherapy administration, depilation and moderately severe temporary pancytopenia (e.g. neutrophil nadir 500–1000/mm³ at days 8–12) as well as specific drug side-effects. During the neutropenic period, fevers, chills or any clinical features suggesting infection require serious attention and perhaps hospital admission; approximately 1%–4% of patients suffer septicaemia during such chemotherapy. Unlike the situation in non-small cell bronchial cancer, the toxicity of drug therapy may be more than outweighed by the improvement in general health and well-being that accompanies tumour regression.

The cytotoxic chemotherapy may induce cytological changes in the non-malignant bronchial epithelium which may confuse cytological interpretation at follow-up of these patients (Fig. 7) (Gazdar et al. 1979; Plowman and Stovin 1980).

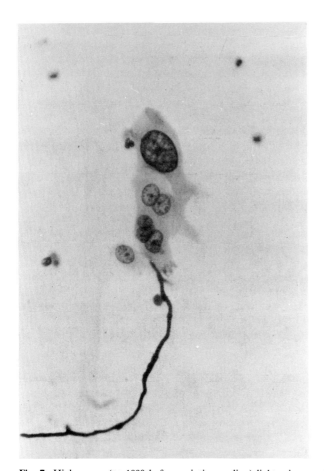

Fig. 7. High-power (× 1000 before printing scaling) light microscopic photograph of non-malignant bronchial epithelial cells following combination chemotherapy (cyclophosphamide, methotrexate and CCNU). Note the 'megaloblastic' nuclear changes probably related to the methotrexate.

The majority of these responding patients will relapse and die of their disease within 18 months, responding poorly to further chemotherapy; this aspect of SCBC is of the greatest interest and is being studied at present. The chest or primary site is the first site of relapse in at least one-third of these patients, and this has led many authors to sandwich primary site radiotherapy into the chemotherapy scheme. The optimum timing of these two modalities has yet to be established. Large masses may respond more effectively to chemotherapy if initially debulked by radiotherapy or if radiotherapy is used concurrently. Alternatively, in some series chemotherapy has been administered prior to irradiation so that both the local lesion and the widespread disease are treated simultaneously. Improvement in local tumour control and a small increase in survival has been reported comparing combined chemotherapy and radiotherapy with chemotherapy alone (Salazar and Creech 1980). However, in 1981 the Medical Research Council Lung Cancer Working Party reported on its results comparing the effectiveness of radiotherapy alone and radiotherapy followed by three drug chemotherapy in the treatment of limited extent small cell carcinoma. The results showed an improved survival at 1 year for the combined treatment but disappointingly little difference in results at 3 years.

Combined modality treatment does result in an increase in complications and toxicity. The action of bleomycin, cyclophosphamide and methotrexate on lung tissue may result in lung fibrosis and this effect is potentiated by radiotherapy; in addition there is an increase in the cardiac toxicity of adriamycin and cyclophosphamide if the mediastinum is irradiated. As a result of combined modality treatment, toxicity to the bone marrow is increased and skin and mucosal reactions are enhanced. A recall of an epithelial reaction due to irradiation may be produced many years later by the administration of chemotherapy. These findings have led to the concept of the Dose Effect Factor and in some series the radiotherapy dose has been reduced when given in combination with chemotherapy. To date the survival of these patients has been short and the possible development of a second malignancy due to combination treatment not a problem..

The brain is a well-known sanctuary site where tumour cells remain uninfluenced by systemic chemotherapy; in acute lymphoblastic leukaemia, prophylactic cranial radiation has decreased the brain relapse rate. In an attempt to prevent SCBC brain relapse, prophylactic cranial radiotherapy has been given to completely responding limited disease patients; while there has been a demonstrable reduction in the brain relapse rate, in most series no improvement in overall survival has been obtained (Hansen 1980, 1982). Unlike acute leukaemia, the control of the SCBC systemic disease is less excellent/durable, and as isolated CNS relapse is uncommon, our current policy is not to administer prophylactic cranial radiotherapy.

Other attempts to improve survival have been directed towards different chemotherapy strategies. The NCI workers examined the effects of intensifying the CMC induction regime, escalating the dose of cyclophosphamide to $1.5-2$ g/m^2 (Cohen et al. 1977, 1979; Vogl and Mehta 1982). These studies demonstrate at best slight improvements in remission rates, and these minor improvements were more than counterbalanced by the extra toxicity. In another study in which methotrexate was administered in high dosage (6 g/m^2 bolus with later folinate rescue) on a CAV-based chemotherapy induction scheme, the high dosage group of patients had neither a higher remission rate nor an improved survival but a more severe rate of mucositis (Hande et al. 1982). Megadosage chemotherapy with autologous bone marrow transplantation as a rescue procedure has been explored but at present does not look a promising approach (Farha et al. 1981).

In general, using moderately aggressive triple drug chemotherapy (e.g. CMC with cyclophosphamide up to 1000 mg/m^2), one would expect to see a good tumour response in the first 6–8 weeks (i.e. after two chemotherapy courses), and if this is not apparent then a change to another regime (e.g from CMC to VP16 – adriamycin – vincristine) has been demonstrated to increase the likelihood of complete response. The major benefit from drug treatment of SCBC in terms of survival occurs in the group of patients achieving complete clinical remission (Cohen et al. 1979), and thus the importance of effective induction chemotherapy is well recognised by all workers and has provided the spur to intensify or alternate drug regimens in the early treatment period. Some workers have, from the outset of treatment, alternated 'non-cross resistant' drug regimes in an attempt to increase the complete remission and survival rates (Cohen et al. 1979; Dombernowsky et al. 1979; Friedman and Carter 1980). Disappointingly, this approach has not achieved its goal, although there is a suggestion of improved results in extensive disease patients.

The other aspect of chemotherapy which is currently of great interest relates to the length of therapy. Although this issue is still full of uncertainties and will change as chemotherapy improves, some studies have suggested that short duration (4–6 months) chemotherapy gives results equal to those obtained by chemotherapy for 1–2 years (Johnson et al. 1978; Maurer et al. 1980). However, this view is not generally accepted at this time.

In conclusion, SCBC is a highly chemoresponsive tumour and the median survival can be considerably prolonged in the majority of patients by combination cytotoxic chemotherapy, which also improves the quality of life in the majority of responding patients. However, the usual pattern of behaviour is for the tumour to relapse again within 12–18 months and for this relapse to be fatal. Despite many attempts to overcome this tendency to relapse, no satisfactory strategy has yet been devised and the number of long-term disease-free survivors remains small.

Conclusion

Historically the results of treatment for bronchial carcinoma were dismal and this led many physicians to adopt a nihilistic approach to therapy. Currently, although chemotherapy has not produced a major breakthrough in terms of cure, nevertheless recent studies are encouraging in that such therapy has prolonged the median survival in patients with small cell carcinoma and provided useful palliation. Unfortunately the results for non-small cell carcinoma are less promising, but combined chemotherapy can result in tumour regression.

We feel that further progress with this modality lies in the continuance of carefully conducted chemotherapy studies in the major oncological centres, which we believe will increase our knowledge and understanding of this distressing disease.

Acknowledgement. We acknowledge with thanks the help of Miss F. Baptiste in the preparation of this manuscript.

References

Aisner J, Hansen H (1981) Current status of chemotherapy for non-small cell lung cancer. Cancer Treat Rep 65:979–986

Bersagel D, Jenkin R, Pringle J, White D, Fetterley J, Klassen D, McDermott R (1972) Lung cancer: Clinical trial of radiotherapy alone versus radiotherapy plus cyclophosphamide. Cancer 30:621–627

British Medical Journal (1971) Study of cytotoxic chemotherapy as an adjuvant to surgery in carcinoma of the bronchus. Br Med J II: 421–428

Broder LE, Policzer S, Meyerson WH et al. (1982) A phase II clinical trial testing the sequential use of two four drug chemotherapy regimes for bronchogenic adenocarcinoma. The World Conference on Lung Cancer, Tokyo, Japan, 17–20, May 1982, p 184 [Abstr 263]

Cohen MH, Creaven PJ, Fossieck BE, Broder LE, Selawry OS, Johnston AV, Williams CL, Minna JD (1977) Intensive chemotherapy of small cell bronchogenic carcinoma. Cancer Treat Rep 61:349–354

Cohen MH, Ihde DC, Bunn PA, Fossieck BE, Matthews MS, Chackney SE, Johnston-Early A, Makuch R, Minna JD (1979): Cyclic alternating chemotherapy for small cell bronchogenic carcinoma. Cancer Treat Rep 63:163–170

Cormier Y, Bergeron D, La Forge J et al. (1982) Benefits of polychemotherapy in advanced non-small cell bronchogenic cancer. Cancer 50:845–849

Dombernowsky P. Hansen HH, Sorenson S, Osterlind K (1979) Sequential versus non-sequential combination chemotherapy using 6 drugs in advanced small cell carcinoma. A comparative trial including 146 patients. Proc Am Soc Clin Oncol 20:277

Eagan RT, Ingle JN, Frytak S et al. (1977) Platinum based polychemotherapy versus dianhydrogalactitiol in advanced non-small cell lung cancer. Cancer Treat Rep 61:1399–1445

Evans WK, Feld R. De Boer G et al. (1981) Cyclophosphamide, doxorubicin and cis-platinum in the treatment of non-small cell bronchogenic carcinoma. Cancer Treat Rep 65:947–954

Farha P, Spitzer G, Valdivieso M et al. (1981) Treatment of small cell bronchial carcinoma (SCBC) with high dose chemotherapy (CT) and autologous bone marrow transplantation (ABMT). Proc Am Soc Clin Oncol [Abstr. C637, p 496]

Fox W, Scadding JG (1973) Medical Research Council comparative trial of surgery and radiotherapy for primary treatment of small cell or oat cell carcinoma of bronchus: Ten year follow up. Lancet II: 63–65

Friedman M, Carter S (1980) Results of the Northern California Oncology Group

Gazdar AF, Cohen MH, Ihde DC, Minna JD, Matthews MJ (1979) Bronchial epithelial changes in association with small cell carcinoma of the lung. In: Muggia F, Rozencweig M (eds) Lung cancer, progress in therapeutic research. Raven Press, New York, pp 167–174

Gralla RJ, Casper FS, Kelsen DP et al. (1982) Trials in non-small cell cancer with regimens combining vindesine and cis-platinum. The World Conference on Lung Cancer, Tokyo, Japan, 17–20 May 1982, p 188 [Abstr. 271]

Greco FA, Oldham RK (1979) Current concepts in cancer: small cell lung cancer. N Engl J Med 301:355–358

Green RA, Humphrey E. Close H et al. (1969) Alkylating agents in bronchogenic carcinoma. Am J Med 46:516–524

Hande KR, Oldham RK, Fer MF, Richardson RL, Greco FA (1982) Randomized study of high dose versus low dose methotrexate in the treatment of extensive small cell lung cancer. Am J Med 73:413–419

Hansen HH (1974) Bone metastases in lung cancer. Munksgarrd, Copenhagen

Hansen HH (1980) Management of small cell anaplastic carcinoma. Proceedings of the 11$_{nd}$ World Congress on Lung Cancer (Copenhagen 1980). Excerpta Medica, Amsterdam Oxford Princeton, pp 113–132

Hansen HH: Management of small cell anaplastic carcinoma 1980-1982. Proceedings of the 111$_{rd}$ World Congress on Lung Cancer (Tokyo 1982), pp 31–54

Itri LM, Gralla RJ, Kelsen DP et al. (1983) Cis-platinum, vindesine and bleomycin (CVB) combination chemotherapy of advanced non-small cell lung cancer. Cancer 51:1050–1055

Johnson RE, Brereton HD, Kent CH (1978) 'Total' therapy for small cell carcinoma of the lung. Ann Thorac Surg 25:509–515

Jones HD, Bleehen NM, Grant RM et al. (1983) Scheduled and unscheduled combination chemotherapy in the treatment of squamous cell lung cancer. (Cyclophosphamide, adriamycin, vincristine and bleomycin, with and without cis-platinum). Anti-Cancer Res 3:235–238

Karnofsky DA, Abelmann WH, Craven LF et al. (1948) The use of nitrogen mustards in the palliative treatment of cancer. Cancer 1:634–656

Kelsen DP, Gralla RJ, Stoopler M et al. (1982) Cisplatin, doxorubicin, cyclophosphamide and vindesine combination chemotherapy for non-small cell lung cancer. Cancer Treat Rep 66:247–251

Knost SA, Greco FA, Hande, KR et al (1981) Cyclophosphamide, doxorubicin and cis-platin in the treatment of advanced non-small cell cancer. Cancer Treat Rep 65: 941–945

Laing AH, Berry RJ, Newman CR, Smith P (1975) Treatment of small cell carcinoma of bronchus. Lancet I:129–132

Livingston RB, Fee WH, Einhorn LH et al. (1976) Bacon (bloemycin, adriamycin, CCNU, oncovin and nitrogen mustard) in squamous lung cancer. Experience in fifty patients. Cancer 37:1237–1242

Livingston RB, Heilbrun L, Lehane D et al. (1977) Comparative trial of combination chemotherapy in extensive squamous carcinoma of lung: A South West Oncology Group Study. Cancer Treat Rep 61:1623–1629

Matthews MJ, Rozencweig M, Staquet MJ, Minna JD, Muggia FM (1980) Long term survivors with small cell carcinoma of the lung. Eur J Cancer 16:527–831

Matthews MJ, Mackay B, Likeman J (1983) The pathology of non-small cell carcinoma of lung. Semin Oncol 10:34–55

Maurer LH, Pajak TF (1981) Prognostic factors in small cell carcinoma of the lung: A cancer and leukaemia group B Study. Cancer Treat Rep 65:767–774

Maurer LH, Tulloh M, Weiss RB, Blom J, Leone L, Glidewell O, Pajak TF (1980 A randomised combined modality trial in small cell carcinoma of the lung: Comparison of combination chemotherapy–radiotherapy versus cyclophosphamide radiotherapy, effects of maintenance chemotherapy and prophylactic whole brain irradiation. Cancer 45:30–39.

Meyer JA, Comiz RL, Ginsberg SJ, Ikins PM, Burke WA, Parker FB (1979) Selective surgical resection in small cell carcinoma of the lung. J Thorac Cardiovasc Surg 77:243–248

Mountain CF (1978) Clinical biology of small cell carcinoma: Relationship to surgical therapy. Semin Oncol 5:272

Plowman PN, Stovin PGI (1980) Chemotherapy induced bronchial epithelial changes. Proceedings of the IInd World Congress on Lung Cancer (Copenhagen 1980). Excerpta Medica, Amsterdam, Oxford, Princeton p 164

Rissanen PM, Tikka V, Holsti LR (1968). Autopsy findings in lung cancer treated with megavoltage radiotherapy. Acta Radiol Ther Phys Biol 7:433–442

Roswit B, Patno ME, Rapp R (1968) The survival of patients with inoperable lung cancer: A large scale randomised study of radiation therapy versus placebo. Radiology 90:688–697

Salazar OM, Creech RH (1980) 'The state of art' toward defining the role of radiation therapy in the management of small cell bronchogenic carcinoma. Int J Radiat Oncol Biol Phys 6:1103–1117

Shore DB, Paneth M (1980) Survival after resection of small cell carcinoma of the bronchus. Thorax 35:819–822

Stanley KE (1980) Prognostic factors for survival in patients with inoperable lung cancer. J Natl Cancer Inst 65:25–32

Trovo MG, Tirelli U, De Paoli A et al. (1982) Combined radiotherapy and chemotherapy with cyclophosphamide, adriamycin, methotrexate, procarbazine (CAMP) in 64 consecutive patients with epidermoid bronchogenic carcinoma. Int J Radiat Oncol Biol Phys 8:1051–1054

Vogl SE, Mehta C (1982) High dose cyclophosphamide in the induction chemotherapy of small cell lung cancer — minor improvements in the rate of remission and in survival. Proceedings of the IIIʳᵈ World Congress on Lung Cancer (Tokyo 1982), p 168 [Abstr. 234]

Chapter 18

Photoradiation for Bronchial Carcinoma

Philip Hugh-Jones

Introduction

Bronchial carcinoma is at present killing six times as many men and women in Britain as are killed on the roads, and in the 55–65 year age group, in which it is most prevalent, no less than 16 times as many (Office of Population Census and Surveys 1979). Although surgery can be curative for a fortunate few who get the disease (mostly those with peripheral squamous cell carcinoma or adenocarcinoma), about 93% of sufferers eventually die from their disease. Much of this toll is preventable simply by ceasing to smoke cigarettes (Royal College of Physicians 1983) but even if that habit were to cease forthwith, which is inconceivable, lung cancer would affect huge numbers of people for the next 20–30 years (Hugh-Jones 1978). Moreover, if young women continue to smoke cigarettes at their present rate, it is predicted in the USA that bronchial cancer will outstrip breast cancer as the commonest cancer among young women by the end of the year 1984. Thus any new treatment for the condition, whether it be merely palliative for the distressing symptoms, or more hopefully, curative, deserves careful assessment and consideration (Grant 1982), especially if that treatment is relatively innocuous to the patient. Such treatment has now come about in the form of photoradiation therapy.

Basis of Photoradiation Treatment

Effect of Light on Cells

The non-ionising radiation which we call 'light', partly visible to the human eye and partly invisible in the ultraviolet (UV) or infra-red (Fig. 1), is relatively non-specific in its effects on cancer or other rapidly growing cells and, in that respect, is unlike the ionising radiation of X-rays, which have a much shorter wavelength. However, ordinary light can destroy or modify any cell by thermal damage or by photochemical activation or destruction of critical enzyme systems within the cell, provided the light energy is absorbed. Ultraviolet light more readily kills cells than visible light, a fact used by bacteriologists for sterilisation, but this is not due to the properties of the light itself, though photons of UV light carry more energy than those of visible light. It is rather because of the properties of light-absorbing

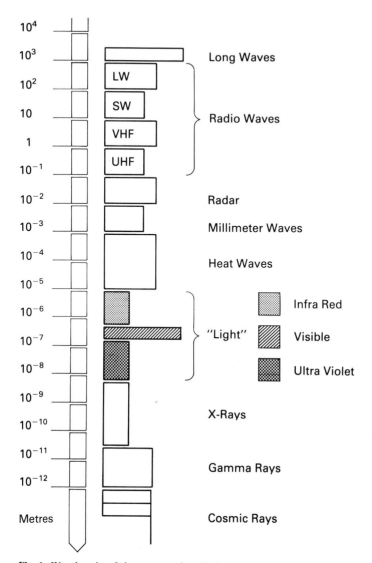

Fig. 1. Wavelengths of electromagnetic radiation.

molecules whose photochemical alteration leads to inactivation of the biological enzyme system (Smith 1979). Thus all wavelengths of light (UV through invisible to infra-red) are active in initiating photochemical reactions provided they are absorbed onto the appropriate molecular system.

Endoscopic Laser Delivery System

It is the almost simultaneous invention of the fibre-optic delivery system and of laser light which has suddenly made it possible to apply endoscopically a light beam to tumour masses with accuracy. There is nothing 'magic' about a laser except that the laser's high intensity, coherence and monochromaticity make it a unique source of photons so that under selected conditions molecular events and subsequent photobiological responses are quantitatively and qualitatively different from those caused by conventional light sources (Parrish 1979). In other words, the use of an endoscopic fibre-optic system with laser light allows a light beam to be accurately applied with the following advantages:

1. A specific wavelength of monochromatic light can be directed onto tumours otherwise reached only by surgery.
2. Precise measurement of power density and time of application is possible.
3. One can apply a uniform field over an area which can be varied by de-focussing.
4. The treatment can be repeated indefinitely, unlike radiotherapy.

If we now add to this spatial selectivity the possibility of photo-activation of radiosensitisers – substances which are differentially retained in malignant tissue and which can be rendered cytotoxic by photo-activation from the appropriate laser – it is obvious we are dealing with a potentially powerful tool for cancer treatment.

In some ways the interest in the use of lasers in medicine and surgery has been bedevilled by the 'James Bond' image of burning. It is true that the uniquely high photon density and possibility of very short pulses of high peak power make it possible to induce photobiological effects from large energy doses locally, which can vaporise cells, and that these effects can be achieved in very short times whereas minutes or hours of light irradiation would be required from other sources. But the coherent property of lasers, with their associated collimated beam and monochromaticity, in addition means that the utterly different, slow photochemical effects can also be achieved as well as the more obvious burning (photoresection). Thus, in summary, the endoscopic use of laser light can be made relatively tumour-specific either (a) spatially, by the accurate direction of the laser, and/or (b) chemically, by the photo-activation to toxicity of a systemically given photo-sensitiser which is differentially retained in the tumour.

Use of Lasers

Principles of Laser Action

Most members of the public know that the term LASER is an acronym for Light Amplification by the Stimulated Emission of Radiation and that these devices produce intense beams of light. The possibility of laser action was postulated by Einstein at the beginning of this century but only achieved in 1960 when Maiman of the Hughes Research Laboratory constructed the first ruby laser (Parsons 1982). Since that time many different substances have been made to 'lase' – using solids, liquids and gases – and these different lasers each have a different wavelength and have revolutionised the use of light in medical research, diagnosis and treatment. Indeed, over the last 5–10 years, the explosion of knowledge about photoradiation in medicine has been almost overwhelming.

Light acts both as a wave and as a particle, or parcel of energy called a 'photon'. The energy of a photon is defined by the equation:

$$E = HV \qquad (1)$$

where V is the frequency of the radiation while H is Plank's Universal Constant. Photons of energy are produced whenever an electron or an atom changes its state of energy and releases enough of that energy to satisfy Eq (1). But unlike the gradual production of heat, an atom produces energy only in discrete 'quanta' or jumps so that:

$$E2 - E1 = HV \qquad (2)$$

where $E2$ is energy at the higher level, whilst $E1$ is energy at the lower level. Since the quantum jumps occur only between certain energy levels, V can only take on certain fixed values and the spectrum of energy released is discrete and monochromatic.

All lasers have a mechanism for producing a 'population inversion' which implies the electrical and/or optical method of pumping atoms to higher energy states ($E2$) (by moving electrons in the outer ring further from the nucleus) and arranging a rapid decay to a lower, but still excited, state ($E1$). If then the decay back to the ground state ($E0$) is somewhat slower than the rate of arrival of particles at the higher state, an accumulation takes place at that level. The other requirement, before the device operates as a laser, is that there is some form of optical feedback. Not all the emitted photons can be removed, but a significant fraction must remain to cause more stimulated emissions of other photons. This is achieved by having two suitable mirrors confining the lasing process, the one reflecting 100% at the desired wavelength, but the other transmitting a fraction of the radiation which falls on it; the latter is the output mirror of the laser to be used (Fig. 2). The laser beam thus produced is collimated (parallel), coherent (predictable and constant because the photons emitted by the stimulating process are in phase with the stimulated photons and hence the coherent output) and almost monochromatic (of single wavelength).

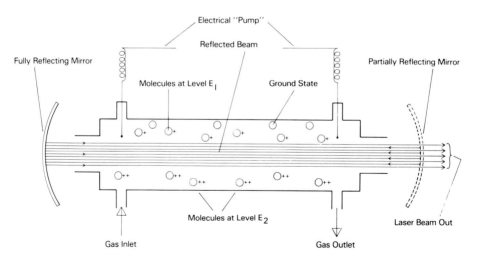

Fig. 2. Diagram of mode of laser action as exemplified by a gas laser.

The biological effect of laser radiation is particular to the wavelength of the light; hence different lasers having different wavelengths are used for different therapeutic purposes. However, dye lasers, produced by pumping a dye (e.g. rhodamine dye) by a given laser (e.g. an argon laser), can be 'tuned' to give light of different wavelengths.

The power output of the laser beam is measured in watts or milliwatts. The beam is then more or less focussed onto the tumour, where its effects depend only only on the wavelength of the particular laser light, but also on the power density measured in watts per cm². Of course, the biological effect also depends on the total energy supplied by the beam, which is a function of time multiplied by power output and is measured in joules. It is this ability both to control time of application and to focus the beam onto a given area (and hence change power density) which makes the laser such a precise tool for medical and surgical use.

Lasers can either produce pulses of light (e.g. when a ruby rod is made to lase, the photons available reach a peak and leave the one mirror during a pulse of abut 0.1 to a few seconds) or produce a continuous beam, which can be used for a precisely controlled time, as with a carbon dioxide gas laser for example. Helium–neon lasers are of low power and used endobronchoscopically to act as light guides for the invisible CO_2 or Nd–YAG (neodymium–yttrium aluminium garnate) laser. The helium–neon guide is exactly co-linear with the visible beam so that it marks the spot which will be treated when the invisible beam is switched on. Dye lasers are used for relatively low-power photochemical effects from the photo-activation of radiosensisiters, in particular haematoporphyrin derivative (HpD).

Effects of Lasers on Living Tissues

When light falls on tissue, four things can happen. It can be reflected from the surface, transmitted through the tissue, scattered within the tissue, or absorbed. The relative importance of each depends both on the tissue and on the light (Bown 1982). The effect of a laser beam on tissue depends on (a) the type of target tissue (how it absorbs or scatters the light), (b) the power density (the power output of the laser in relation to the spot size of the focus beam), (c) the duration of application (the power multiplied by the duration determines the total energy supply) and (d) the wavelength of the laser light.

At very low light intensity cells can be stimulated (e.g. hair growth may increase and healing of wounds may be hastened). As the light intensity is increased, it first inhibits the cells and then kills them. Still at relatively low energy levels coagulation of proteins takes place so that bleeding is stopped (especially, for example, when the blue–green light of an argon laser is absorbed onto the red haemoglobin). Then, if the energy is increased still further, destruction of tissue occurs and, finally, vapourisation. This last effect is the principle of the 'light-knife', which is the main use of a CO_2 laser. Except at very low light intensity most of the effects are thermal (Table 1).

Apart from the intensity of the light, its wavelength is of crucial importance in relation to its biological effects. Each laser operates at a specific wavelength so that to change from one wavelength to another entails the use of a different laser, except in the case of dye lasers where the laser can be tuned or the dye can be changed.

Table 1. Heating effects of lasers on living tissue

Temperature (°C)	Effect
44	Photochemical effects
	Photoactivation of dyes
44	Normal cells survive,
	some tumour cells killed
60	Cell death
70–80	Collagen denaturation
100	Loss of water
250	Carbonisation
350	Vapourisation

Types of Laser Used for the Treatment of Bronchial Carcinoma

The different lasers which have been used for the phototherapy of bronchial carcinoma are shown in Table 2. Because of their different wavelengths, each has a different effect on biological tissue. This is illustrated in Fig. 3, where it is seen that the CO_2 laser causes local tissue vapourisation but very little heating of the surrounding tissue. The latter increases with an argon laser, and is at its maximum with

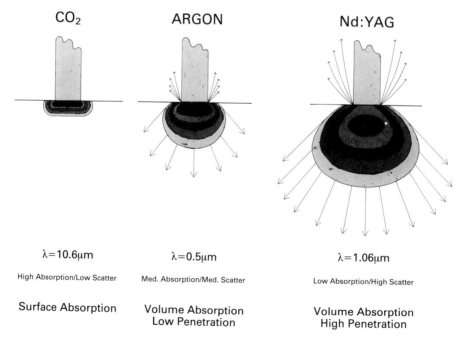

CO₂   ARGON   Nd:YAG

$\lambda = 10.6\mu m$ $\lambda = 0.5\mu m$ $\lambda = 1.06\mu m$

High Absorption/Low Scatter   Med. Absorption/Med. Scatter   Low Absorption/High Scatter

Surface Absorption   Volume Absorption   Volume Absorption
                       Low Penetration   High Penetration

Fig. 3. The effect of three different lasers on biological tissue. (Diagram supplied by Barr and Stroud Ltd.)

Table 2. Lasers of different wavelength used for treatment of bronchial carcinoma

Type of laser	Wavelength	Use
1. Carbon dioxide (CO_2)	10 600 nm (invisible — far infra-red)	Cutting
2. Neodymium–yttrium aluminium garnate (Nd–YAG)	1060 nm (invisible — near infra-red)	Deep heating
3. Argon-ion (A)	488 and 514 nm (visible — blue–green)	Heating — fluorescence
4. Krypton-ion (KR)	405 nm (visible — red)	Fluorescence
5. Helium–neon (He–Ne)	633 nm (visible — red)	Low-power guide for invisible lasers
6. Dye	Variable (rhodamine dye: 630 nm visible — red)	Photochemical activation
7. Gold vapour	628 nm (visible — red)	Photochemical activation

the Nd–YAG laser. Carbon dioxide, argon-ion and Nd–YAG are the lasers most commonly used for their thermal effect. With all these three lasers if sufficient energy is absorbed at the surface, the superficial cells are destroyed and further application bores a hole in the tissues. But the difference lies in the volume of tissue heated before burning destruction of the superficial cells occurs. The CO_2 laser is mainly absorbed by water in the tissue and the cell damage below the surface is only about 0.1 mm. The blue–green argon laser is absorbed into the red haemoglobin so that at least 1 mm is heated by the start of superficial burning. With the Nd–YAG laser the radiation is more deeply absorbed and scattered so that up to 10 mm of tissue may be affected (Fig. 3).

It is the very localised effect of the CO_2 laser which makes it a 'light-knife', for only the cells immediately under the beam are destroyed with virtually no damage to adjacent cells. The argon laser could be used for this purpose, but the Nd–YAG would be quite unsuitable. By contrast, the argon and the Nd–YAG lasers shrink tissue by heating larger volumes and hence can be used better to control bleeding. The volume heated by a CO_2 laser is so small that it is of little use for this purpose.

The Carbon Dioxide Laser

As yet there is no light guide which will transmit a CO_2 laser, so the beam must be used directly. This is achieved (a) by an articulated arm with a hand-piece for using the laser as a surgical knife at thoracotomy or (b) by fitting the laser head to a laryngoscope or a bronchoscope and directing the beam precisely with a joystick control via a long focal length (400 mm for the larynx) dissecting microscope either onto the larynx itself or down the bronchoscope (Fig. 4).

The beam emitted by the CO_2 laser is in the invisible far infra-red (10.6nm), but there is a helium–neon light guide. An optical resonator ensures maximum focussing capability with minimum beam divergence and peak power at the beam centre. In this way the beam-tissue interaction is highly localised; the absorbed energy raises the temperatuire of water content of the tissue to boiling point so that the manufac-

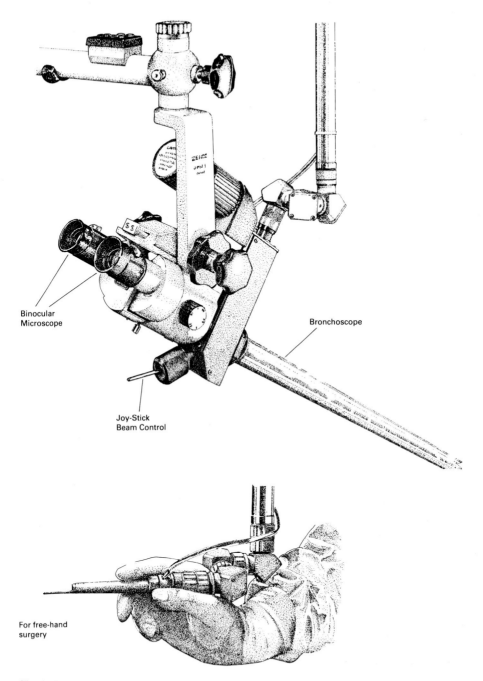

Binocular
Microscope

Bronchoscope

Joy-Stick
Beam Control

For free-hand
surgery

Fig. 4. Carbon dioxide laser for bronchoscopic work or free-hand surgery. (Reproduced by courtesy of Sharplan CO_2 lasers)

turers claim that a beam of constant power across 1 mm^2 will vapourise to a depth of 1 mm with a 20-Watt pulse of 0.1/s. In the thin layer of cauterised tissue surrounding the vapourised zone, the small vessels of the lymphatics are sealed, resulting in a relatively bloodless cut, although this laser is not as haemostatic as the argon or Nd–YAG laser. The CO_2 has been used for laparoscopy (Tadir et al. 1982) and for de-bulking large tumour masses (Nogoret et al. 1982). Little swelling or erythema of adjacent tissue and little postoperative pain is claimed, with good wound healing (Das Gupta et al. 1982; Carruth 1982). The minimal tissue damage has made it useful as a surgical knife, for example in mastectomy, and Kaplan (1982) and Christensen (1982) claim that at thoracotomy there is less bleeding and fewer postoperative drains are needed.

The accuracy of remote control of the CO_2 laser beam provides easy surgical access to lesions in deep and narrow cavities such as the upper air or food passages, where malignancies can be resected with reduction of intra- and postoperative bleeding and absence of postoperative oedema and pain. Thus the CO_2 laser is excellent for fine resection of laryngeal tumours (Freche 1982) and has been used for the palliative resection of advanced bronchogenic carcinoma since it is now possible to remove obstruction of the trachea or main bronchus by advanced cancer without opening the thorax (Kullman 1980). A full account of the use of the CO_2 laser is given in the book edited by Andrews and Polanyi (1982).

The Nd–YAG Laser

Bronchoscopic Use

The Nd–YAG laser, like the CO_2 laser, is in the invisible infra-red and hence it also needs the helium–neon light guide, but, unlike the former, it can be transmitted down a quartz fibre inserted through the biopsy channel of a fibre-optic broncho-scope. The beam emerging from the fibre-guide diverges and can be focussed to give a larger or smaller area, according to the distance from the end of the light guide to the tumour mass (Fig. 5). Care has to be taken with anaesthesia to ensure that burning does not take place, so the laser is either used with transnasal bronchoscopy under a local anaesthetic, or via a rigid bronchoscope but by ventilation with air or, at the most, 50% oxygen. The operator's eyes must be protected and, if the laser is removed from the bronchoscope without switching off, the eyes of all those in the operating theatre must be protected.

Animal Experiments

By using intradermally transplanted non-immunising carcinomata of mice measur-ing 3–55.5 mm in diameter, Gardner et al. (1982) were able to test the effects of different times of exposure and energy densities on this highly malignant tumour. A clear dose–response relationship was found. Below a given dose threshold (2 J per mm^2) the tumours continued to grow at the same rate as the controls, though the effect of the radiation could be seen histologically. Above this threshold the tumour

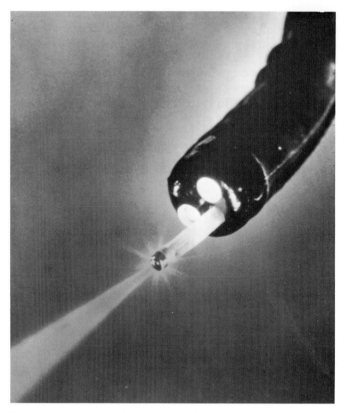

Fig. 5. End of fibre-optic bronchoscope, showing He-Ne laser beam diverging from end of fibre and acting as a high-guide for invisible Nd-YAG beam (Photograph supplied by Barr and Stroud Ltd.)

disappeared but by 10–14 days started to re-grow. At the highest dose (5.5. J per mm^2) there was complete regression and skin healing and no evidence of local recurrence or metastases 6 months later. The Nd–YAG laser provided a more controlled and certain method of eradication than quite wide surgical excision. These results were obtained below the burning level; hence it seemed justified to try to achieve similar effects in man with inoperable squamous carcinoma of the bronchus. It appeared that, apart from the effect of photoresection, the general heating also killed malignant cells. However, much more experimental work is needed at critical temperatures of about 44°C for longer durations, to see if the laser can produce a differential lethal effect preferentially on malignant cells, such has been reported in work using other methods of heating (Marmor et al. 1978; Giovanella et al. 1979; Kim and Hahn 1979).

Clinical Application

Suitable Nd–YAG lasers for clinical use are now manufactured in Britain by Barr and Stroud and in Germany (the Medilas laser) by Messerschmidt.

Following the successful use of an Nd–YAG laser to obliterate bladder cancer (Hofstetter and Frank 1980), the Nd–YAG laser has been widely used for the palliative treatment of advanced carcinoma of the bronchus in man. Toty et al. (1981) reported in 164 cases treated in 317 sessions using a power of 50–90 W to treat 72 cancers, 21 benign or malignant tumours and 44 iatrogenic stenoses. Bleeding was readily controlled and the main problem was with the advanced condition of the patients, sometimes in acute asphyxia. They were referred for laser treatment when all else failed, including radiotherapy, especially when the tumours affected the trachea or main bronchi. Hetzel et al. (1983) reported a similar result and concluded that the treatment was essentially palliative and suitable for relatively few patients — those with predominantly endobronchial growth and symptoms mainly of obstruction or haemoptysis. Good palliation was obtained in just over half the cases of partial obstruction of the trachea or main bronchi, but best results were when the tumour mass was in the trachea or at the main carina. Re-expansion of collapsed lung was achieved in some cases, but with a considerable risk of pneumonia. They found that patients tolerated the treatment better than chemotherapy or radiotherapy and that it was a useful adjunct for such palliative treatment. Dumon et al. (1982) reported 200 treatments on 111 patients in Marseilles with similarly good palliative results.

In summary, the present place of the Nd–YAG laser is entirely palliative, by photoresection of tumour masses; it is especially used in this way when radiotherapy has nothing more to offer, usually in advanced cases of squamous cell carcinoma or adenocarcinoma of the lung. It is most successful for rapidly providing an airway, especially with cancer affecting the trachea or main bronchi, and for stopping haemoptysis. It is possible, in future, that an alternative method of use would be by slow heating of tumour masses with or without the prior use of such drugs as misonidazole which are differentially retained by tumours and made cytotoxic by heat. However, much animal experimental work first needs to be done to check critical heating and the effects of heat sensitisation of radiosensitisers.

Photo-activation of Haematoporphyrins

History and Basis of HpD

The first attempt to use photosensitisation to treat cancer was made in 1903 when von Tappeiner and Jesionek used topical eosin and sunlight to treat skin tumours (von Tappeiner and Jesionek 1903; Jesionek and von Tappeiner 1904). Although they claimed some success, no further interest was shown in the subject until it was realised that a number of radiosensitisers, dyes preferentially retained in tumours, existed. The perfect radiosensitiser would be non-toxic, taken up only by malignant cells, and activated by specific wavelength light to then become locally cytotoxic. No such perfect substance exists though many have promise. Thompson et al. (1974) showed that acridine orange activated by an argon laser could treat epithelial tumours of a mouse. Many other dyes have been selectively used either for diagnosis or for treatment of cancer, such as fluoresceins (Moore 1953), tetracyclines (Rall et al. 1957) etc., but especially porphyrins and metallo-porphyrins (Figge and Weiland 1948).

Haematoporphyrin is of low toxicity and can be given systemically. It appears to be selectively retained in malignant tissue and its derivative HpD is even more selective (Lipson et al. 1961). Although the dye has no therapeutic effect for treating cancer, it can be photo-activated in the presence of oxygen to become highly cytotoxic locally (Dougherty et al. 1975).

Much work has been done on why HpD is relatively specific for tumour tissue, but the reason is not fully known. It may be a cellular property or tissue factor such as vascular permeability, lack of lymphatic drainage, and non-specific binding of serum protein to stromal elements (Bugelski et al. 1981). What appears more certain is that once it is deposited in maligant tissue, it seems to be cleared more rapidly from normal tissue so that the optimum therapeutic ratio is attained at about 72 h after its systemic injection. It can be activated by photons of light to produce singlet oxygen which is locally highly cytotoxic (Dougherty et al. 1976; Weishaupt et al. 1976). Recently it has been suggested that both heat and light may cause the death of malignant cells with HpD photo-activation (Svaasand and Doiron 1983).

Localisation of Bronchial Carcinoma with HpD Photoradiation

One use of HpD for the treatment of bronchial cancer is to detect early and to determine the extent of tumours within the bronchial tree. Doiron et al. (1979), after injecting 2.5 mg/kg of HpD and originally illuminating the bronchial tree with a mercury vapour lamp, but more recently, and better, with a krypton-ion laser and a photomultiplier within the bronchoscope, claimed to be able to detect a tumour only 100 μm thick. They were not only able to detect the site of the lung cancer in sputum-positive but X-ray-negative patients, but also much better able to delineate more advanced cancer and hence better determine operability. Kinsey et al. (1978) have similarly used HpD photofluorescence while Hyata et al. (1982a) report similar success in 17 patients, 16 of whom had bronchogenic carcinoma while one had severe squamous metaplasia in the bronchus. All four major histological types of cancer fluoresced (Fig. 6).

Photoradiation Treatment (PRT) with HpD

For treatment of endobronchial carcinoma the HpD is injected intravenously (3–5 mg/kg) and 72 h later (when the dye has been shown to give the optimal differential between tumour and normal tissue) the patient undergoes bronchoscopy using a fibre-optic instrument with local anaesthesia. The tumour can then be illuminated by passing redlight either from a gold-vapour laser (628 nm) or, more usually, from a rhodamine-B dye laser (630 nm) down a suitable fibre passed through the biopsy channel of the bronchoscope. The light is either directed to cover the surface of the tumour or, if an appropriate scintered-end fibre is available, this can be inserted into the tumour mass to illuminate the tumour from within. The whole tumour mass is flooded with red light for about 15 min, the exact time depending on the power density required. In principle any source of light of the appropriate spectrum (about 580–640 nm) and power output could be used for HpD activation. Originally a quartz-halogen lamp was used to provide the light, but the high-power density and small beam diameter of a fibre-transmitted laser gives better light realisation, tissue penetration and absorption.

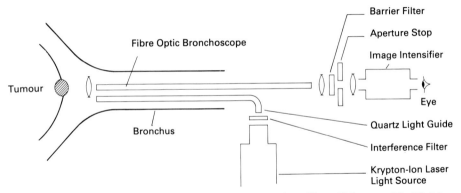

Fig. 6. Diagram of apparatus used for photofluorescent detection of bronchial cancer. (Modified from Hyata et al. 1982a)

HpD treatment, initially introduced by Dougherty et al. (1978, 1979), was extended to treatment of various different kinds of tumours by Forbes et al. (1980). Recently Hyata et al. (1982b) have treated 13 lung cancer patients by this technique and have shown that it is capable of relieving obstruction by tumours in the trachea and bronchus within a day, making it excellent palliative treatment in selected cases — especially as it can be used after radiotherapy has failed. Another important advance was the demonstration that some patients who were not suitable for surgery before HpD phototherapy became candidates for potentially curative surgery after it. Even more interesting are the results in early cases. Hyata and Kato (1983) reported complete remission, with no histological evidence of any recurrence of tumour over 2 years, in all eight cases of early squamous bronchogenic cancer treated. They got similarly good results in early oesophageal and gastric cancer and concluded 'excellent therapeutic results were obtained in early stage cancer cases with PRT, especially in lung cancer'.

Cortese and Kinsey (1982) report a study on ten patients with advanced tracheal-bronchial carcinoma; there was complete response in four superficial carcinomata, partial response in five larger carcinomata, but also two deaths. These deaths were from fatal bleeding, but in patients with advanced invasive cancer. It is evident that if tumour stroma is removed by treatment when it was supporting blood vessels, then this problem of bleeding will arise and must be anticipated.

Apart from this risk of bleeding in very advanced cases, complications from PRT using HpD seem few and not serious. Light sensitisation of the skin is perhaps the most tiresome, but can be avoided over the ensuing 2–3 weeks by keeping the patient indoors and by using light-barrier lotions (such as Spectra-Ban-15) on exposed skin; in sunny climes the sleep rhythm can be reversed so that the patient sleeps in the day and is awake at night. Diarrhoea has occasionally been reported from the HpD, but is rare and not serious.

Laser Safety

Now that this new exciting field for the treatment of lung cancer has come about it is essential that careful safety regulations be established and used. It is obvious, for example (and especially with invisible lasers), that eye damage to the operator, theatre staff or patients must be rigorously avoided. Again, the fire damage with an Nd–YAG laser or, more especially with a CO_2 laser, is a very real hazard. Recently the British Medical Laser Association (BMLA) has been formed which, it is hoped, will help to maintain safety standards through dissemination of knowledge about phototherapy and to train potential laser users. The Natural Radiation Protection Board (McKinley and Harlen 1983) has given standards for maximum permissible laser exposure.

Outlook in Photoradiation Treatment

One criticism of the use of HpD made hitherto was that the HpD is a mixture of porphyrins and, to some extent, variable in photo-activity (Bonnett et al. 1983) so that while the active component remained unidentified the treatment was empirical. Now, however, it is claimed that the main active component of HpD has been isolated by gel electrophoresis (Dougherty 1983) and has been found to consist of two porphyrin molecules linked by an ether bond. Dougherty has suggested the name of di-haematoporphyrin ether, or DHE. This substance is to be marketed as 'Photofrin-11' as opposed to the commercial preparation of HpD, which is known as 'Photofrin-I'. DHE is more than twice as active as HpD, so that less of the substance is needed to give a therapeutic level in the tumour, and (the temporary) skin light sensitisation, found with HpD, is reduced because of the improved therapeutic ratio between tumour and normal tissues. As soon as DHE is freely available, HpD will presumably become obsolete, and better therapeutic results can be anticipated.

Actually the ether bond between the two porphyrin molecules of the DHE can be made in a number of different ways so that a series of similar compounds are possible and for each there are a number of optical isomers. Thus, there are a large number of potentially useful molecules and it is by no means certain that the present form of DHE will prove to be the most photo-active. Moreover, not only the chemical structure but also the aggregation state of the molecule and the nature of the micro-environment affect the mechanism and efficiency of porphyrin photo-sensitisation (Truscott 1983), so that the whole subject of porphyrin physical chemistry is complex and many future developments in it can be anticipated. It is for this reason that a dye laser system seems preferable to a gold-vapour laser. The latter is less expensive but is of fixed wavelength; by contrast a dye laser can not only be tuned but the dye changed for a different wavelength as different compounds become available. Suitable dye lasers are manufactured by Coherent, Lexel-Cooper and Spectra-Physics.

Another interesting finding (Dougherty 1983) is that DHE can be activated not only by light but also by heat to some extent. The two effects appear additive. A rhodamine-B dye laser ensures light activation, but is not a good way of putting in heat; thus it has been suggested that in future light activation by dye laser might be followed by heat enhancement using sub-hyperthermic effects from an Nd-YAG laser run to give rather low power density. Earlier this year, 1983, El-Far and Pimstone stated that they found uro-porphyrin-I to be superior to other porphyrins as a selective tumour localiser and suggested its superiority for treatment as well. But

Dougherty (1983), while conceding that it localises in tumours, denies its usefulness for specific treatment as he found it not to be made toxic by light and concluded any apparent tumour death that these two workers found was simply from non-specific local heating because of the high laser power that they used.

Although the palliative and curative results so far reported from clinical use, even with crude HpD, seem promising, much chemical and biological experimental work is needed to determine the mechanisms of action and the optimum types of photo-sensitiser. Meanwhile much can be discovered about the present place for this new type of endobronchoscopic treatment for non-small cell lung cancer and how it fares as a sole treatment or in combination with surgery or radiotherapy. For example, Hyata and Kato (1983) stated that another use of PRT was '. . . widening the indications for surgery'. They gave PRT to five patients deemed to be inoperable, of whom only one remained inoperable; it was possible, subsequent to the PRT, to do a successful sleeve resection in two cases, a pneumonectomy in one and a tracheo-plasty in the fourth; these cases remained disease-free at 12 to 27 months.

The technique of light dosimetry of the tumours needs elaborating, as does whether the treatment is tolerated better under local anaesthesia with a flexible bronchoscope or with one or more fibres down a rigid bronchoscope, and general anaesthetic with adequate ventilation. Certainly the ventilation must be with air and not 100% oxygen — one fatality from fire has been reported when 100% oxygen was used. It appears that the present place for PRT with the available HpD is for palliation in cases of non-small cell carcinoma, especially in those in whom radio-therapy has failed. Potentially operable patients whose prior general condition precludes operation are another obvious choice. If non-small cell bronchogenic cancer can be diagnosed early enough, then bronchoscopic PRT might even become a curative treatment of choice. Obviously its potential is great, but it is as yet too early to know.

What is now needed, first, are some trials to establish the clinical efficacy of photochemotherapy for bronchogenic carcinoma by determining what proportion of patients show complete or partial regression of their tumours, as judged by the change in tumour volume estimated from measurements on bronchoscopic photo-graphs, radiographs, or CAT scan. Then, if the results from such trials are satisfactory, further more extensive and controlled trials are needed to determine the place of photochemotherapy in relation to other established treatments. Were it to be of proven value then it might place a premium on the very early diagnosis of lung cancer by such means as radio-immunodetection and localisation by external photo-scanning (Ranking and McVie 1983), possibly in combination with bronchoscopic staging by porphyrin fluorescence.

In summary, photoresection or vapourisation with an Nd–YAG or CO_2 laser and photochemotherapy by light activation of photosensitisers seem to be new forms of local treatment for bronchogenic carcinomata, but their precise place in relation to other treatment modalities has yet to be established.

References

Andrews AH, Polyani TG (1982) Microscopic and endoscopic surgery with the CO_2 laser. Wright, Boston Bristol London

Bonnett R, Berenbaum MC, Kaup H (1983) Chemical and biological studies on haematoporphyrin derivative. Proceedings of an international symposium on porphyrins in tumour phototherapy. Milan, Italy

Bown SG (1982) Interaction of laser light with living tissue. In: Proceedings of the first British conference on lasers in medicine and surgery. British Medical Laser Association

Bugelski PJ, Porter CW, Dougherty TJ (1981) Autoradiographic distribution of haematoporphryin derivative in normal and tumour tissue of the mouse. Cancer Res 41:4606–4612

Carruth JAS (1982) Resection of the tongue with the carbon dioxide laser. J Laryngol Otol 96:529–543

Christensen J (1982) The use of the CO_2 laser in thoracic surgery. In: Proceedings of the first congress of the European Laser Association. Cannes, 7–8 October 1982

Cortese DA, Kinsey JH (1982) Endoscopic management of lung cancer with haematoporphyrin derivative phototherapy. Proc Mayo Clin 57:543–547

Das Gupta AR, Frome JW, Rhys Evans PH, Dalton GA (1982) The CO_2 laser in the management of oral pre-malignant lesions. In: Proceedings of the first congress of the European Laser Association. Cannes, 7–8 October 1982

Doiron DR, Profio E, Vincent RG, Dougherty TJ (1979) Fluorescence bronchoscopy for detection of lung cancer. Chest 76:27–32

Dougherty TJ, Grinday GB, Fiel R et al. (1975) Photoradiation therapy: cure of animal tumours with haematoporphyrin and light. J Natl Cancer Inst 55:115–121

Dougherty TJ, Gomer CJ, Weishap MR (1976) Energetics and efficiency of photoactivation of murine tumour cells containing haematoporphyrin. Cancer Res 36:2300–2333

Dougherty TJ, Kaufman JE, Goldfarb A et al. (1978) Photoradiation therapy for the treatment of malignant tumours. Cancer Res 38:2628–2635

Dougherty TJ, Lawrence G, Kaufman JH et al. (1979) Photoradiation in the treatment of recurrent breast cancer. J Natl Cancer Inst 62:231–237

Dougherty TJ (1983) Proceedings of an international symposium on porphyrins in tumour phototherapy. Milan, Italy

Dumon JF Reboud E, Garbe L et al. (1982) Treatment of tracheo-bronchial lesions by laser photoresection. Chest 81:278–284

El-Far MA, Pimstone NR (1983) Superiority of uroporphyrin I over other porphyrins in selective tumour localisation. Proceedings of conference on medical uses of lasers. Santa Barbara, California

Figge FHJ, Weiland GS (1948) The affinity of neoplastic, embryonic and traumatised tissue for porphyrins and metalloporphyrins. Anat Rec 100:659

Forbes IJ, Cowled PA, Leong AS et al. (1980) Phototherapy of human tumours using haematoporphyrin derivative. Med J Aust 2:489–493

Freche C (1982) Experience du laser CO_2 dans les synechies et stenoses du larynx a propos de 150 cm^2. In: Proceedings of the first congress of the European Laser Association. Cannes, 7–8 October 1982

Gardner WN, Hugh-Jones P, Caroll MA et al. (1982) A quantitative analysis of the effect of Nd–YAG laser of transplanted mouse carcinomas. Thorax 37:594–597

Giovanella BC, Stehlin JS, , Shepard RC (1979) Hyperthermia treatment of human tumours heterotransplanted in nude mice. Cancer Res 49:2236–2241

Grant IWB (1982) Laser photoradiation for lung cancer (L.A.). Br Med J 2:323

Hetzel MR, Millard FJC, Ayes R et al. (1983) Laser treatment for carcinoma of the bronchus. Br Med J 286:12–18

Hofstetter A, Frank F (1980) The Nd–YAG laser in urology. Roche, Basel

Hugh Jones P (1978) Report of the address on lung cancer to British Association. The Times, 13 June

Hyata Y, Kato H (1983) Photoradiation therapy in early stage cancer cases. Proceedings of an international symposium on porphyrins in tumour phototherapy. Milan, Italy

Hyata Y, Kato H, Ono J et al. (1982a) Fluorescence fibre-optic bronchoscopy in the diagnosis of early stage lung cancer. Cancer Res 82:121–130

Hyata Y, Kato H, Konaka C, Ono J, Takizania N (1982b) Haematoporphyrin derivative and laser photoactivation in the treatment of lung cancer. Chest 81:269–277

Jesionek A, von Tappeiner H (1904) Behandlung der Hautcarcinome mit fluorescierenden Stoffen. Dtsch Arch Klin Med 82:223–227

Kaplan I (1982) Current CO_2 laser surgery. Plast Reconstr Surg 69:552–555

Kim JM, Hahn EW (1979) Chemical and biological studies of localised hyperthermia. Cancer Res 39:2258–2261

Kinsey JH, Cortese DA, Sanderson DR (1978) Detection of haematoporphyrin fluorescence during fibre-optic bronchoscopy to localise early bronchogenic carcinoma. Proc May Clin 53:594–599

Kullman GL (1980) Laser palliation of bronchogenic carcinoma. J Fla Med Assoc 67:566

Lipson R, Baldes E, Olsen A (1961) The use of a derivative of haematoporphyrin in tumour detection. J Natl Cancer Inst 26:1–8

Marmor JB, Pounds D, Hahn N, Hahn GM (1978) Treating spontaneous tumours in dogs and cats by ultrasound induced hyperthermia. J Radiat Oncol Biol Phys 4:967–978

McKinlay AF, Harlen F (1983) Biological bases of the maximum permissible exposure levels of the UK laser standard BS 4803. Nat Rad Protection Bd R 153, Didcot, Oxon

Moore GE (1953) Diagnosis and localization of brain tumours. Charles Thorac, Springfield, Illinois.

Nogoret JM, Lejeune F, Pector JC, Mattheiem W, Fruhling J, Gerard A (1982) Indications for CO_2 laser knife in malignant tumours. In: Proceedings of the first congress of the European Laser Association. Cannes, 7–8 October 1982

Office of Population Census and Surveys (1979) DH2, No. 6. HMSO, London

Parrish JA (1979) Potentials for lasers. In: Pratesi R, Sacchi CA (eds) Lasers in photomedicine and photobiology. Springer, Berlin Heidelberg New York

Parsons RJ (1982) Introduction to laser physics. In: Proceedings of the first British conference on lasers in medicine and surgery. British Medical Laser Association

Rall DP, Loo TL, Lane M et al. (1957) Appearance and persistence of fluorescent material in tumour tissue after tetracycline administration. J Natl Cancer Inst 19:79–84

Rankin EM, McVie JG (1983) Radioimmunodetection of cancer. Br Med J 287: 1402–1404

Royal College of Physicians (1983) Health or smoking? Follow-up Report from Royal College of Physicians, Pitman, London

Smith KC (1979) Common misconceptions about light. In: Lasers in photomedicine and photobiology. Springer, Berlin Heidelberg New York

Svaasand LO, Doiron DR (1983) On the probability for simultaneous action of hyperthermal and photodynamic effects during photoradiation therapy for malignant tumours. Proceedings of an international symposium on porphyrins in tumour phototherapy. Milan, Italy

Tadir Y, Kaplan I, Zukerman Z, Edelstein T, Ovadia J (1982) New instrumentation and technique for laparoscopic CO_2 laser operations. In: Proceedings of the first congress of the European Laser Association. Cannes, 7–8 October 1982

Thompson SH, Emmett EA, Fox SH (1974) Photodestruction of mouse epithelial tumours after oral orange and argon laser. Cancer Res 34:3124–3127

Toty L, Personne C, Colchen A, Vouch G (1981) Bronchoscopic management of tracheal lesions using the Nd–YAG laser. Thorax 36:175–178

Truscott TG (1983) Excited state properties of haematoporphyrin. In: Proceedings of an international symposium on porphyrins in tumour phototherapy. Milan, Italy

von Tappeiner H, Jesionek A (1903) Zur Behandlung der Hautcarcinome mit fluorescierenden Stoffen. Münch Med Wochenschr 1:2042–2044

Weishaupt KR, Gomer CJ, Dougherty TJ (1976) Identification of singlet oxygen as the cytotoxic agent in photo-activation of a murine tumour. Cancer Res 36:2326–2329

Subject Index

TNM-Atlas

Illustrated Guide to the Classification of Malignant Tumors

Published in cooperation with the UICC
Edited by **B. Spiessl**, Basel, **O. Scheibe**, Stuttgart,
G. Wagner, Heidelberg
Illustrations by U. Kerl
1982. 311 figures. XII, 229 pages.
ISBN 3-540-11429-7

"In its tough flexible cover, this booklet is designed for the pocket of the practising doctor rather than for the bookshelf of the academic taxonomist. It is a contribution to clinical oncology of which the authors may well be proud, which will be surely valued and which, at the same time, may be considered a tribute to the "inventor" of the TNM system." **M. Harmer**, *UICC Bulletin*

Manual of Clinical Oncology

Edited under the auspices of the International
Union Against Cancer
3rd fully revised edition. 1982. 44 figures. XV,
346 pages. ISBN 3-540-11746-6

The continuing success of the UICC's *Clinical Oncology*, the refinement of their educational objectives for medical students and young practioners, and the siginificant advances scored over the last few years in cancer research all led to the decision to publish a third edition of this manual. It presents students and practioners with a concise summary of essential knowledge.
"... this well-prepared compact volume fulfills admirably its roles as an aid to the understanding of malignant disease for all sections of the medical community." *British Journal of Surgery*

The Histology of Borderline Cancer

With Notes on Prognosis

by **W. W. Park**, Dundee
With the collaboration of J. W. Corkhill
1980. 314 figures. XIV, 471 pages.
ISBN 3-540-09792-9

"The is book can be seen as the culmination of the work of a lifetime of a distinguished pathologist, as a new form of the art of teaching at its best, as a philosophical treatise on cancer or as an exposition of what collaboration between workers in different disciplines can achieve in the way of correct management of the patient. ... It should be bought read, brooded over and savoured by the pathologist who has got through the hurdles of artificial examinations and has begun to confront the problems of real life as they are seen in a real hospital and affect real patients." **J. G. Azzopardi**, *Histopathology*

Histopathology of Non-Hodgkin's Lymphomas

by **K. Lennert**, Kiel
(Based on the Kiel Classification)
In Collaboration with H. Stein
Translated from the German by M. Soehring,
A. G. Stansfeld
1981. 68 figures, some in color. IX, 135 pages.
ISBN 3-540-10445-3

"Professor Lennert and his collaborators are to be congratulated on producing such an excellent monograph on a difficult topic in which advances in immunological techniques have produced rapid changes in recent years. I recommend this book to all concerned with the diagnosis and management of patients with non-Hodgkin's lymphomas, in particular to histopathologists. There is, to my knowledge, no better illustrated account of the non-Hodgkin's lymphomas on the market today." **D. H. Wright**, *Cancer Topics*

Functional Partial Laryngectomy

Conservation Surgery for Carcinoma of the Larynx

Edited by **M. E. Wigand, W. Steiner**, Erlangen and
P. M. Stell, Liverpool
1984. 211 figures, 88 tables. XVII, 328 pages.
ISBN 3-540-13175-2

Internationally recognized laryngologists, pathologists and radiologists from 16 countries have combined their efforts in this book to provide a comprehensive survey of current diagnostic and surgical methods for cancer of the larynx. Their contributions reflect the state of the art in their particular fields and provide the oncologic surgeon with authoritative coverage of all important aspects of laryngeal function preservation.

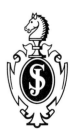

Springer-Verlag
Berlin
Heidelberg
New York
Tokyo

Pathology of the Esophagus

by **H. Enterline**, Philadelphia, and
J. Thompson, Portland

1984. 185 figures, 10 in color. IX, 192 pages
ISBN 3-540-90896-X

This volume provides a comprehensive source of
information regarding the anatomy, embryology,
and histology of the esophagus as well as the
clinical presentation and pathology of esophageal
diseases. With its unique balance of clinical, radiologic and pathologic information, the book offers a
practical, well-illustrated guide to current concepts
of both common and unusual diseases of the
esophagus, including epithelial and non-epithelial
tumors and squamous cell tumors.

Manual of Pulmonary Surgery

by **Edward W. Humphrey**, Minneapolis;
Deanne Lawrence McKeown, Medical Illustrator

1982. 215 figures (190 in full color). XI, 259 pages
(Comprehensive Manuals in Surgical Specialties)
ISBN 3-540-90732-7

This comprehensive volume covers all aspects of
surgery on the lung and related structures. It
includes a surgeon's-eye-view of the anatomy, indications for pulmonary resection, a step-by-step
discussion of preferred operative techniques for the
lung, mediastinum, diaphragm, and chest wall, and
advice on how to manage – or avoid – postoperative
complications. **Manual of Pulmonary Surgery**
contains over 200 illustrations – more than 150 of
them in full color – and is based on the author's
more than 20 years of experience in thoracic
surgery.

A Manual of Morphometry in Diagnostic Pathology

by **J. P. A. Baak**, Delft, and **J. Oort**, Amsterdam

1983. 90 figures. XIV, 205 pages.
ISBN 3-540-11431-9

The use of morphometry in diagnostic pathology
offers the advantages of objectivity, reproducibility
and the detection of minor differences between
structures. This technique can help overcome the
serious problem of interobserver variability, of
special interest in oncology where patient treatment
often depends on the assessment of "grade" and
"prognosis probaility". This manual, written in a
methodological "cookery book" style, will help in
the application of morphometry in daily diagnostic
work. Such aspects as numerical probability state-
ments are clearly described, and practical examples
and many illustrations are provided.

Diseases of the Lymphatic System

Diagnosis and Therapy

Edited by **D. W. Molander**, New York City
1984. 111 figures. XVIII, 340 pages.
ISBN 3-540-90850-1

Diseases of the Lymphatic System was written with
the practicing oncologist in mind. This comprehensive reference source contains chapters by leading
clinicians covering such lymphatic disorders as
Hodgkin's disease, non-Hodgkin's lymphomas, and
the acquired immune deficiency syndrome (AIDS).
The authors provide detailed information on
biochemical abnormalities, radiological findings and
treatment, as well as psychological issues to
consider when treating patients with these malignant diseases.

Biological Rhythms and Medicine

by **A. Reinberg**, Paris, and **M. H. Smolensky**,
Houston
With contributions by H. v. Mayersbach, J. E. Pauly,
L. A. Scheving, L. E. Scheving, T. H. Tsai

1983. 148 figures. XIII, 305 pages. (Topics in Environmental Physiology and Medicine).
ISBN 3-540-90791-2

Biological Rhythms and Medicine is both an authoritative introduction to the field of chronobiology as
well as a guide to the integration of bioperiodic
effects into disease management and physiologic
studies. Its coverage includes the investigative
methodology of chronobiology, the chronobiology
of cellular morphology and proliferation and its
implications for oncology and cancer chemotherapy, human chronopathology, clinical chronophar-
macology, and the chronobiologic aspects of nutrition.

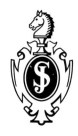

Springer-Verlag
Berlin
Heidelberg
New York
Tokyo